Wrist Surgery

Tricks of the Trade

Indian Edition by

Vitasta

Vitasta Publishing Pvt. Ltd.
New Delhi

Thieme

Wrist Surgery

Tricks of the Trade

Mark E. Baratz, M.D.
Professor and Vice Chairman
Department of Orthopaedic Surgery
Director, Division of Upper Extremity Surgery
Residency and Fellowship Program Director
Drexel University College of Medicine
Allegheny General Hospital
Pittsburgh, Pennsylvania

Melvin P. Rosenwasser, M.D.
Professor
Department of Orthopaedic Surgery
Columbia University College of Physicians and Surgeons
Director, Orthopaedic Hand Trauma Service
New York–Presbyterian Hospital
New York, New York

Brian D. Adams, M.D.
Professor
Director, Hand Surgery Fellowship
Department of Orthopaedics
University of Iowa College of Medicine
University of Iowa Hospitals and Clinics
Iowa City, Iowa

Scott H. Kozin, M.D.
Associate Professor
Department of Orthopaedic Surgery
Temple University School of Medicine
Director, Upper Extremity Surgery
Philadelphia Shriners Hospital
Philadelphia, Pennsylvania

Thieme
New York • Stuttgart

Thieme Medical Publishers, Inc.
333 Seventh Ave.
New York, NY 10001

Executive Editor: Esther Gumpert
Associate Editor: Owen Zurhellen IV
Vice President, Production and Electronic Publishing: Anne T. Vinnicombe
Production Editor: Print Matters, Inc.
Sales Manager: Ross Lumpkin
Chief Financial Officer: Peter van Woerden
President: Brian D. Scanlan
Compositor: Thomson Digital
Printer: Maple-Vail

Library of Congress Cataloging-in-Publication Data

Wrist surgery : tricks of the trade / Mark E. Baratz ... [et al.].
p. ; cm.
Includes bibliographical references and index.
ISBN 1-58890-217-X (US-HC) – ISBN 3-13-139011-5 (GTV)
1. Wrist–Surgery. 2. Wrist–Wounds and injuries–Surgery. I. Baratz, Mark.
[DNLM: 1. Wrist Injuries–surgery. 2. Wrist Joint–surgery. 3. Orthopedic Procedures–methods. WE 830 W9559 2006]
RD559.W755 2006
617.5′74–dc22

2005055992

Important note: Medical knowledge is ever-changing. As new research and clinical experience broaden our knowledge, changes in treatment and drug therapy may be required. The authors and editors of the material herein have consulted sources believed to be reliable in their efforts to provide information that is complete and in accord with the standards accepted at the time of publication. However, in view of the possibility of human error by the authors, editors, or publisher of the work herein or changes in medical knowledge, neither the authors, editors, or publisher, nor any other party who has been involved in the preparation of this work, warrants that the information contained herein is in every respect accurate or complete, and they are not responsible for any errors or omissions or for the results obtained from use of such information. Readers are encouraged to confirm the information contained herein with other sources. For example, readers are advised to check the product information sheet included in the package of each drug they plan to administer to be certain that the information contained in this publication is accurate and that changes have not been made in the recommended dose or in the contraindications for administration. This recommendation is of particular importance in connection with new or infrequently used drugs.

Printed in the United States

5 4 3 2 1

TMP ISBN 1-58890-217-X
GTV ISBN 3 13 139011 5

I dedicate this book to my wife, Arlene, and my children, Katie, Chris, and Chelsea.

—*Mark E. Baratz*

I dedicate this book to my wonderful wife, Phoebe, and our children, Ted, Chuck, Kate, and Allie, who make my days happy.

—*Melvin P. Rosenwasser*

My contribution to this book is dedicated to the memory of Jayasankar "Jay" Menon, M.D., who was instrumental in developing new ideas to make total wrist replacement a real possibility for many of our patients.

—*Brian D. Adams*

I dedicate this book to our children, Bryan and Samantha, for their everlasting supply of joy and wonder; to my wife, Louise, for her ongoing support, partnership, and love; and to my parents, William and Roni, for their countless lessons of life and family.

—*Scott H. Kozin*

Contents

Foreword

In *Wrist Surgery: Tricks of the Trade,* four seasoned hand surgeons provide technical insight into the application of a variety of surgical procedures for the treatment of wrist disorders. The beauty of this text lies in the uniform outline for each chapter (indications, technique, pearls and pitfalls, alternatives, postoperative care, and suggested readings), liberal use of high-quality illustrations to supplement the text, and the concise nature of each chapter.

The text focuses on the major problem areas that the orthopaedic hand surgeon faces on a daily basis. These include individual chapters regarding the surgical management of distal radius fractures and reconstruction; the distal radioulnar joint, including instability, management of abutment, and arthroplasty; scaphoid fractures, both acute and nonunions; degenerative conditions of the carpus; Kienböck disease; and disorders of the thumb trapeziometacarpal joint.

There are no black and white answers for the management of many of the domains outlined above. For example, in the section on scapholunate ligament disruption, the reader is presented with the spectrum of procedures to manage this difficult problem. Because of the succinct nature of each chapter, a surgeon, in short order, can read all the chapters on a topic, such as on scapholunate ligament reconstruction, and decide which procedure best addresses the problem of their particular patient.

The liberal use of illustrations and pitfalls and pearls helps to demystify the described procedures. The format highlights the nuances of each procedure, permitting even experienced surgeons to improve their care.

When I first started reading the book, I thought the intended audience should be hand fellows. Upon completion, however, it was clear that the book has something for everyone. For the resident, surgical approaches and anatomy will be beneficial, and for the attending physician, pearls and pitfalls will prove invaluable.

We are indebted to these authors for a pithy, well-illustrated text that will facilitate our surgical decision-making and management of wrist disorders.

Peter J. Stern, M.D.
Normal S. and Elizabeth C. A. Hill Professor and Chairman
Department of Orthopaedic Surgery
University of Cincinnati College of Medicine
Cincinnati, Ohio

Preface

The wrist positions the hand for tasks that require the precision of a surgeon, the force of a fighter, and the explosive velocity of a pitcher. Wrist dysfunction arises from congenital differences, trauma, and aging. For many wrist problems we have solutions; for some, particularly wrist instability, we have procedures that moderate but rarely cure the associated pain. With over 70 years of combined practical experience, we have learned what procedures work. In this text, we describe a variety of approaches to treating wrist dysfunction that we have found successful. Most surgeons are visual learners who rely on images of anatomy, surgical approaches, and techniques. For this reason have constructed a book where each of 72 wrist operations is presented with an outline of indications, technique, postoperative care, and alternative techniques. Liberally illustrated with line drawings, the book is designed to be a resource for all practicing surgeons, residents, and fellows who need a quick reference when treating the ailing wrist.

Mark E. Baratz, M.D.

Acknowledgments

I would like to acknowledge the considerable contributions of Jodie Fowler, Kim Avolio, Lorenda Layne, and Eric Mullins, M.D.

Mark E. Baratz

I would like to acknowledge my hand fellow Ryan Beekman, M.D., for his invaluable assistance.

Melvin P. Rosenwasser

Section I

Overview of Distal Radius Fractures

1 Closed Reduction and Percutaneous Pin Fixation of Distal Radius Fractures

Indications

- Dorsally angulated fracture with palmar cortex that is not comminuted
- Indications for surgery are based on radiographic parameters. The indications vary with the patient's age and the demands to be placed on the wrist. Consider surgery for:

    1. Dorsal angulation beyond neutral
    2. Shortening > 4 mm

■ Pearl

Check for acute carpal tunnel in all patients with a distal radius fracture. If the patient has numbness and abnormal two-point discrimination, consider carpal tunnel release.

Technique

- Close reduce fracture. Check reduction with intraoperative radiograph.
- If fracture reduced:

    1. Create 1 to 2 cm incision centered over the radial aspect of the radial styloid (**Fig. 1–1**).
    2. Identify and protect sensory nerves. Expose the radial styloid dorsal to the tendons of the first extensor compartment (**Fig. 1–2**).
    3. Insert two or more 0.062 in. wires across fracture fragments (**Fig. 1–3A,B**). Make a small incision over fragments that will be pinned via a dorsal approach. Retract and protect the extensor tendons.

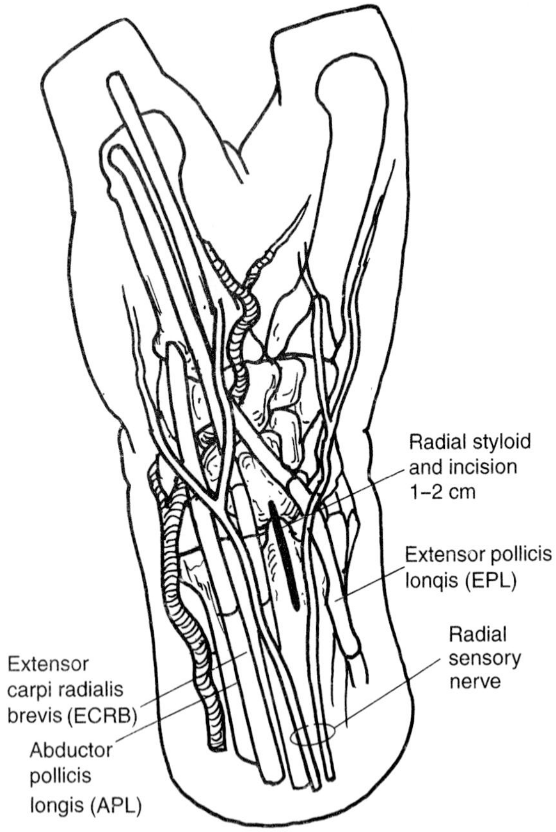

Figure 1–1

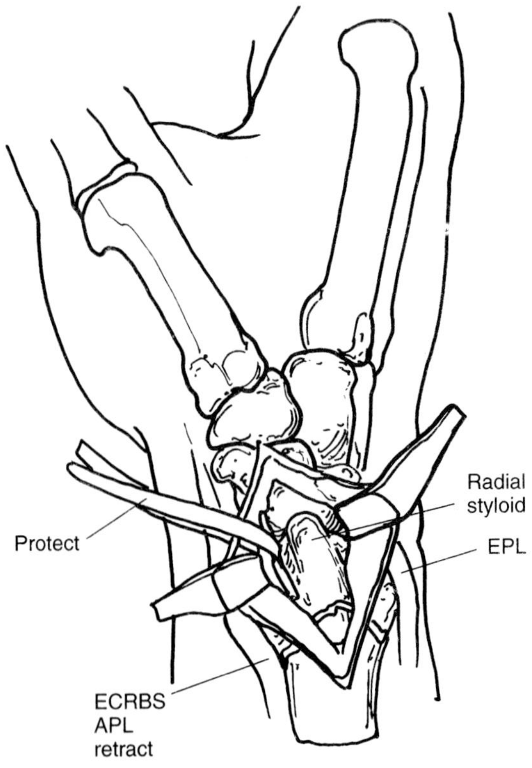

Figure 1–2

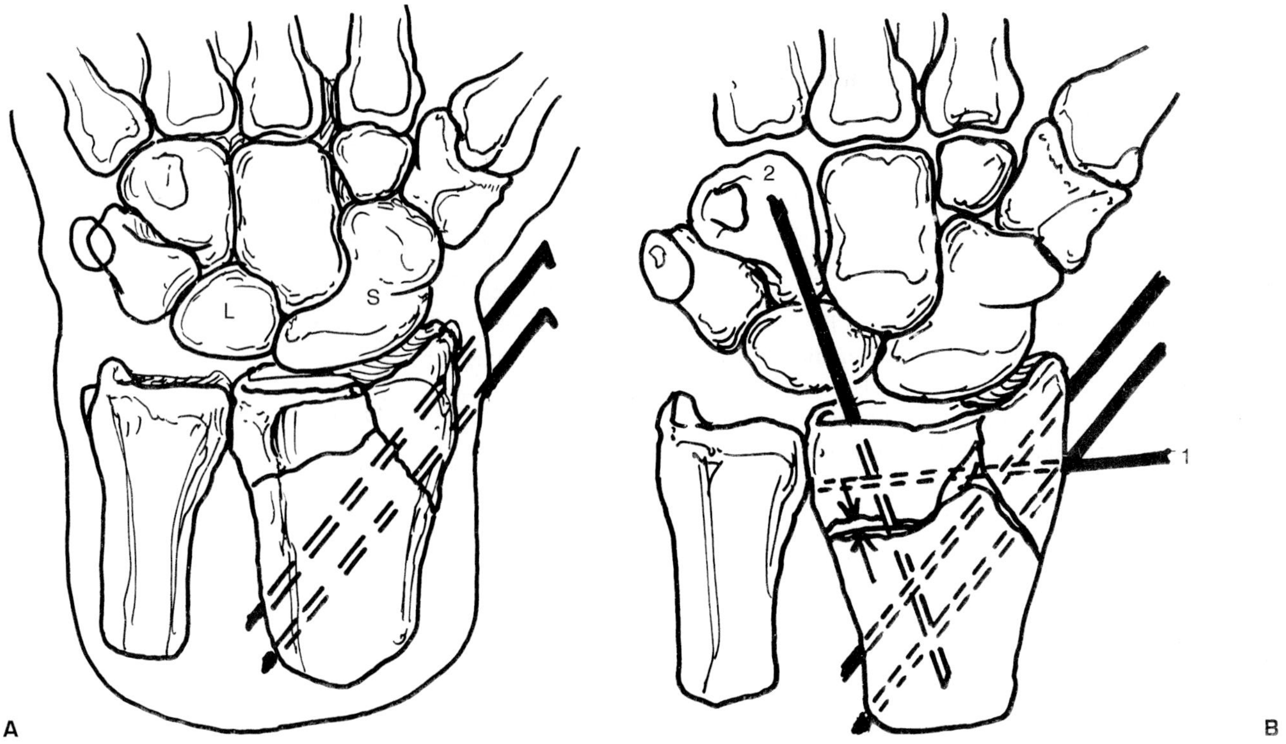

Figure 1–3

- If fracture not reduced after attempted closed reduction:
    1. Use fluoroscopy to localize the fracture on a lateral projection.
    2. On AP projection localize two points along the fracture line: one beneath the scaphoid(S) fossa, the second beneath the lunate(L) fossa. Make two 1 cm incisions at these points.
    3. Spread through incisions to dorsal cortex with curved hemostat.
    4. Insert, without power assist, 0.062 in. wires into the fracture site to, but not through, the palmar cortex. Verify position with fluoroscopy (**Fig. 1–4**).
    5. Place wire driver on wire and move driver distally until pin is ~45 degrees to the long axis of the radius (**Fig. 1–5**). Check reduction with fluo-

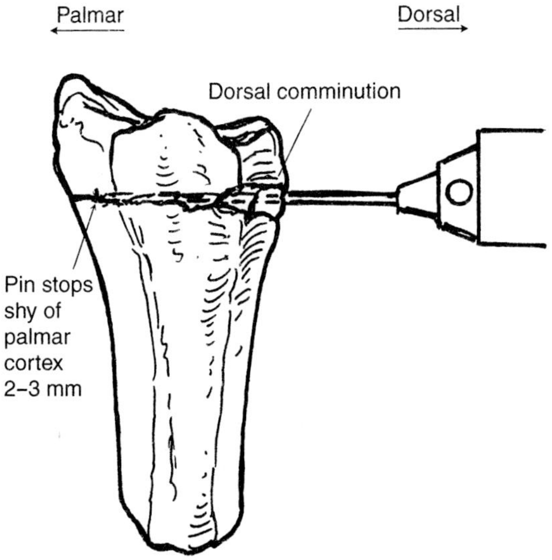

Figure 1–4

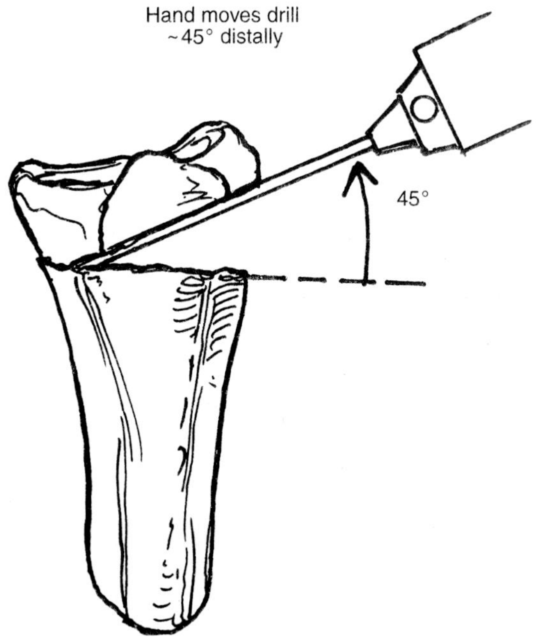

Figure 1–5

roscopy. Advance pin through palmar cortex (**Fig. 1–6**). Place second pin in similar fashion.

6. Augment dorsally placed pins with two 0.062 in. pins inserted through the radial styloid (**Fig. 1–3A**).

■ Pearl

A small drill guide can be used when placing pins to protect sensory nerves and tendons.

■ Pitfalls

If you encounter unexpected comminution of the dorsal cortex with intra-articular extension consider augmenting fracture stabilization with an external fixator (see Chapter 2).

If the palmar cortex displaces during fracture reduction consider placing a palmar plate (see Chapter 2).

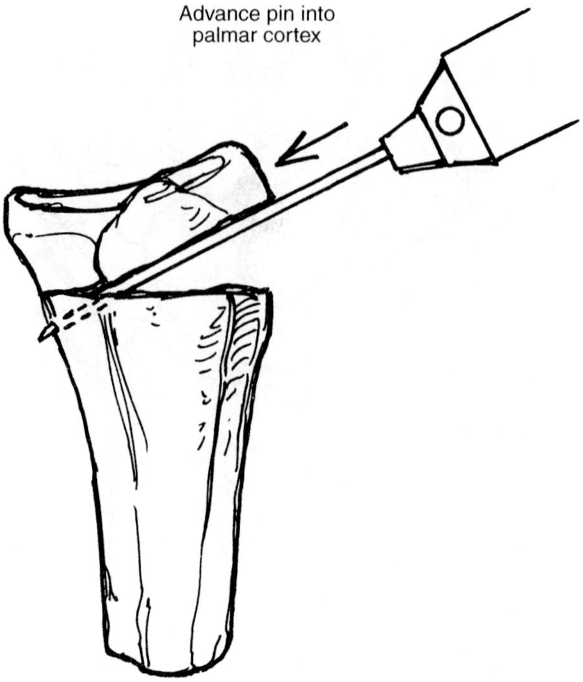

Figure 1–6

Postoperative Care

- Splint wrist in neutral position.
- Encourage finger motion; 20 times an hour.
- Short arm cast applied at 2 weeks.
- Remove pins when there are clinical and radiographic signs of healing; usually 4 to 6 weeks.

Suggested Readings

Hede JS, Lindblad BE, Mikkelsen SS, Knudsen HM. Comparison of intramedullary fixation and percutaneous pinning of displaced and comminuted Colles' fractures: a prospective and consecutive study. Scand J Plast Reconstr Surg Hand Surg 2000;34:161–166

Trumble TE, Wagner W, Hanel DP, Vedder NB, Gilbert M. Intrafocal (Kapandji) pinning of distal radius fractures with and without external fixation. J Hand Surg [Am] 1998;23:381–394

2 Limited-Open Reduction and Percutaneous Pin Fixation with External Fixation of Distal Radius Fractures

Indications

Displaced, intra-articular fracture of the distal radius without palmer comminution

Technique

- Expose the dorsoradial aspect of the index metacarpal identifying and protecting radial sensory nerves.
- Predrill and place two external fixation pins at a 45 degree angle from the dorsum of the hand. Place the proximal pin at the proximal metaphyseal flare (**Fig. 2–1**).
- Expose the dorsoradial aspect of the radius just proximal to the strap muscles. Identify the radial sensory nerve as it emerges from between the brachioradialis and extensor carpi radialis longus. Develop the interval between the extensor carpi radialis longus (ECRL) and extensor carpi radialis brevis (ECRB). Predrill and place two pins in the radial shaft. Check pin placement in the metacarpal and radial shaft with fluoroscopy.
- Assemble fixator. As a temporary measure, distract the wrist to help reduce the fracture and tighten the fixator. It may be necessary to supinate, flex, and place the wrist in ulnar deviation to effect a good reduction. Check the reduction with fluoroscopy.
- Make a 2 to 3 cm incision on the dorsal aspect of the distal radius (**Fig. 2–2**).

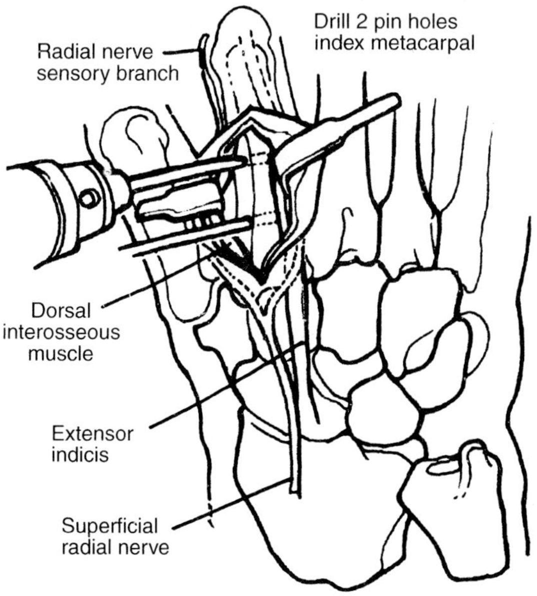

Figure 2–1

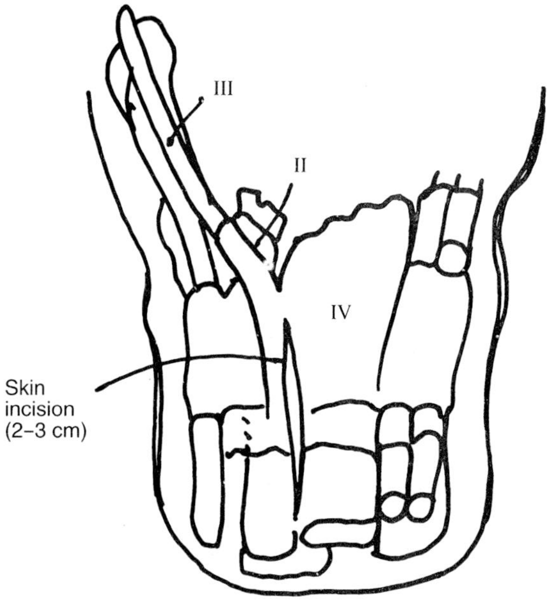

Figure 2–2

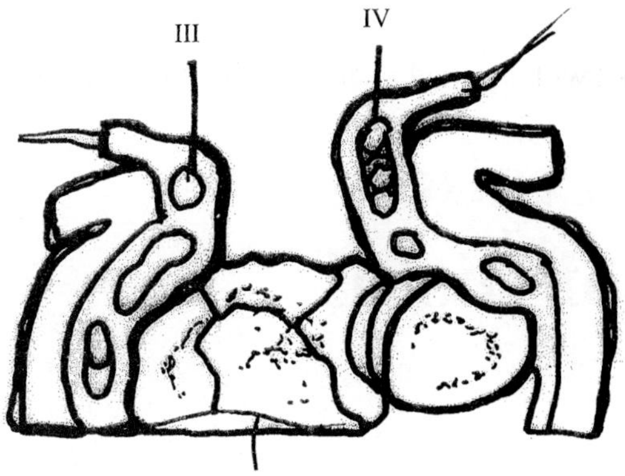

Figure 2–3

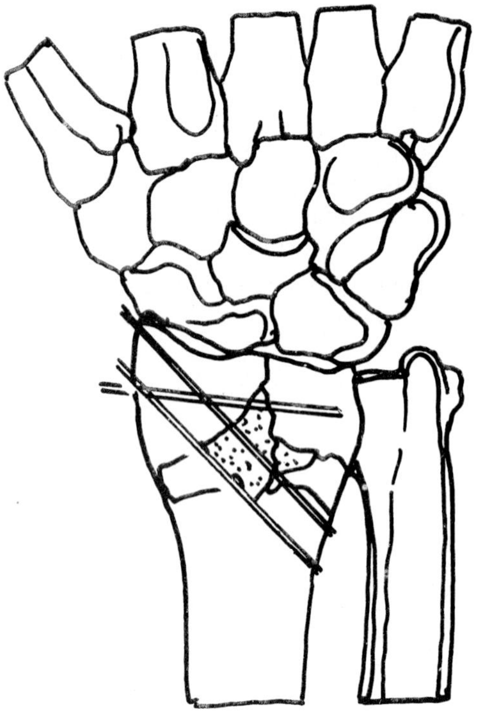

Figure 2–4

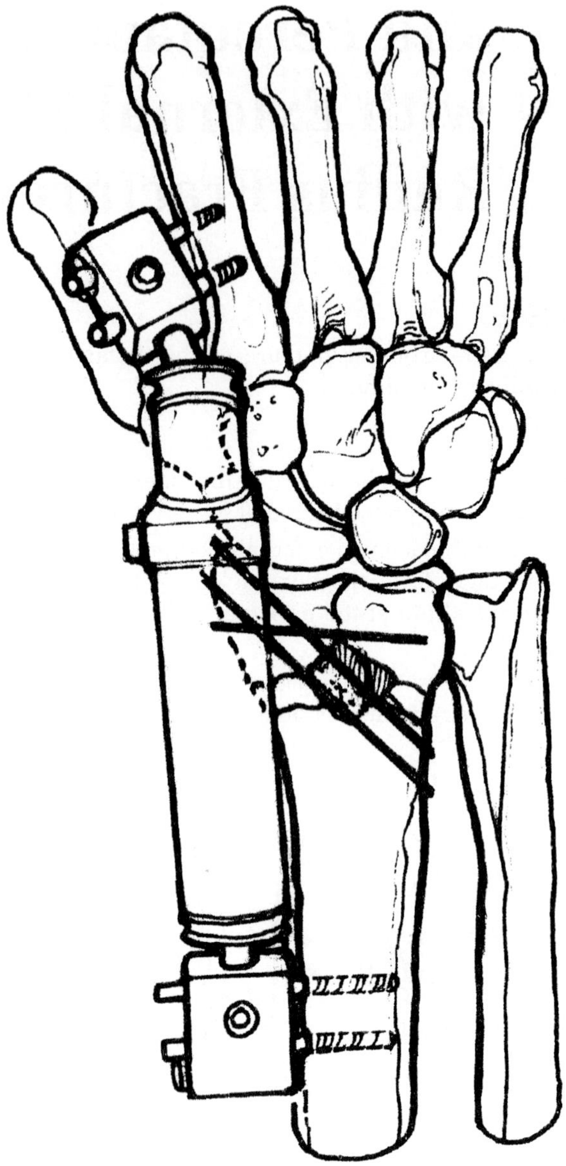

Figure 2–5

- Release extensor pollicis longus (EPL) tendon from third compartment and retract radially. Elevate tendons of fourth extensor compartment to expose only the comminuted portion of the radius fracture (**Fig. 2–3**).
- Make a 2 cm incision just radial to the radial styloid. Expose tip of styloid dorsal to the first extensor compartment. Protect sensory nerves.
- Elevate and pin articular components of the fracture. Then pin reassembled articular surface to the intact proximal radius (**Fig. 2–4**).
- Check fracture and pin position with fluoroscopy. Place bone graft in the metaphyseal defect.
- Relieve the distraction on the wrist. Place the wrist in neutral position with only slight distraction and retighten the fixator (**Fig. 2–5**). Check wrist position with fluoroscopy.
- Before wound closure check the stability of the distal radoulnar joint (DRUJ) with the forearm in neutral, supination, and pronation. An unstable DRUJ should be managed with either closed pinning, repair of the triangular fibrocartilage complex (TFCC), or open reduction internal fixation (ORIF) of an associated ulnar styloid fracture.

■ Pearls

After final positioning of the wrist with the external fixator:

- The wrist should rest in a natural position.
- The fingers, especially the index finger, should have normal passive flexion at the metacarpophalangeal and interphalangeal joints.
- The radiocarpal and midcarpal joints should look normal or only slightly widened on intraoperative fluoroscopy.

■ Pitfall

Intra-articular fractures with palmer comminution cannot be managed with external fixation without a palmer plate.

Postoperative Care

- Splint wrist in neutral position.
- Encourage finger motion; 20 times an hour.
- Pin care twice a day with alcohol or dilute peroxide
- Fixator removal is dictated by the stability of the fracture after grafting and percutaneous pin fixation and evidence of healing. Most fixators are removed in 4 to 6 weeks.

Suggested Readings

Dunning CE, Lindsay CS, Bicknell RT, Patterson SD, Johnson JA, King GJ. Supplemental pinning improves the stability of external fixation in distal radius fractures during simulated finger and forearm motion. J Hand Surg [Am] 1999;24:992–1000

Trumble TE, Wagner W, Hanel DP, Vedder NB, Gilbert M. Intrafocal (Kapandji) pinning of distal radius fractures with and without external fixation. J Hand Surg [Am] 1998;23:381–394

3 Intra-articular Fractures of the Distal Radius Treated with Dorsal Plate

Indications

Displaced intra-articular fractures with dorsal cortical comminution, minimal displacement, and no comminution of the palmar cortex.

Technique

- Dorsal approach to the distal radius
- Open the retinaculum over the second (II) through fourth (IV) extensor compartments as two opposing flaps (**Fig. 3–1A,B**).
- Reduce the articular surface starting with sigmoid notch and lunate fossa. Attempt indirect reduction of the joint with the assistance of fluoroscopy. If the reduction does not appear adequate, the joint can be exposed through a transverse arthrotomy.

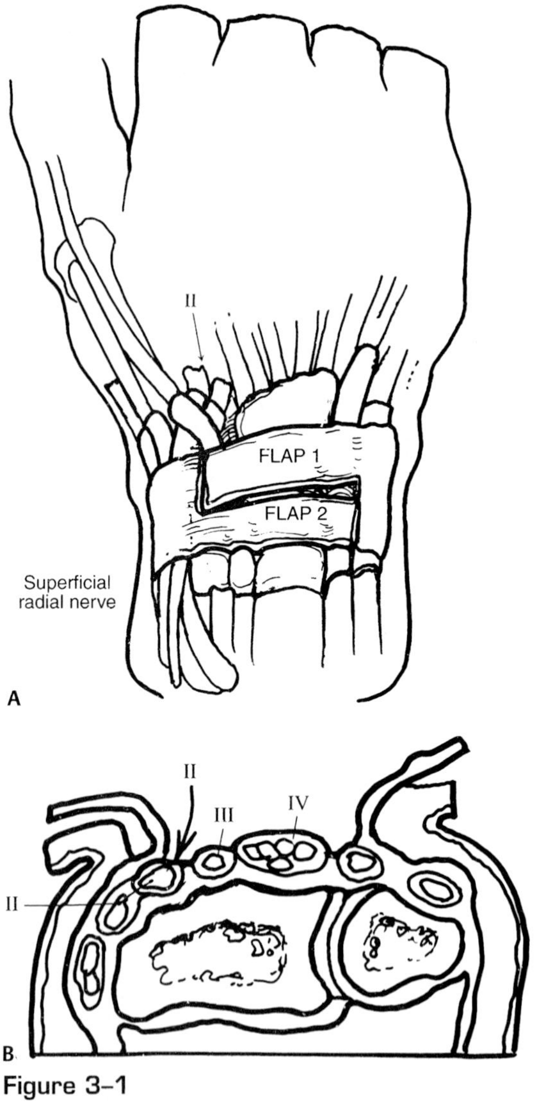

Figure 3–1

■ Pearl

If the distal fragment is malrotated, reduction may be facilitated by releasing the brachioradialis.

- Hold the reduction with 0.045 in. wire(s) placed through the radial styloid.
- Graft metaphyseal defects with autogenous or banked bone.
- Apply dorsal plate and place screws in radial styloid and in radial shaft.
- Check reduction with intraoperative radiograph.
- Fill remaining holes in the plate as the fracture pattern permits. A dorsal plate that accommodates smooth pins or screws with heads that thread into the plate converts the implant to a fixed-angle device. The pins can serve as a buttress for comminuted portions of the subchondral plate (**Fig. 3–2**).

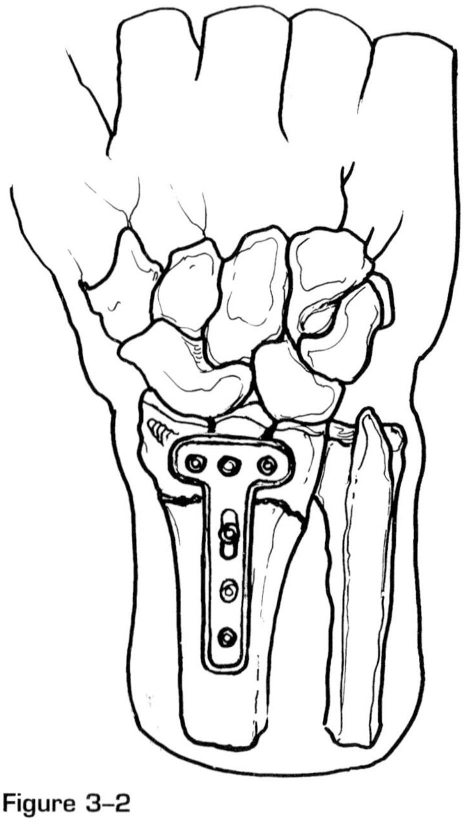

Figure 3–2

■ **Pearl**

Comminuted fragments of the lunate fossa may be supported by pins placed transversely from the radial styloid to beneath the subchondral bone of the lunate fossa.

- Place one flap of retinaculum over plate, beneath extensors. Suture the flap in place. Place the second flap over the extensors and suture in place (**Fig. 3–3A,B**). Leave extensor pollicis longus free in the subcutaneous tissues.

■ **Pearl**

If fracture is still not stable, augment the fixation with external fixator.

Postoperative Care

- Immediate active range of motion of fingers
- Splint 2 weeks
- Cast 2 to 6 weeks depending on clinical and radiographic evidence of healing

■ **Pitfall**

Follow patients for evidence of extensor tendonitis from the plate. Irritation of the radial wrist extensors is common.

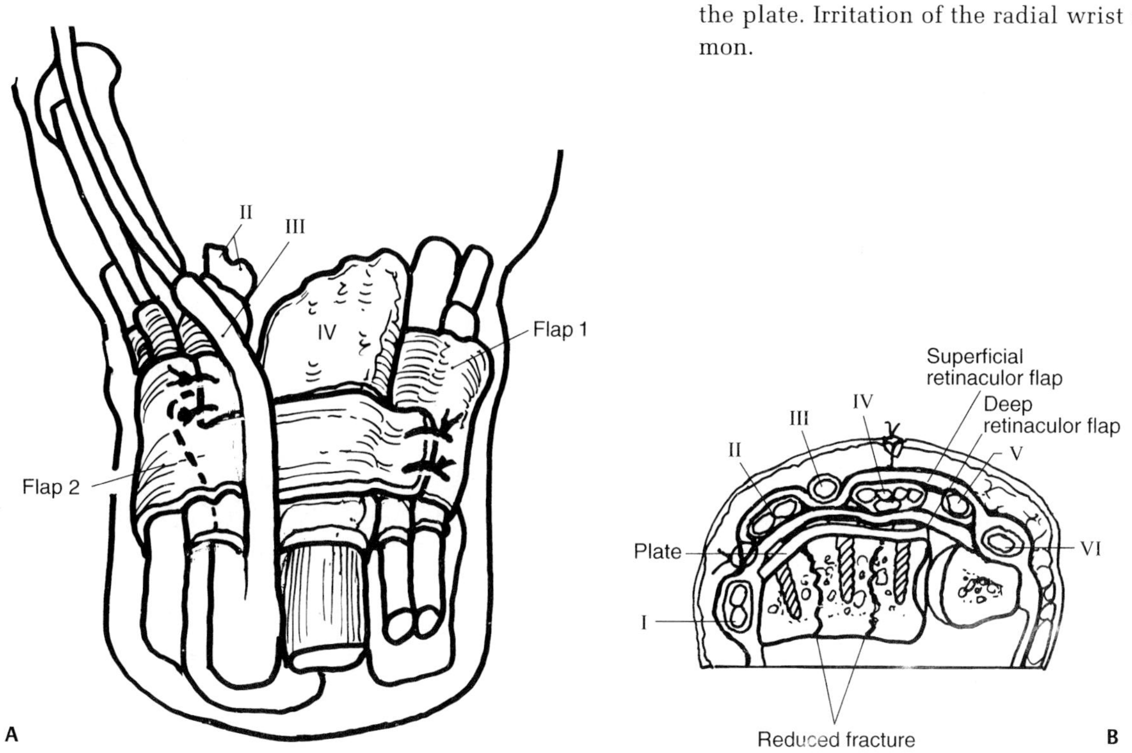

Figure 3–3

Suggested Readings

Chiang PP, Roach S, Baratz ME. Failure of a retinacular flap to prevent dorsal wrist pain after titanium plate fixation of distal radius fractures. J Hand Surg [Am] 2002;27:724–728

Rozental TD, Beredjiklian PK, Bozentka DJ. Functional outcome and complications following two types of dorsal plating for unstable fractures of the distal part of the radius. J Bone Joint Surg Am 2003;85-A:1956–1960

4 Palmar Fracture/Subluxation of the Distal Radius

Indications

Displaced intra-articular fracture of the distal radius with palmar subluxation of the carpus on lateral radiograph

Technique

- Palmar approach via zigzag incision over flexor carpi radialis (FCR) sheath. (**Fig. 4–1**)

■ Pitfall

Don't stray radial to the FCR in superficial dissection, which will risk injury to the palmar cutaneous branch of the median nerve.

- Retract FCR radially.
- Incise floor of FCR sheath.
- Elevate pronator quadratus off of radius by subperiosteal dissection working from radial to ulnar (**Fig. 4–2A**).
- Elevate the brachioradialis off the radial styloid.

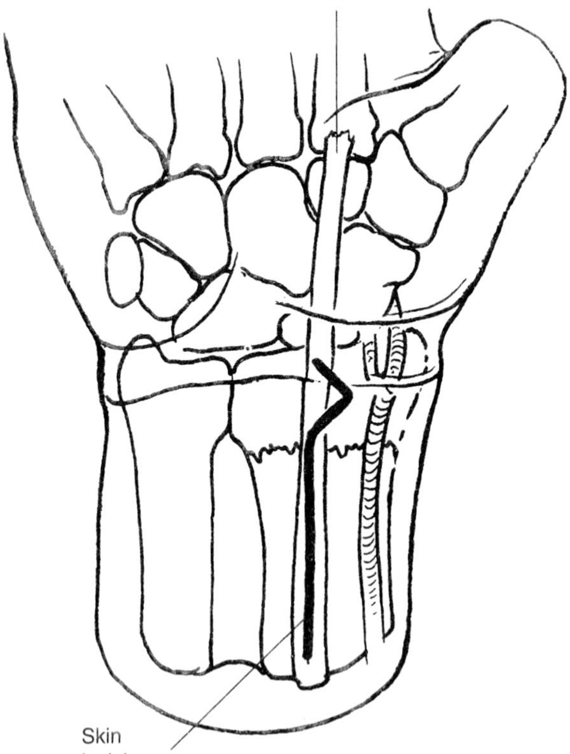

Figure 4–1

- Debride fracture site, elevate palmar cortical fragments to access and reduce impacted articular surface (**Fig. 4–2B**).

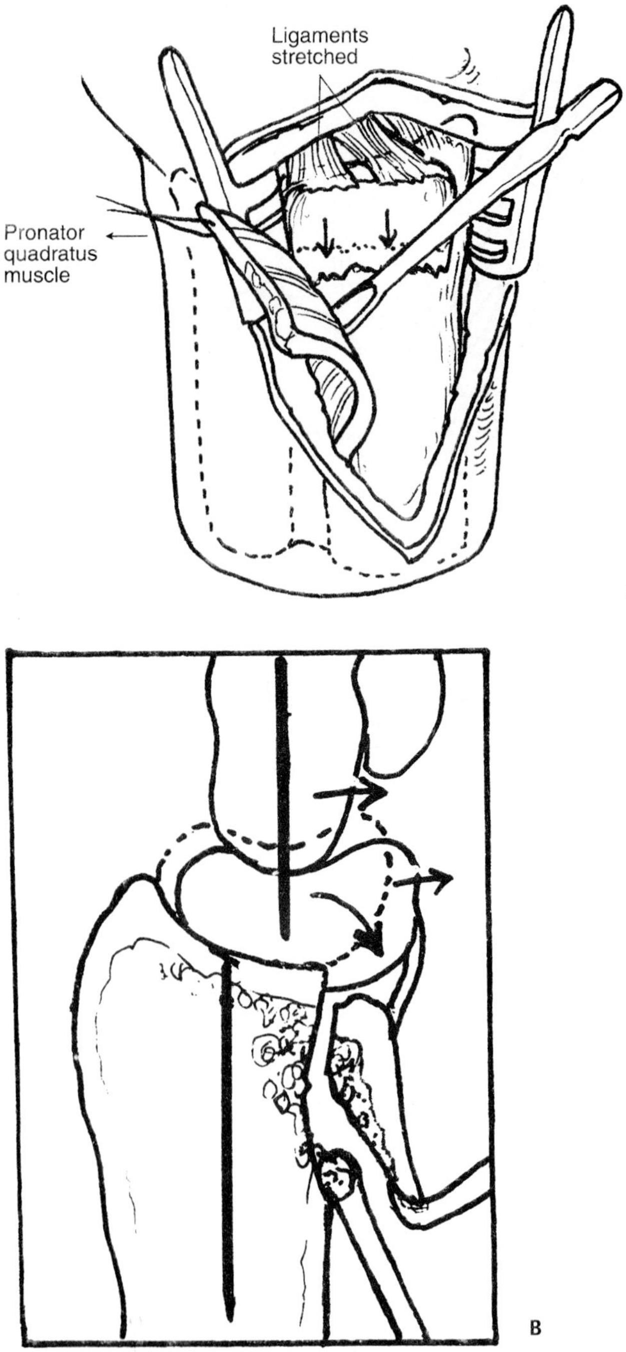

Figure 4–2

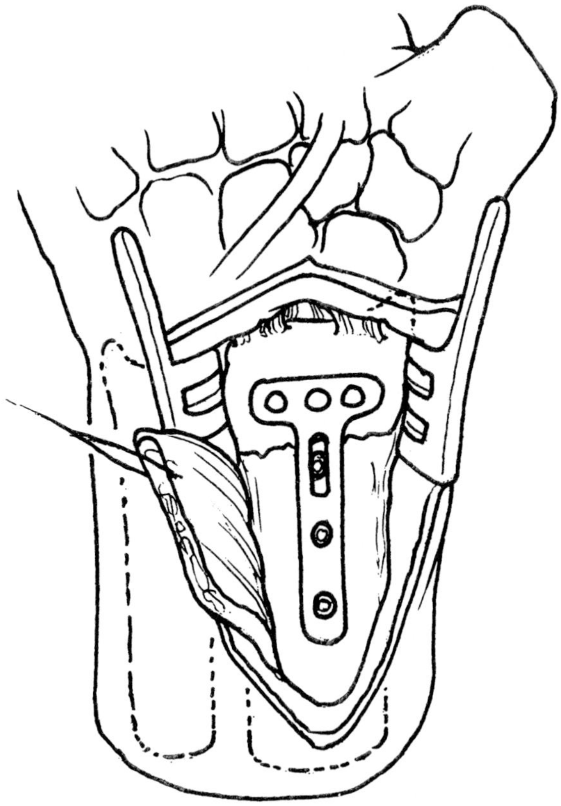

Figure 4–3

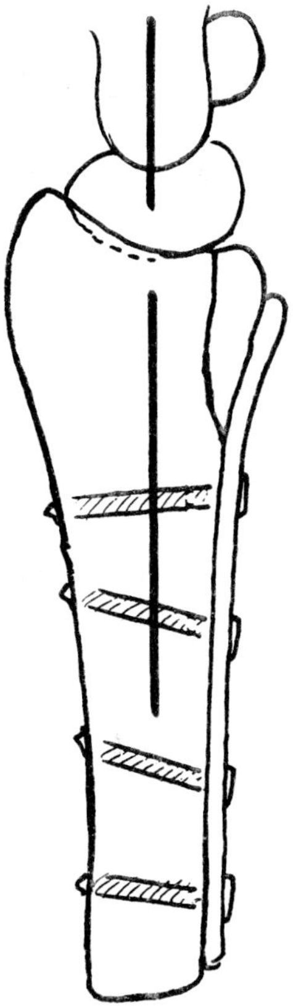

Figure 4–4

■ **Pearl**

Displacement in distal radius fractures is frequently a combination of angulation and malrotation. Malrotation is apparent in the offset seen along the fracture line through the palmar cortex. Angulation is usually corrected when the distal fragment is tightly applied to a properly positioned palmar plate.

- Apply palmar plate by placing one screw in shaft (proximal fragment) (**Fig. 4–3**).
- The shape of the plate will help guide reduction.
- Locking screws are inserted where there is intact dorsal cortex. Locking pins are used to buttress areas of articular comminution.
- The adequacy of the reduction and the position of the hardware are confirmed with intraoperative fluoroscopy (**Fig. 4–4**).
- Place pronator quadratus over plate. Close skin.

■ **Pearl**

A 20 degree "tilt lateral" will help visualize the articular surface to ensure that no pins or screws have penetrated the joint. A lateral image is obtained with the wrist angled 20 degrees in a radial direction.

Postoperative Care

- Immediate finger motion
- Short arm splint for 2 weeks
- Short arm cast for 2 weeks

■ **Pitfall**

Check for evidence pre- and postoperatively for acute carpal tunnel syndrome. If the patient is numb and has abnormal two-point discrimination, consider carpal tunnel release.

Suggested Readings

Geissler WB, Freeland AE. Arthroscopically assisted reduction of intraarticular distal radial fractures. Clin Orthop June 1996(327):125–134

Trumble TE, et al. Intra-articular fractures of the distal aspect of the radius. Instr Course Lect 1999;48: 465–480

Trumble TE, et al. Factors affecting functional outcome of displaced intra-articular distal radius fractures. J Hand Surg [Am] 1994;19: 325–340

5 Open Treatment of a Distal Radius Fracture with a Fixed Angle Palmar Plate

Indications

Any displaced fracture of the distal radius

■ Pitfall

Intra-articular fractures, particularly those with displaced intra-articular fragments, require experience with this implant.

■ Pearl

Review technique manuals for specifics regarding the various implants currently available on the market.

Technique

- Palmar approach via zig-zag incision over flexor carpi radialis (FCR) sheath (**Fig. 5–1**)
- Retract FCR radially.
- Incise floor of FCR sheath.
- Elevate pronator quadratus off of radius by subperiosteal dissection working from radial to ulnar (**Fig. 5–2**).
- Release brachioradialis tendon from radial styloid.

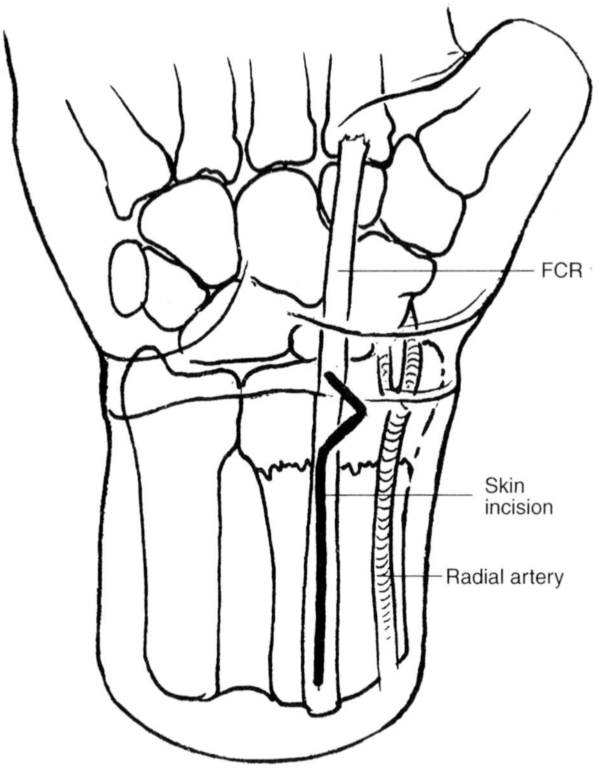

Figure 5–1

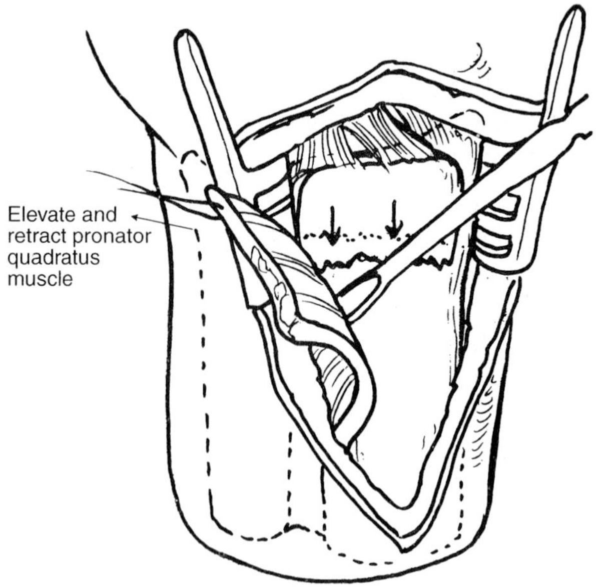

Figure 5–2

■ Pitfall

The brachioradialis tendon forms the floor of the first extensor compartment. Take care to avoid injury to the abductor pollicis longus (APL) tendon.

- Debride fracture site and attempt provisional reduction.

■ Pearl

Malposition of a distal radius fracture is usually a combination of malrotation and dorsal angulation of the distal fragment. Malrotation can be corrected by realigning the palmar cortex. Angulation is corrected by tightly securing the distal fragment against an appropriately positioned and anchored palmar plate.

- Apply palmar plate by placing one screw in oval hole (proximal fragment) (**Fig. 5–3**).
- Maintain fracture reduction with palmarly directed force over wrist and distal fragment using bump (**Fig. 5–3**).
- Check plate and fracture position with intraoperative radiographs.
- Gently screw drill guide into radialmost hole.
- Advance a 0.045 in. wire through guide and into styloid; use finger pressure on dorsal cortex to maintain reduction of distal fragment.
- Check pin position with an AP, lateral, and "20 degree tilt lateral."
- Remove wire and exchange for a screw directed into the radial styloid (**Fig. 5–4**).
- Adjust reduction as necessary.
- Pay careful attention to the reduction of the lunate articular surface and sigmoid notch during fixation into ulnarmost hole (**Fig. 5–4**).
- Fill remaining holes. Place screws where dorsal cortex provides sufficient purchase; use pins with threaded heads where dorsal cortex is comminuted (**Fig. 5–5**).

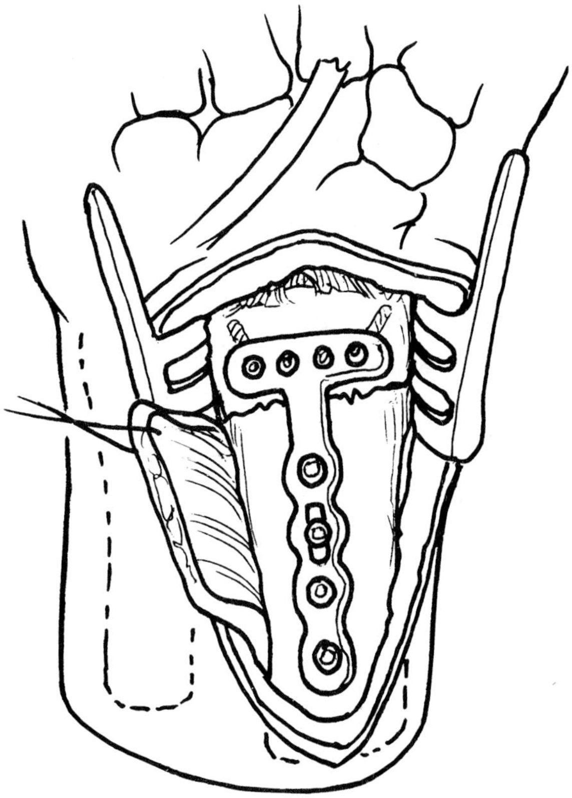

Figure 5–4

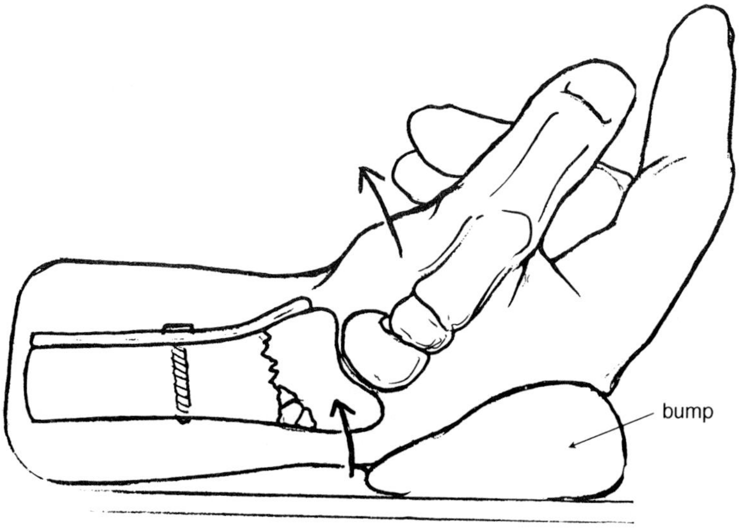

Figure 5–3

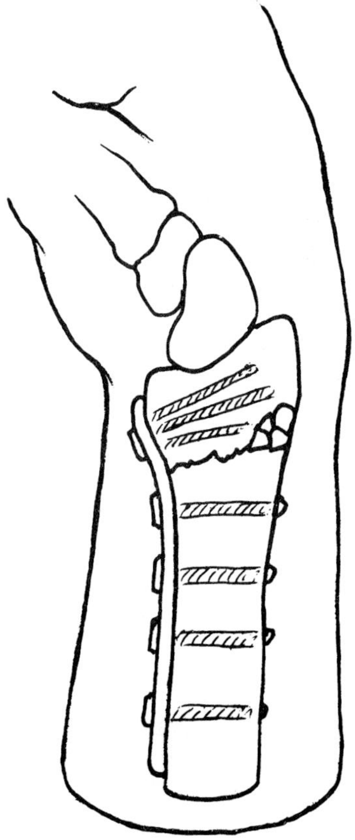

Figure 5–5

- Screws without threaded heads can be used to secure fragments that require drilling at an angle other than possible with the fixed-angle holes in the T portion of the plate.
- Recheck plate and screw position with intraoperative radiographs.
- Place pronator quadratus over plate. Close skin.

Postoperative Care

- Immediate finger motion and forearm rotation
- Short arm plaster splint and bulky bandage for 2 weeks
- Short arm molded plastic for 2 weeks. If the fixation is stable, the splint can be removed for gentle wrist motion.

Suggested Readings

Orbay JL, Fernandez DL. Volar fixation for dorsally displaced fractures of the distal radius: a preliminary report. J Hand Surg 2002;27A:205–215

Orbay JL, Fernandez DL. Volar fixed angle plate fixation for unstable distal radius fractures in the elderly patient. J Hand Surg 2004;29A:96–102

6 Open Treatment of Galeazzi Fractures

Indications

Any displaced fracture of the distal radius with an associated dislocation of the distal radioulnar joint (DRUJ) (**Fig. 6–1**)

Technique

- Palmar approach via zigzag incision over flexor carpi radialis (FCR) sheath (**Fig. 6–2**)
- Retract FCR radially.
- Incise floor of FCR sheath.
- Elevate pronator quadratus off of radius by subperiosteal dissection working from radial to ulnar.
- Extend the dissection proximally, elevating and retracting the fibers of the flexor pollicis longus in a radial direction.

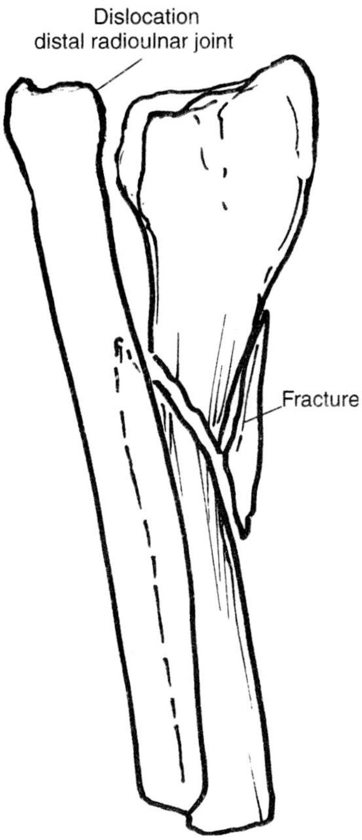

Figure 6–1

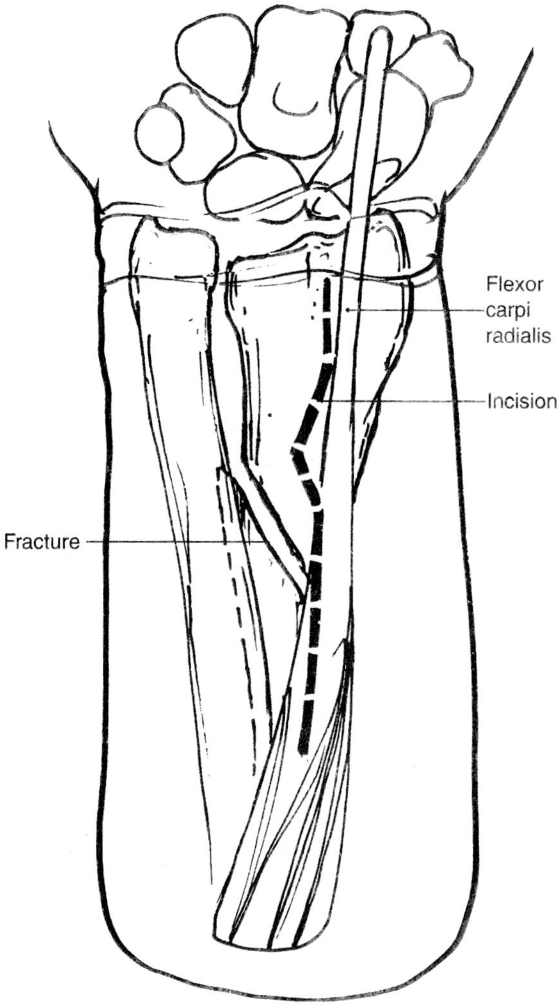

Figure 6–2

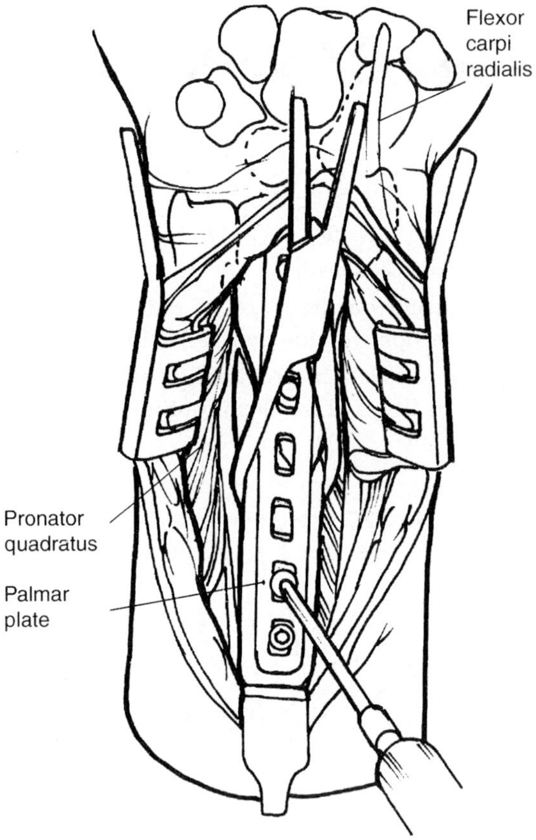

Figure 6–3

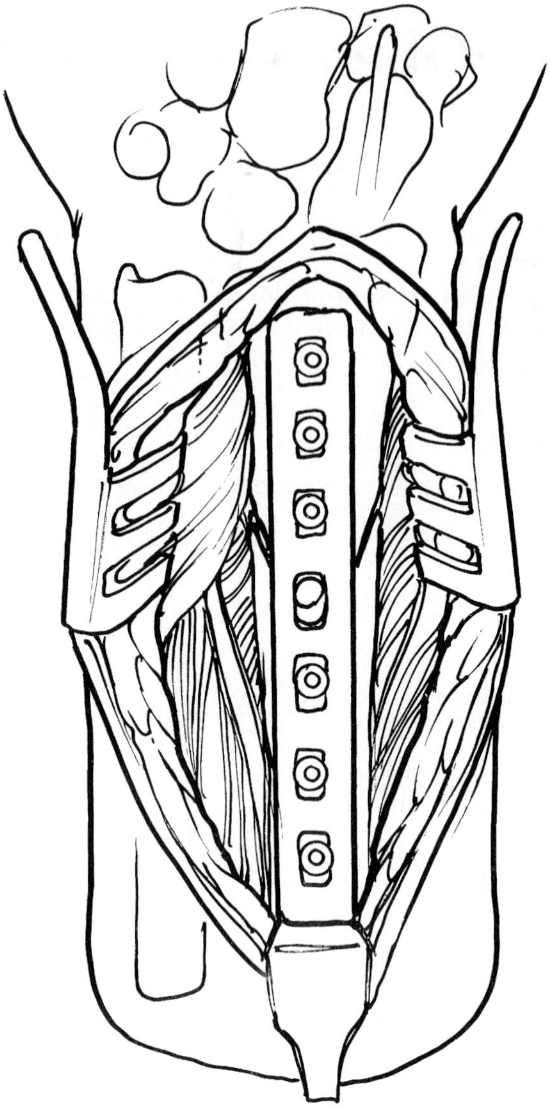

Figure 6–4

- Debride fracture site and attempt provisional reduction.
- Apply palmar plate with provisional fixation: 2 screws distally and 2 screws proximally (**Fig. 6–3**).
- Check plate and fracture position with intraoperative radiographs.

■ Pitfall

Check the position of the distal ulna on the lateral radiographs. Check the forearm rotation. If the ulna is not colinear with the radius on a lateral projection, or if there is a block to forearm rotation, carefully check the alignment of the radius. The most common reason for lack of forearm rotation is malalignment of the radius.

- Fill remaining holes in the plate. Recheck alignment of the radius and hardware placement (**Fig. 6–4**).
- Check the stability of the distal radioulnar joint with the forearm supinated, pronated, and in a neutral position (**Fig. 6–5**).
- If the ulna is stable in supination, consider immobilizing the forearm in supination.

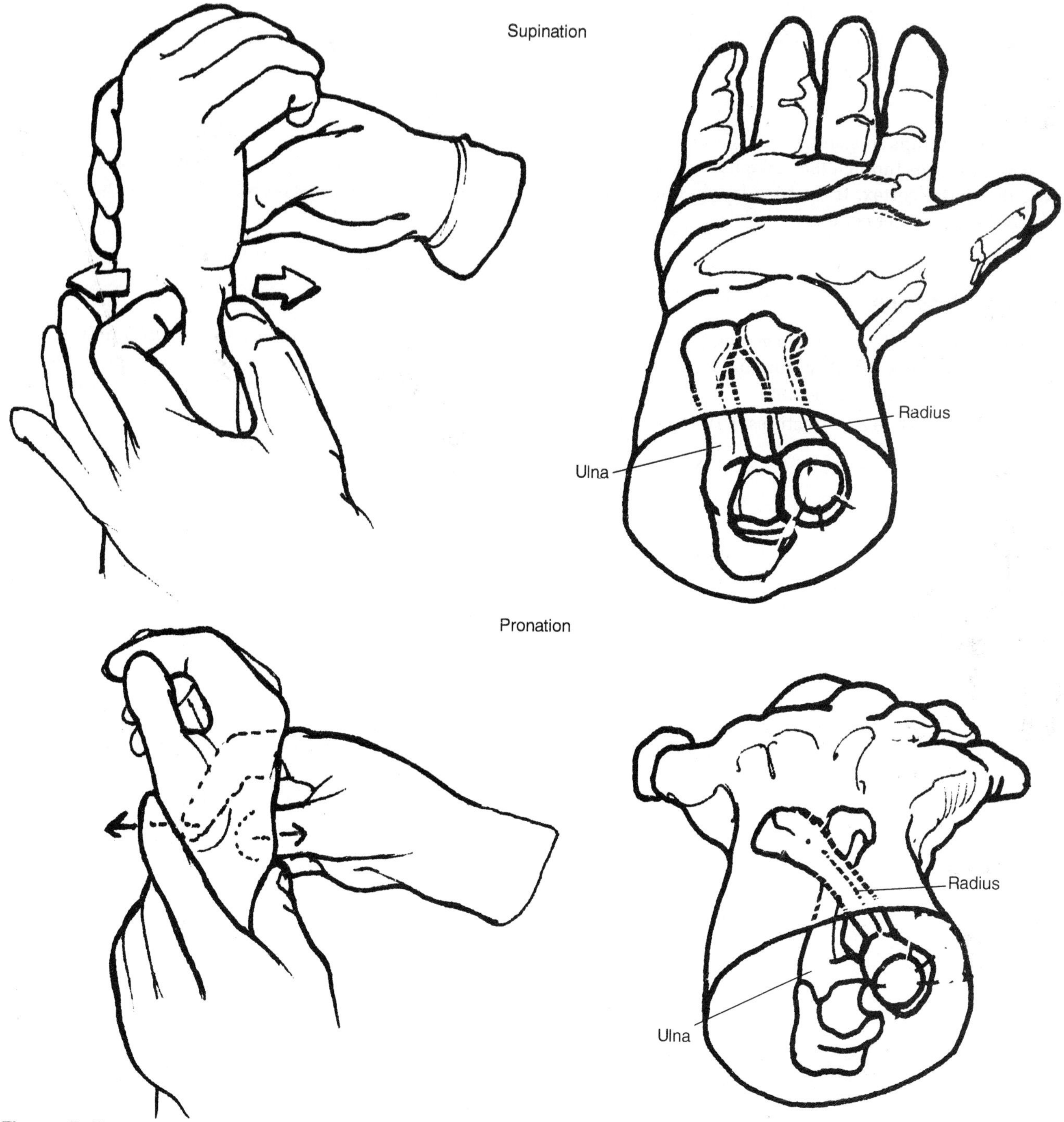

Figure 6–5

- If the ulna is unstable in all positions, consider pinning the distal radioulnar joint with the forearm in neutral.

■ Pearl

Use two 0.62 in. pins to stabilize the distal radial ulnar joint. Insert the pins through the metaphysis of the radius exiting the radial cortex. If the pins break, they can be retrieved through either cortex.

Postoperative Care

- Immediate finger motion and forearm rotation
- Long arm splint in supination if pins are not used and in neutral if pins are placed
- Begin forearm rotation at 4 weeks.
- Use static progressive splinting for limited forearm rotation once there is radiographic evidence that the radius has healed.

Suggested Readings

Faierman E, Jupiter JB. The management of acute fractures involving the distal radioulnar joint and distal ulna. Hand Clin 1998;14:213–229

Kraus B, Horne G. Galleazzi fractures. J Trauma 1985;24: 1093–1095

Strehle J, Gerber C. Distal radioulnar joint function after Galleazzi fracture-dislocation treated by open reduction and internal plate fixation. Clin Orthop 1993;293: 240–245

Section II

Distal Radius Malunions and Nonunions

7 Extension Osteotomy for the Malunited Distal Radius

Indications

- Wrist pain, limited wrist motion (especially flexion), and limited forearm rotation
- Deformity of the radius (**Fig. 7–1**)
- Loss of radial length due to dorsal tilt of articular surface

Preoperative Evaluation

- Template: must decide whether to correct dorsal tilt alone or correct dorsal tilt and lengthen dorsal and palmar cortex
- Prepare the patient for the possibility of a resection of the distal ulna if a block to forearm rotation persists after restoring the shape of the radius, or if there is arthritis of distal radioulnar joint (DRUJ).

Technique

- Use dorsal approach to the radius.
- Remove the extensor pollicis longus (EPL) from the third compartment and retract radially.
- Z-lengthen the retinaculum of the fourth compartment and retract the extensor digitorum communis (EDC) tendons ulnarly (**Fig. 7–2**).

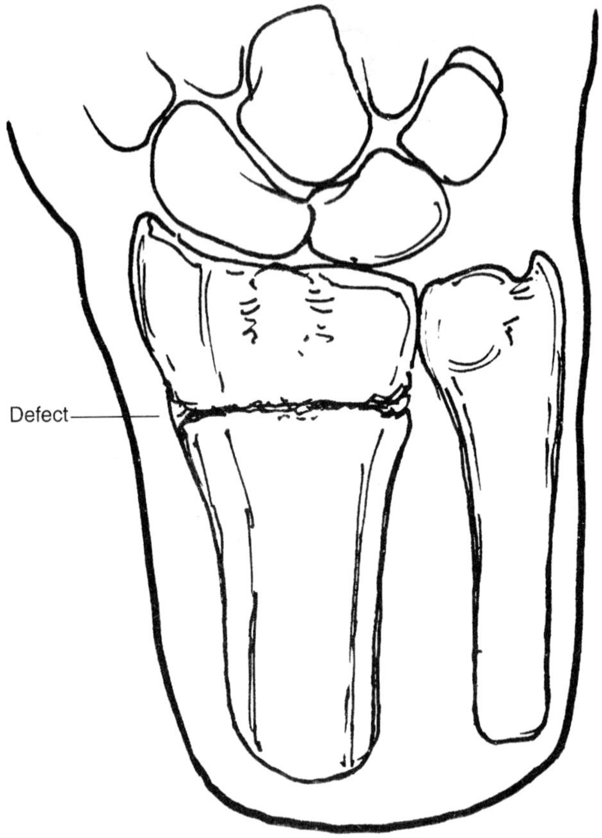

Figure 7–1

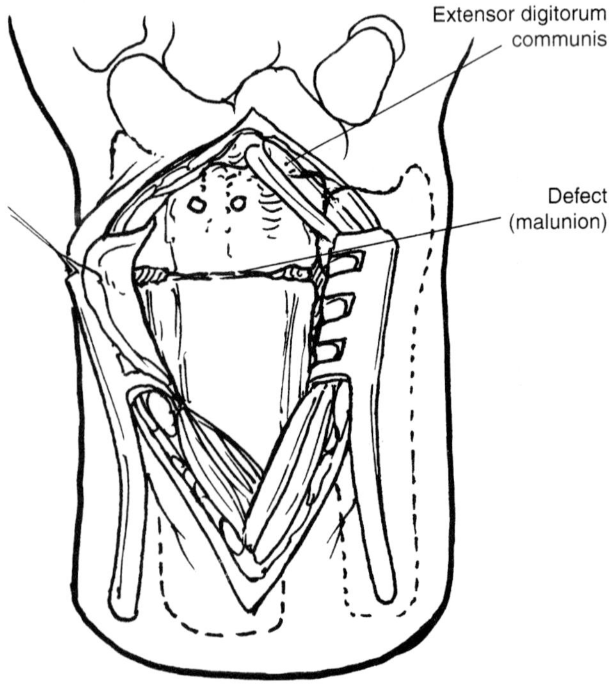

Figure 7–2

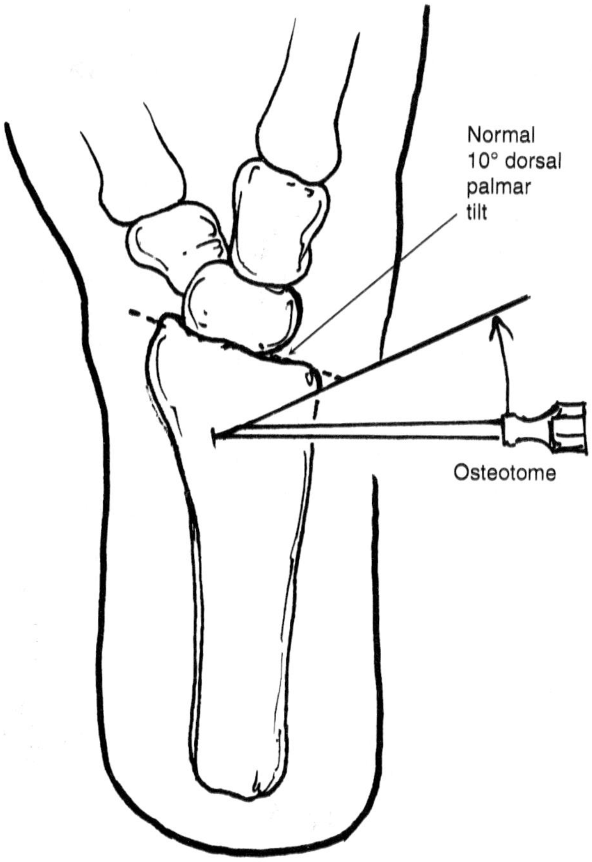

Figure 7–3

- Place spinal needle into radiocarpal joint to show plane of the articular surface.
- Drill K-wire into dorsal aspect of radius at expected level of osteotomy parallel to spinal needle. Check position with fluoroscopy (**Fig. 7–3**).

■ Pearl

The osteotomy should be

- Parallel to the joint
- In the metaphysis; preferably through the original fracture line of the distal fragment
- Proximal enough to allow adequate fixation
- Complete the osteotomy in line with K-wire using osteotome or oscillating saw with generous irrigation.

■ Pearl

Do not violate the palmar cortex if length can be restored by osteotomy of the dorsal cortex alone. An intact palmar cortex adds to the stability of the osteotomized bone. This allows the use of narrow, low-profile plates to stabilize the dorsal cortex.

- Correct malposition. Maintain corrected position with Gelpy retractors ± K-wires (**Fig. 7–2**). Check position with intraoperative imaging.
- Harvest iliac crest bone graft (ICBG) tricortical graft to match size of defect and additional cancellous bone.
- Press fit ICBG to defect.
- Check position with intraoperative image.
- Stabilize with dorsal plate: place distal and proximal screw. Check position with intraoperative imaging (**Fig. 7–4**).

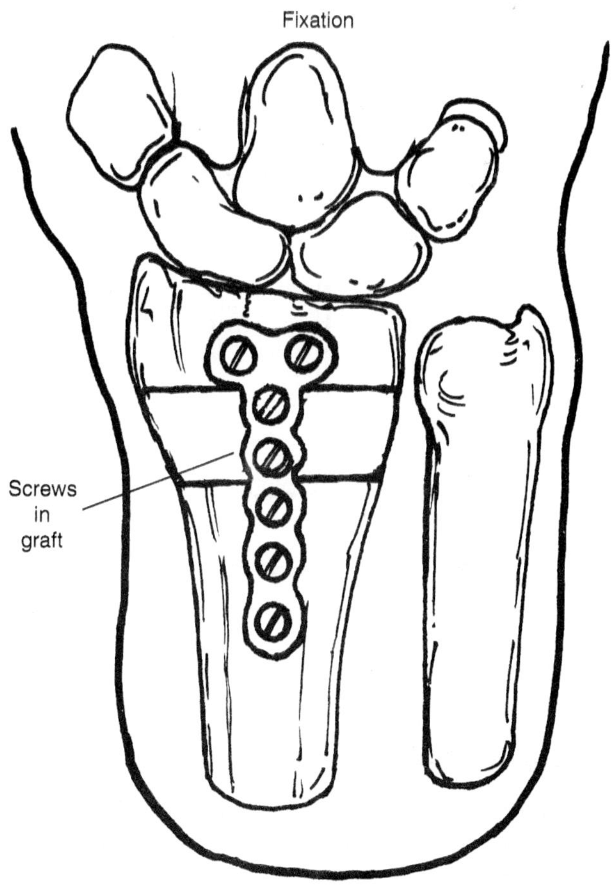

Figure 7–4

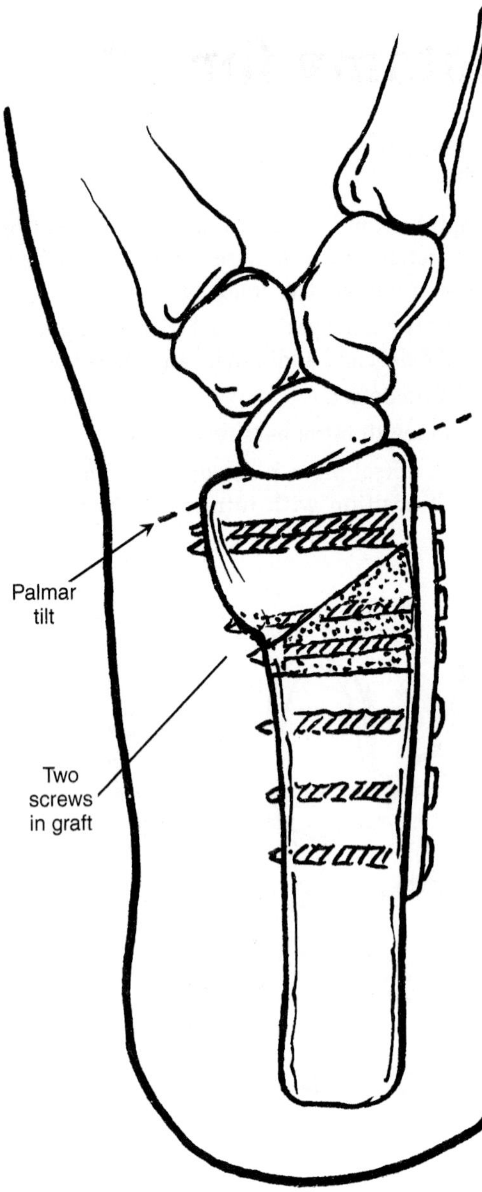

Figure 7–5

■ Pearl

When the EPL tendon is transposed there is an ~1 cm space between the extensor carpi radialis tendon and the EDC tendons. If the palmar cortex is intact and the press fit ICBG creates a stable radius, a 2.0 or 2.4 mini fragment plate can be used to stabilize the radius and secure the graft. If, following plating, the construct does not appear secure use a larger plate or supplement the fixation with two 0.062 in. pins inserted from the radial styloid.

- Fill remaining screws. Check appearance of DRUJ and quality of rotation. If radius is reduced and there is a block to rotation or coexisting arthritis of the DRUJ, consider Darrach resection in older, low-demand patient; hemiresection of the distal ulna in a younger, high-demand patient. (**Fig. 7–5**)
- Close, laying one flap of retinaculum over plate and one over tendons.

Postoperative Care

- Short arm splint for 2 weeks
- Short arm cast until the osteotomy has healed

Alternative Techniques

- Corrective, extension osteotomy of the distal radius can be performed through a palmar approach using palmar plate with locking screws.
- In malunions treated within the first few months it is often possible to use banked bone instead of iliac crest bone graft.

Suggested Readings

Fernandez DL. Reconstructive procedures for malunion and traumatic arthritis. Orthop Clin North Am 1993;24: 341–363

Ladd AL, Huene DS. Reconstructive osteotomy for malunion of the distal radius. Clin Orthop 1996;327: 158–171

8 Dorsal and Palmar Osteotomy for Malunion of Distal Radius with Iliac Crest Bone Graft

Indications

- Wrist pain, limited wrist motion (especially flexion), and limited forearm rotation
- Deformity of radius
- Dorsal tilt of articular surface
- Loss of radial length due to shortening from *both dorsal tilt of the radius and shortening of the palmar cortex*

Preoperative Evaluation

Template: must decide whether to correct dorsal tilt alone or correct dorsal tilt and lengthen dorsal and palmar cortex

Discuss the possibility that the radius cannot be restored to its anatomical length. This may create the need to perform a resection of the distal ulna to restore forearm rotation.

Technique

- Dorsal approach between third and fourth extensor compartment internal via Z-lplasty of retinaculum (**Fig. 8–1**)

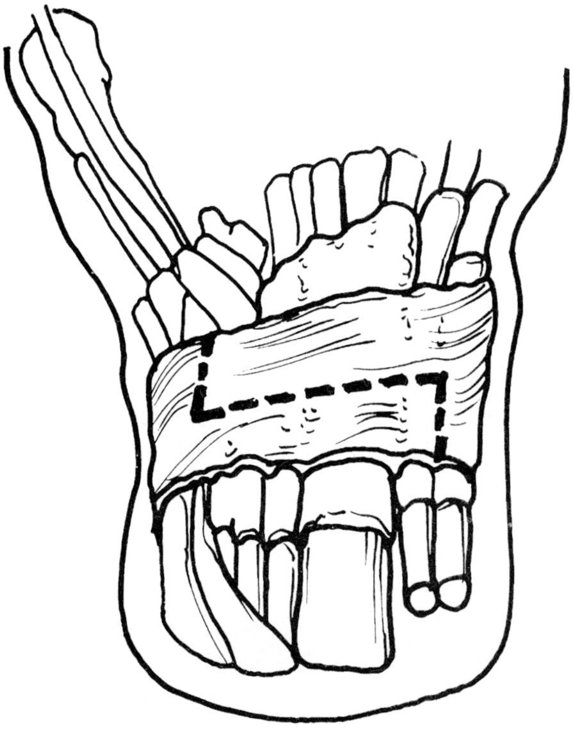

Figure 8–1

- Place spinal needle into radiocarpal joint to show plane of the articular surface.
- Drill K-wire into dorsal aspect of radius at expected level of osteotomy parallel to spinal needle. Check position with fluoroscopy.

Pearl

The osteotomy should be

- Parallel to the joint
- In the metaphysis; preferably through the original fracture line of the distal fragment
- Proximal enough to allow adequate fixation
- Complete the osteotomy in line with the K-wire using an osteotome or an oscillating saw with generous irrigation.
- Correct malposition. Maintain corrected position with Gelpy retractor ± K-wires (**Fig. 8–2**). Check position with intraoperative imaging.
- Harvest iliac crest bone graft (ICBG) tricortical graft to match size of defect. Harvest additional cancellous bone to supplement tricortical graft.

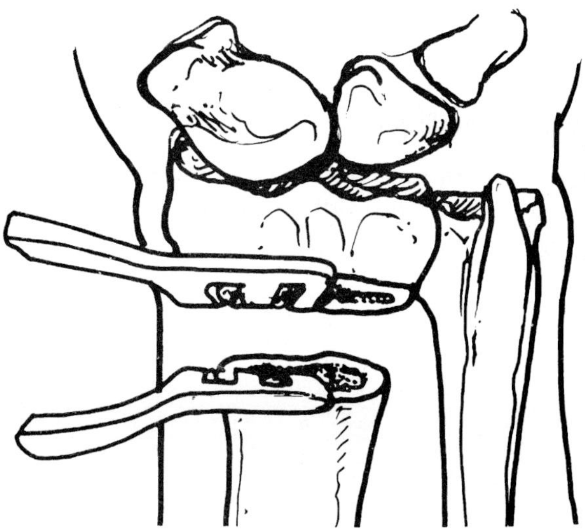

Figure 8–2

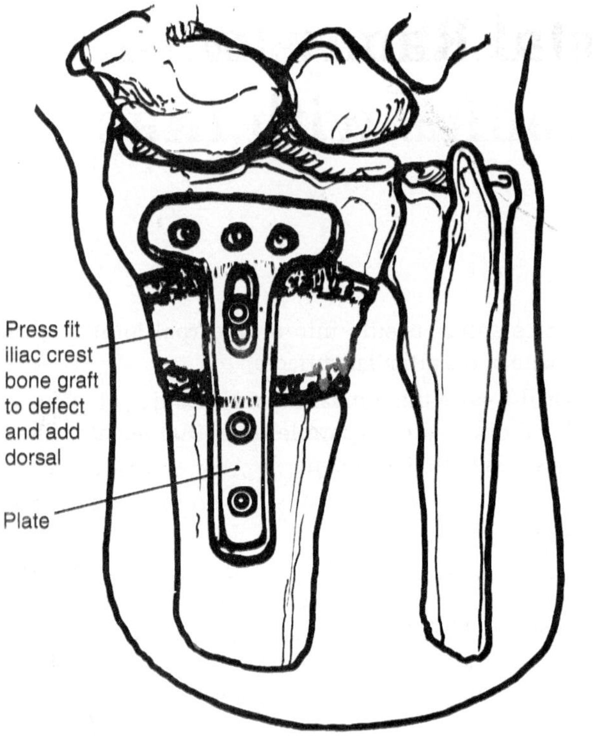

Figure 8–3

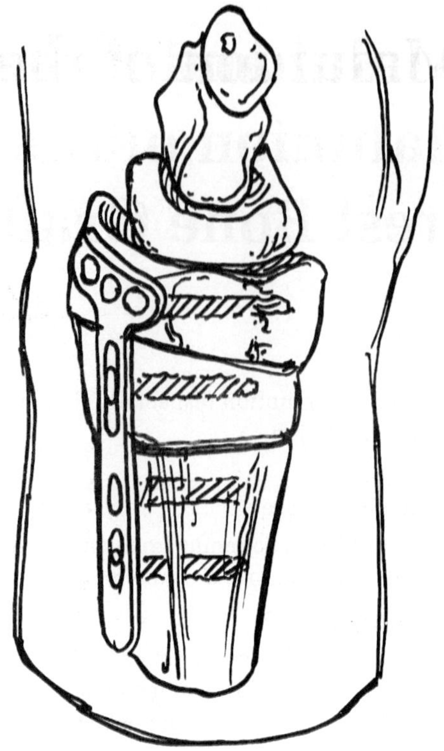

Figure 8–4

- Press fit ICBG to defect (**Fig. 8–3**).
- Check position with intraoperative image.
- Stabilize with dorsal plate: place distal and proximal screw. Check position with intraoperative imaging.
- Fill remaining screws. Check appearance of distal radioulnar joint (DRUJ) and quality of rotation. If radius is reduced and there is a block to rotation or coexisting arthritis of the DRUJ, consider a stabilized Darrach resection (**Fig. 8–4**).
- Close, laying one flap of retinaculum over plate and one over tendons.

Postoperative Care

- Short arm splint for 2 weeks
- Short arm cast until there is radiographic evidence of healing

Alternative Technique

- Palmar plate fixation can be used in conjunction with both a dorsal and a palmar osteotomy.
- A dorsal approach in addition to the palmar approach facilitates placement of the ICBG.

Suggested Readings

Fernandez DL. Reconstructive procedures for malunion and traumatic arthritis. Orthop Clin North Am 1993;24: 341–363

Ladd AL, Huene DS. Reconstructive osteotomy for malunion of the distal radius. Clin Orthop 1996;327: 158–171

9 Malunion of the Distal Radius with Palmar Translation of the Articular Surface

Indications

Fractures with disruption of the palmar cortex that have healed with palmar subluxation of all or a portion of the articular surface.

■ Pearl

Scrutinize the preoperative radiographs for evidence of posttraumatic arthritis of the distal radioulnar joint (DRUJ). A CT scan is often helpful when a definitive diagnosis cannot be made on the basis of plain radiographs.

Technique

- Palmar approach via zigzag incision over flexor carpi radialis (FCR) sheath. Retract FCR radially (**Fig. 9–1**).
- Incise floor of FCR sheath. Elevate pronator quadratus off of radius by subperiosteal dissection working from radial to ulnar.
- Elevate the brachioradialis off the radial styloid.
- Identify the plane of the previous fracture with an osteotome (**Fig. 9–2**). Check with intraoperative fluoroscopy.
- Separate and elevate the palmarly translated fragment from the surrounding soft tissues and bone. Preserve the palmar radiocarpal ligaments.

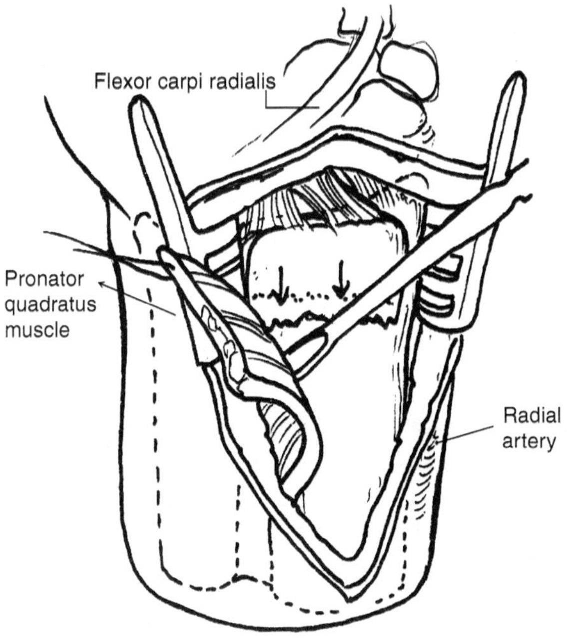

Figure 9–1

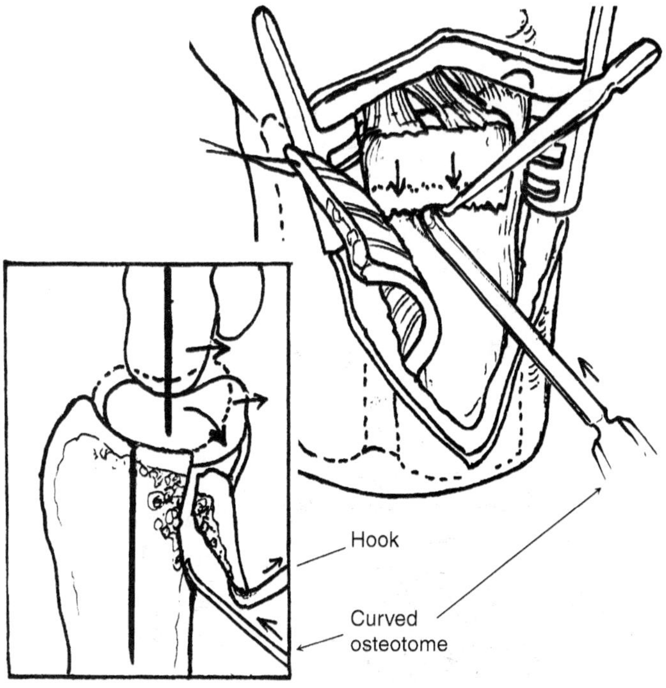

Figure 9–2

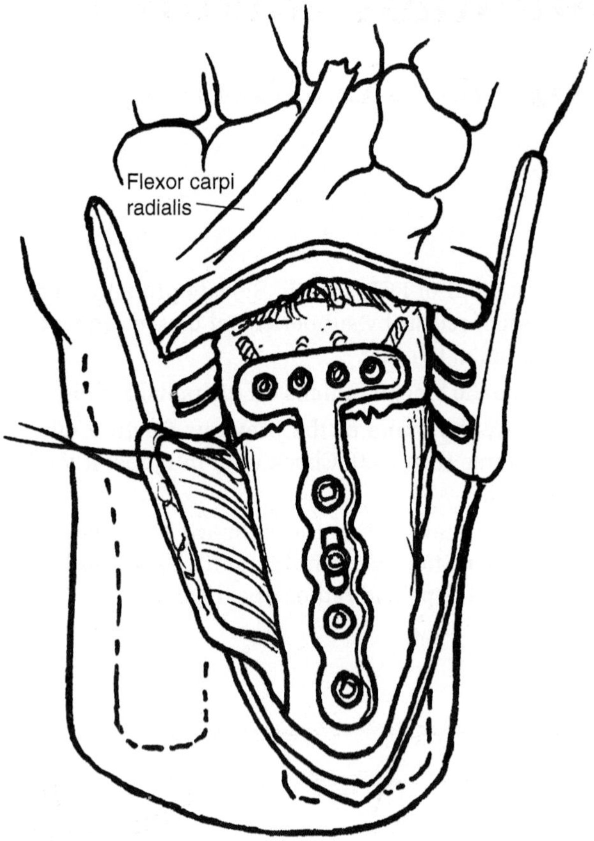

Figure 9–3

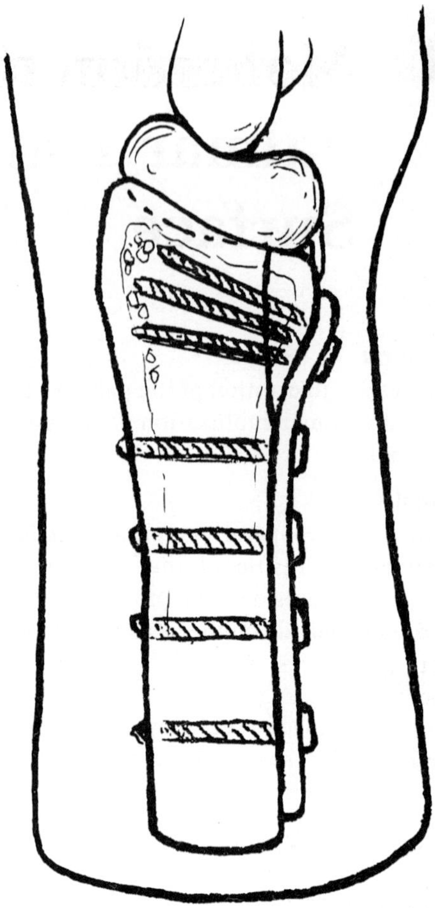

Figure 9–4

■ Pearl

If there seems to be a block to reducing the fragment, the articular surface can be inspected by dorsiflexion of the wrist combined with palmar retraction of the displaced fracture fragment.

- Reduce the fracture and apply palmar plate by placing one screw in the shaft (**Fig. 9–3**).
- Assess fracture reduction and plate placement with fluoroscopy.
- Place the remaining proximal and distal screws.
- Check wrist motion and forearm rotation.
- Use the 20 degree "tilt lateral" view with fluoroscopy as described and illustrated in Chapter 4 to assess the reduction of the fracture and the placement of the distal screws (**Fig. 9–4**).

■ Pitfall

A persistent loss of forearm rotation usually means that the fracture has been inadequately reduced. If the reduction appears adequate, release of the DRUJ capsule may improve forearm rotation. In cases where reduction of the radius is not attainable it may be necessary to perform a resection of the distal ulna through a separate dorsal incision (see Chapter 12).

Postoperative Care

- Immediate finger motion and forearm rotation
- Short arm splint for 2 weeks
- Short arm cast for 2 weeks

■ Pearl

If the fracture fixation is solid, the patient can be placed in a removable splint and allowed gentle wrist motion.

Suggested Readings

Fernandez DL. Reconstructive procedures for malunion and traumatic arthritis. Orthop Clin North Am 1993;24: 341–363

Ladd AL, Huene DS. Reconstructive osteotomy for malunion of the distal radius. Clin Orthop 1996;327: 158–171

10 Nonunion of Distal Radius Fractures

Indications

Nonunited fractures of the distal radius. These fractures commonly have little cancellous bone. Nonunion commonly follows failed treatment with external fixation and percutaneously placed pins.

■ Pearl

Inspect the distal radioulnar joint (DRUJ) on preoperative radiographs. If the DRUJ appears salvageable prepare to use tricortical iliac crest bone graft to help fill the defect created by distal translation of the distal fragment. If the DRUJ does not appear salvageable, prepare the patient for distal ulna resection. In this case the radius can be shortened and grafted with cancellous bone.

Technique

- Use a dorsal approach to the distal radius.
- Open the retinaculum over the second through fourth extensor compartments as two opposing flaps (see Chapter 3, **Fig. 3–1A,B**).
- Remove fibrous tissue and devascularized bone between the fracture fragments. Release the brachioradialis and any soft tissue attachments that may limit reduction of the fragment. Avoid stripping the radiocarpal ligaments (**Fig. 10–1**).
- Decide whether the distal ulna can be preserved or should be resected. We recommend the surgeon consider stabilization of the resected distal ulna as described in Chapter 22.

■ Pearl

If the nonunion extends to the subchondral bone or into the joint, it may be necessary to open the dorsal capsule. A small window in the capsule can aid in reduction of the malunited fragment and confirm that hardware does not enter the radiocarpal joint.

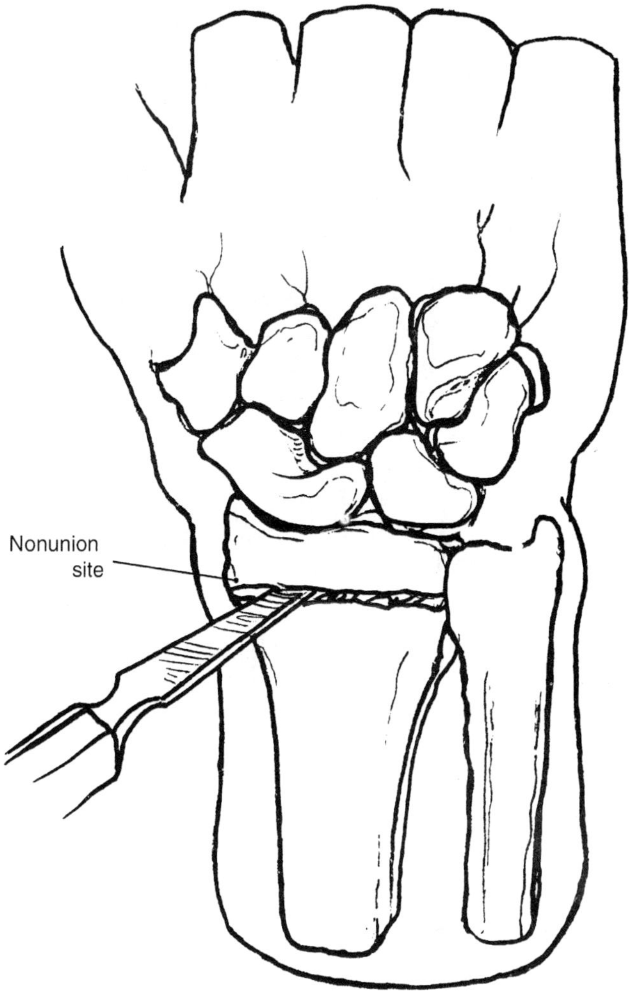

Figure 10–1

■ Pitfall

The most difficult nonunion to manage is the very distal fracture that leaves little bone in the distal fragment. Fixation is a challenge in these instances. It is important

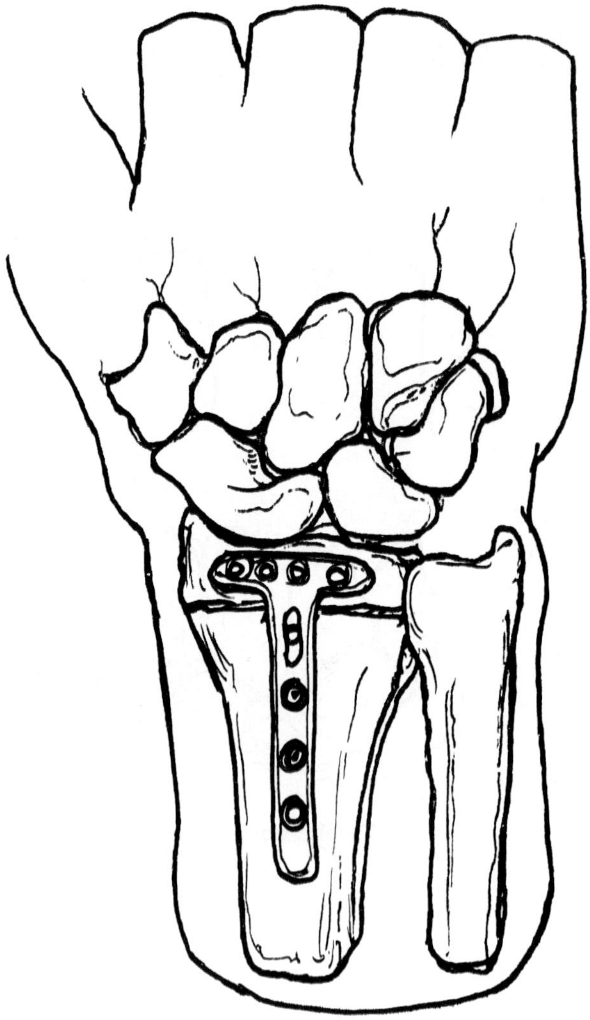

Figure 10–2

to have a variety of fixation devices available, including a distal radial plating system, a mini fragment set, and pins.

- Apply dorsal plate and place screws in radial styloid and in radial shaft (**Fig. 10–2**).
- Check reduction with intraoperative imaging.
- Fill remaining holes in the plate as the fracture pattern permits. A dorsal plate that accommodates smooth pins or screws with heads that thread into the plate converts the implant to a fixed angle device. The pins can serve as a buttress for portions of the subchondral plate that have no metaphyseal bone.
- Use cancellous or tricortical crest graft as necessary to fill voids.
- Place one flap of retinaculum over plate, beneath extensors. Suture the flap in place. Place the second flap over the extensors and suture in place. Leave extensor pollicis longus free in the subcutaneous tissues.

Postoperative Care

- Immediate active range of motion of fingers
- Splint 2 weeks
- Cast 2 to 6 weeks depending on clinical and radiographic evidence of healing

■ Pitfall

Follow patients for evidence of extensor tendonitis from the plate. Irritation of the radial wrist extensors is common.

Alternative Techniques

Nonunions of the distal radius can be managed with locked palmar plates. The same principles apply: remove the sclerotic margins of the nonunion; restore length of the radius by using intercalary iliac crest bone graft. Mobilization of the distal fragment is enhanced by release of the brachioradialis. This relieves a deforming force and gives access to the dorsal aspect of the distal radius. The plate is fixed to the distal fragment first. Pins can be inserted through the plate to determine plate position. The pins should be directed parallel to the joint surface; pin position should be confirmed using intraoperative fluoroscopy. After the plate is fixed to the distal fragment, the plate is brought down and provisionally fixed to the radial shaft through an oblong hole. Length can be adjusted, as needed, with the assistance of intraoperative fluoroscopy. Corticocancellous bone can be inserted from the radial aspect of the radius. If necessary, a small dorsal incision can be used to gain access to the interval between the third and fourth extensor compartments. A wedge of iliac crest can be placed through this dorsal incision.

Suggested Readings

Segalman KA, Clark GL. Un-united fractures of the distal radius: a report of 12 cases. J Hand Surg 1998;23A:914–919

Smith VA, Wright TW. Nonunion of the distal radius. J Hand Surg 1999;24B:601–603

Section III

Distal Ulna Fractures

11 Open Reduction and Internal Fixation of an Ulnar Styloid Fracture

Indications

- Fracture of the distal radius and ulna with instability of the distal radioulnar joint (DRUJ)

Technique

- a linear incision is made along ulnar border of the hand and wrist. The incision begins 1 cm distal to the ulnar styloid and extends to the subcutaneous border of the ulna, palmar to the extensor carpi ulnaris (ECU) tendon sheath (**Fig. 11–1**).

■ Pitfall

Avoid the dorsal cutaneous branch of ulnar nerve that passes obliquely between the ulnar styloid and pisiform.

- Expose with subperiosteal dissection the ulnar aspect of the styloid and the ulnar head. Do not open the ECU subsheath (**Fig. 11–2**).
- Reduce the styloid and insert two parallel 0.35 in. pins through the tip and into the ulnar head.
- Advance the pins so that they barely perforate the medial metaphysis of the ulnar neck.

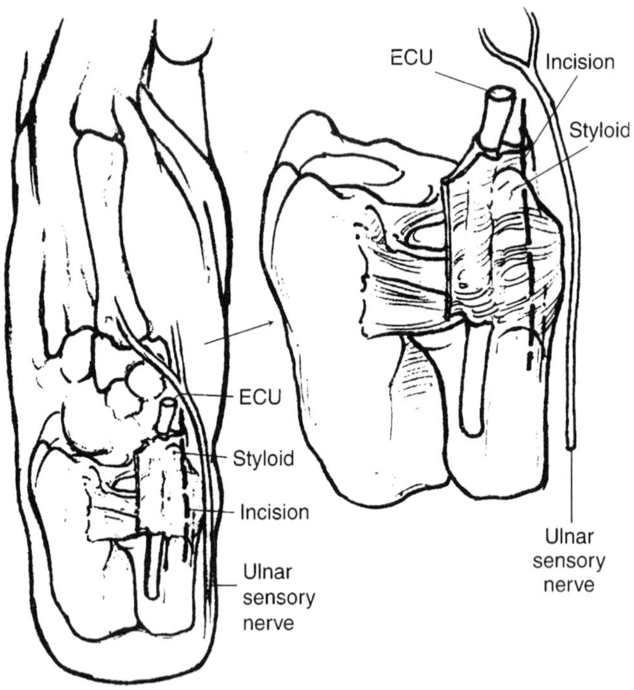

Figure 11–1

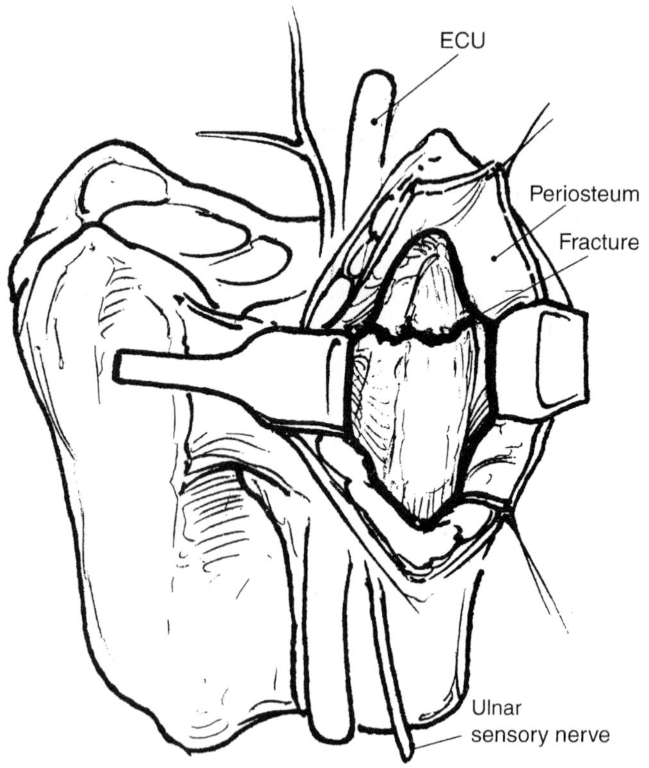

Figure 11–2

■ Pitfall

Pointed bone holding forceps can split the styloid fragment.

■ Pearl

A dental pick used with gentle pressure can help maintain reduction of the fragment while pins are being inserted.

- Make two connecting bone holes at the level of the ulnar neck (**Fig. 11–3**).
- Pass a 26 gauge wire or a 2–0 braided polyester suture through the holes and around the wires in a figure-of-eight configuration (**Fig. 11–4**).
- Bend the two pins into sharp U shapes. Cut the ends on an angle to create a sharp point.
- Rotate the pins so the U shape faces the joint capsule.
- Tap the pins to bury the tips into the ulnar head adjacent to the fovea.
- Check position of the fracture and hardware with intraoperative imaging.
- Check forearm rotation.
- Close joint capsule, subcutaneous tissues, and skin.

■ Pearl

- Using a nonabsorbable suture instead of wire and burying the pin tips may prevent hardware irritation (**Fig 11–5**).

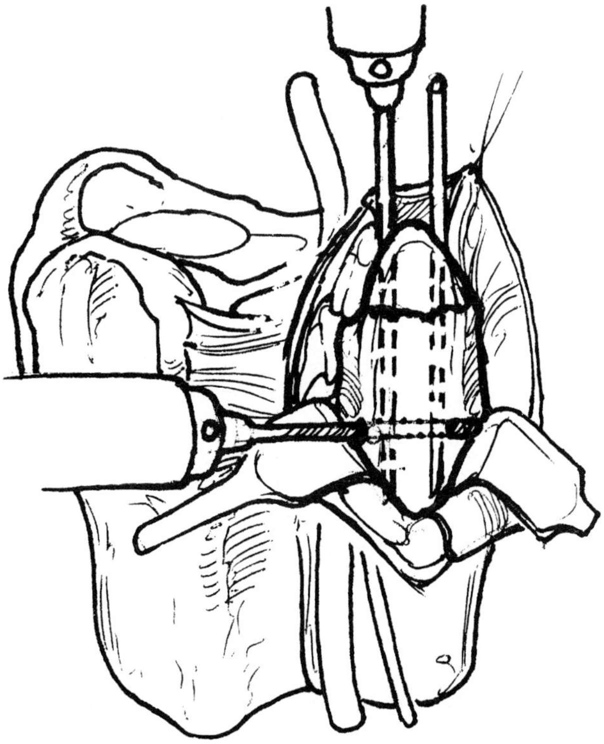

Reduce styloid; insert K-wires

Figure 11–3

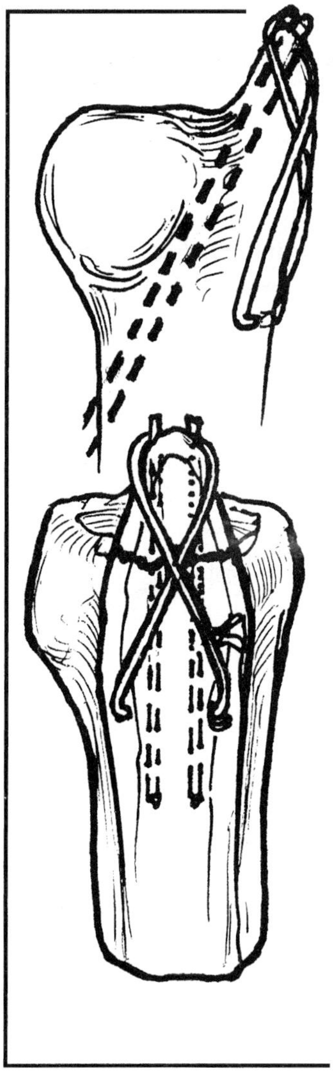

Figure 11–4

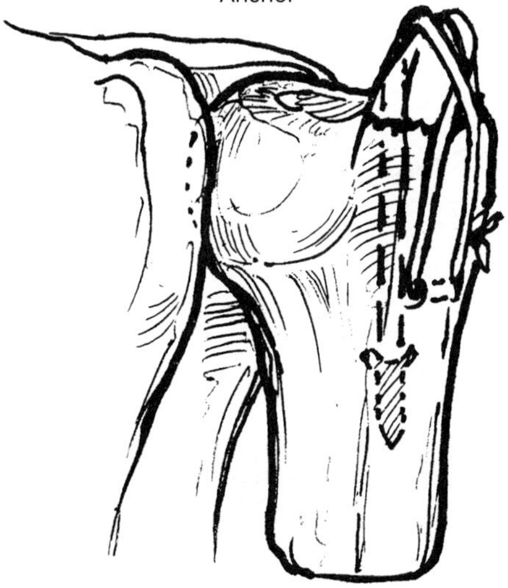

Figure 11–5

Postoperative Care

- Long-arm cast with the forearm in neutral rotation for 4 weeks
- Short-arm cast until the fracture is united

Alternative Technique

- Place a suture anchor into the head of the ulna. The attached sutures are passed either through the styloid fragment if it is large enough or around the fragment if is small. Make two connecting bone holes at the level of the ulnar neck. Create a figure-of-eight tension band using the sutures and the bone holes in the neck **(Fig. 11–5)**.

Suggested Readings

Aulicino PL, Siegel JL. Acute injuries of the distal radioulnar joint. Hand Clin 1991;7:283–293

Trumble TE, Culp R, Hanel DP, Geissler WB, Berger RA. Intra-articular fractures of the distal aspect of the radius. J Bone Joint Surg Am 1998;80-A:582–600

12 Fractures of the Ulnar Head

Indications

- Fractures extending from the fovea to the radial cortex of the ulnar head metaphysic

■ Pitfall

These fractures may be comminuted such that fixation is not possible. Prepare the patient for both fixation of the fracture and either hemiresection or Darrach-type resection of the distal ulna.

■ Pearl

If reduction and fixation of the fracture is chosen, the fixation must be sufficiently secure to permit immediate forearm rotation.

Technique

- Several forms of fixation should be available, including mini fragment plates, screws, and interosseous wire.
- Incision is a gentle curve extending from the base of the fifth metacarpal to the extensor carpi ulnaris (ECU), ~2 cm proximal to the distal radioulnar joint (DRUJ) (**Fig. 12–1A,B**).
- Expose the dorsal aspect of the DRUJ through fifth extensor compartment.
- Create ulnarly based rectangular capsular flap to expose the ulnar head.
- Assess comminution and the attachment of the triangular fibrocartilage complex (TFCC).

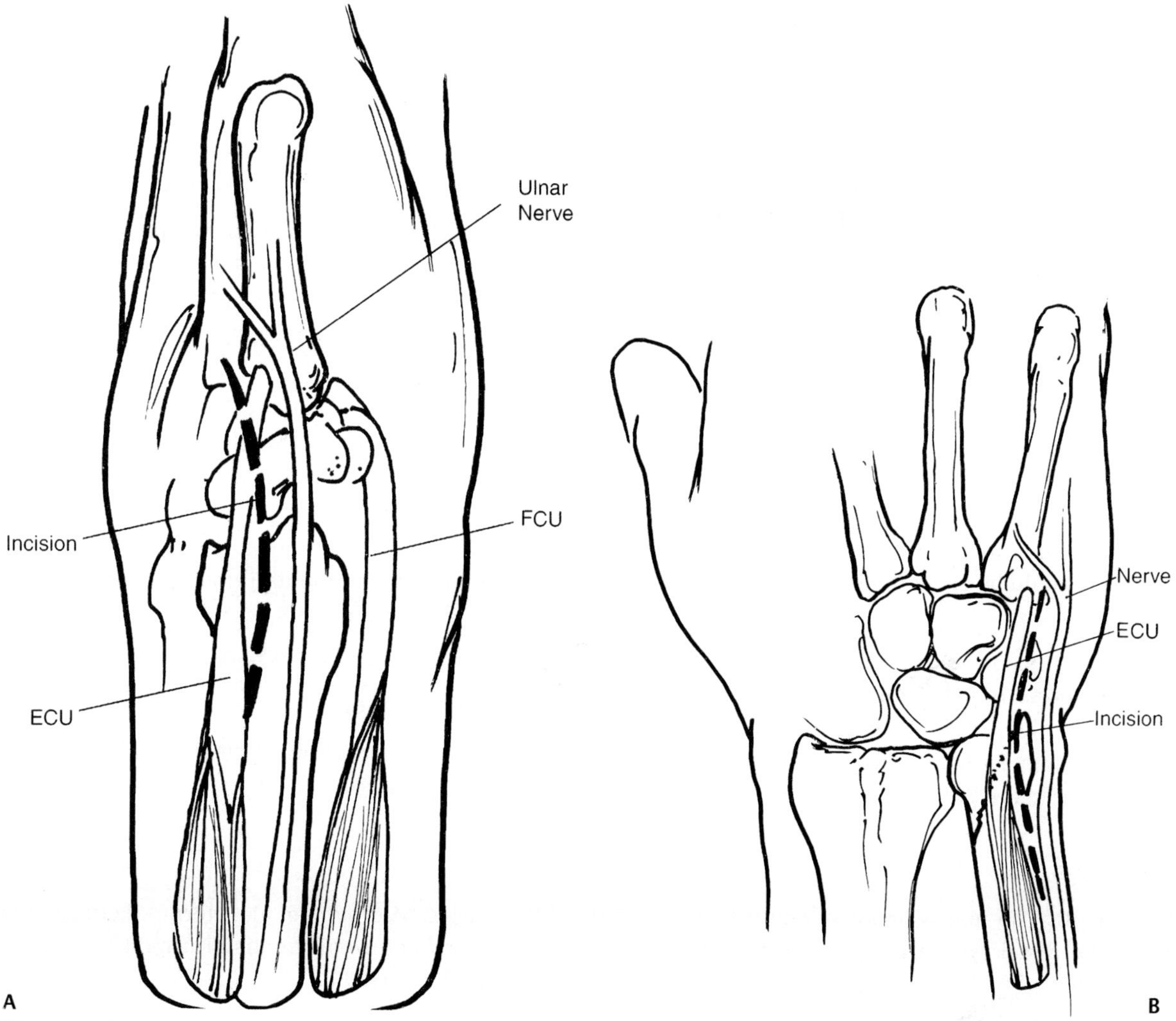

Figure 12–1

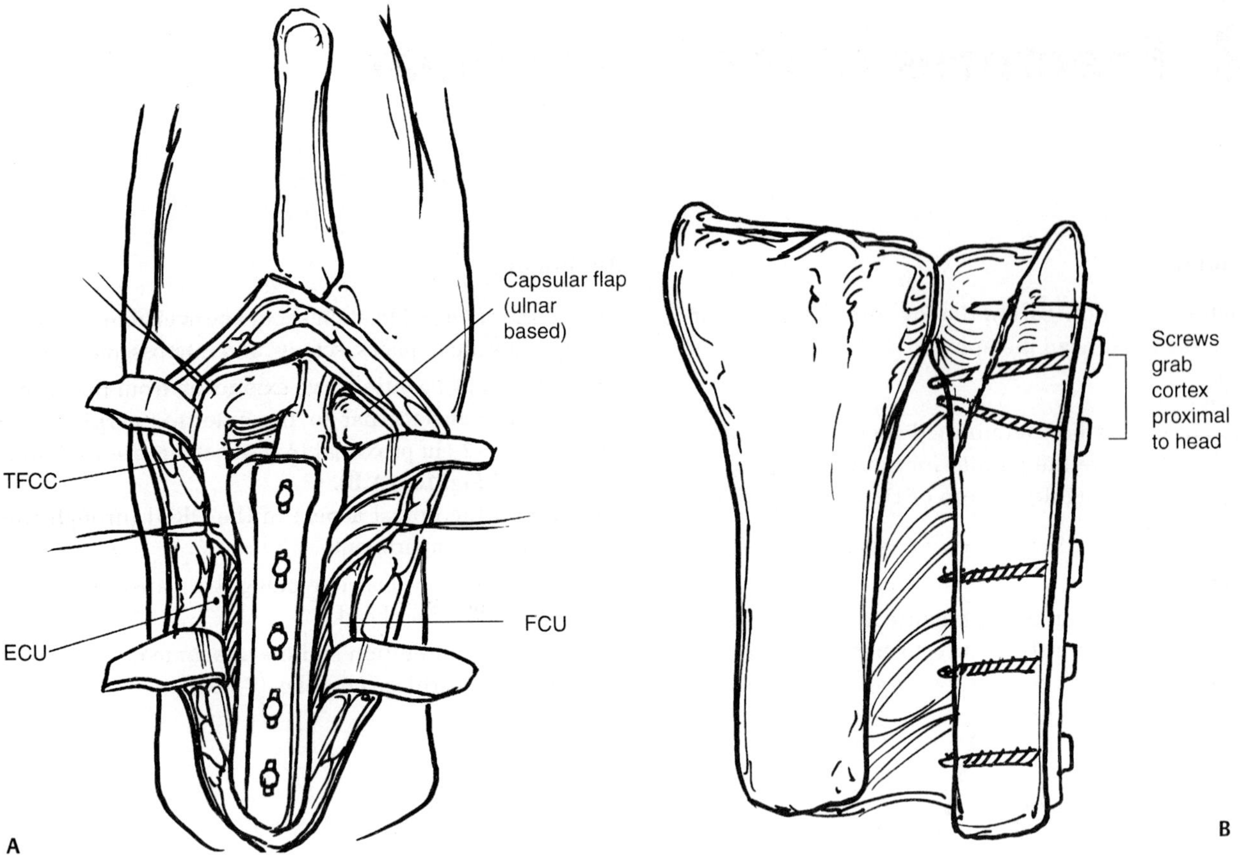

Figure 12–2

- Reduce and provisionally stabilize the fracture with a tenaculum and pins, as needed.
- Elevate the ulnar skin flap exposing the distal ulna in the interval between the ECU and flexor carpi ulnaris (FCU).

■ Pearl

The only opportunity for bicortical fixation of this fracture is between the intact ulnar cortex of the distal ulna and the radial metaphyseal fragment that is often attached to the head fragment. If bicortical fixation is not possible strong consideration should be given to performing a distal ulna resection.

- Attempt to place at least one countersunk lag screw from the ulnar cortex into the radial metaphyseal fragment attached to the head fragment.
- Place a mini fragment T-plate or blade plate on the ulnar cortex palmar to the ECU sheath.
- Attempt to place at least one screw from the plate to the radial metaphyseal fragment (**Fig. 12–2A,B**).
- Check the fracture reduction and hardware placement with intraoperative imaging.
- Rotate the forearm.
- Close the dorsal capsule and retinaculum, leaving the Extensor digiti quinti (EDQ) superficial to the retinaculum.

Postoperative Care

- Short arm immobilization until fracture healed
- Immediate finger motion
- Gentle, active, assisted forearm rotation

Alternative Techniques

- Hemiresection arthroplasty of the distal ulna
- Darrach procedure

Suggested Readings

Faierman E, Jupiter JB. The management of acute fractures involving the distal radioulnar joint and distal ulna. Hand Clin 1998;14:213–229

Jakab E, Ganos DL, Gagnon S. Isolated intra-articular fracture of the ulnar head. J Orthop Trauma (U.S.) 1993;7:290–292

Solan MC, Rees R, Molloy S, et al. Internal fixation after intra-articular fracture of the distal ulna. J Bone Joint Surg Br 2003;85:279–280

13 Fractures of the Ulnar Neck

Indications

- Unstable fractures through the neck of the distal ulna

■ Pitfall

Fractures with metaphyseal comminution are particularly difficult to manage.

■ Pearl

If reduction and fixation of the fracture is chosen, the fixation must be sufficiently secure to permit immediate forearm rotation.

Technique

- Incision is a gentle curve extending from the base of the fifth metacarpal to the extensor carpi ulnaris (ECU), ~2 cm proximal to the distal radioulnar joint (DRUJ) (**Fig. 13–1A,B**).
- Expose the dorsal aspect of the ulnar head through the fifth extensor compartment.
- Initial fixation via plate placed in the interval between the flexor carpi ulnaris (FCU) and extensor carpi ulnaris (ECU) just proximal to ulnar styloid (**Fig. 13–2**).

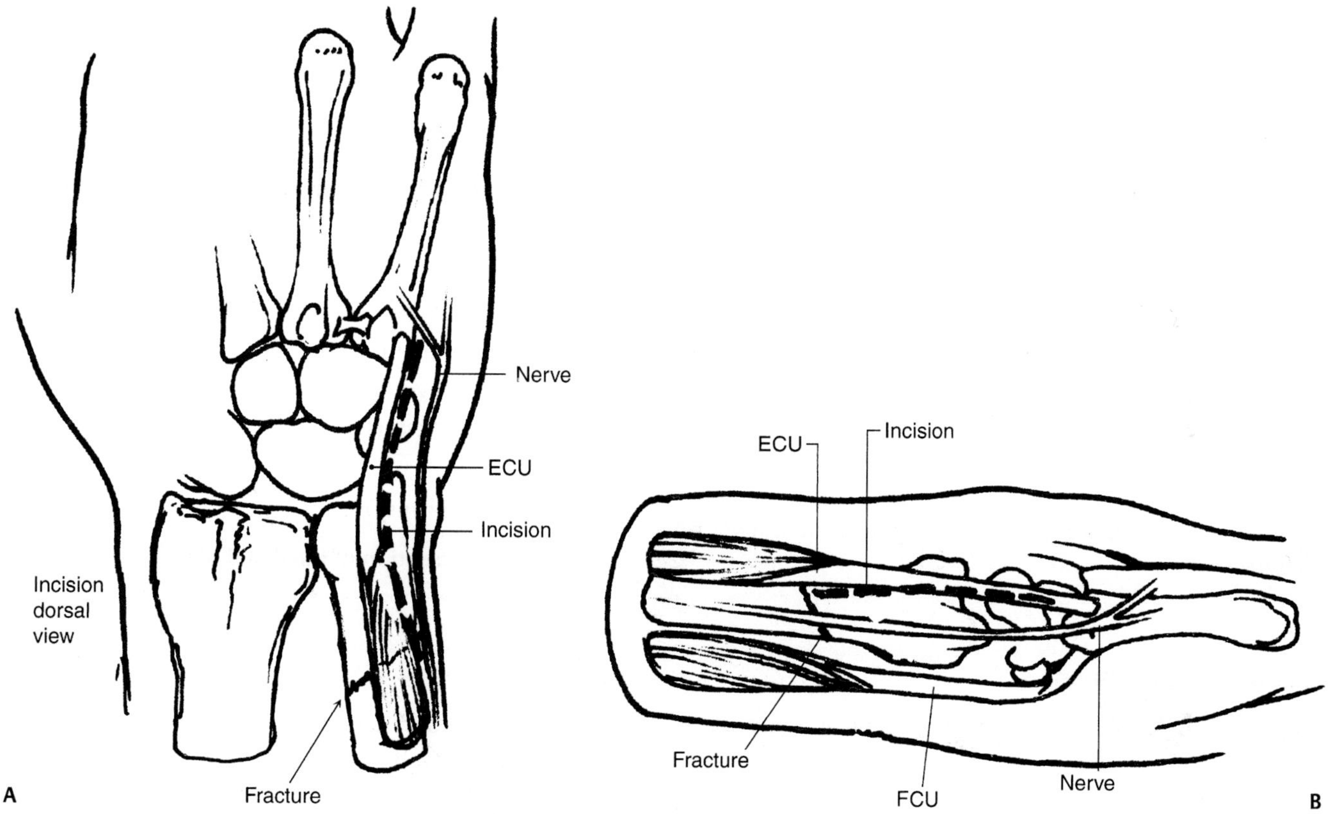

Figure 13–1

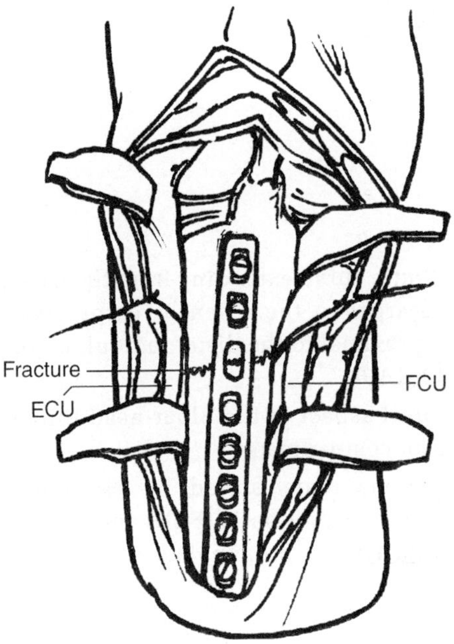

Figure 13–2

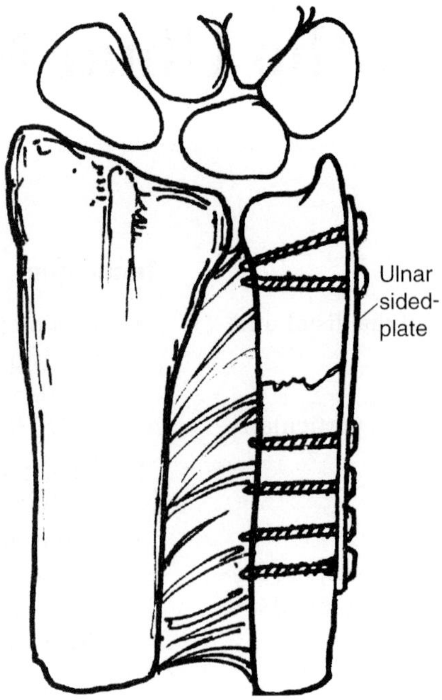

Figure 13–3

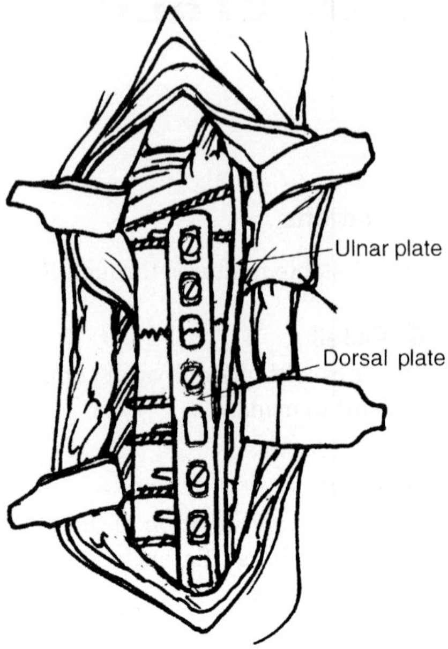

Figure 13–4

- Ensure distal screw placement does not enter distal radioulnar joint using operative fluoroscopy (**Fig. 13–3**).
- Span the fracture with a second plate placed 90 degrees to the first, on the dorsal surface of the distal ulna (**Fig. 13–4**).
- Check the fracture reduction and hardware placement with intraoperative imaging.
- Close the dorsal retinaculum over the dorsal plate, leaving the Extensor digiti quinti (EDQ) superficial to the retinaculum.

■ Pearl

Distal fractures can be managed using the T-plates with two distal holes or the blade plate. More proximal fractures can be stabilized with the mini dynamic compression plate placed on the dorsal cortex and a T-plate on the ulnar cortex.

■ Pearl

If stable, dual plate fixation is not possible, consider performing a distal ulnar resection with some form of tendon stabilization.

Postoperative Care

- Short arm immobilization until fracture healed
- Immediate finger motion
- Gentle, active, assisted forearm rotation

Alternative Techniques

- Stabilized resection of the distal ulna

Suggested Readings

Faierman E, Jupiter JB. The management of acute fractures involving the distal radioulnar joint and distal ulna. Hand Clin 1998;14:213–229

Ring D, McCarty LP, Campbell D, et al. Condylar blade plate fixation of unstable fractures of the distal ulna associated with fracture of the distal radius. J Hand Surg [Am] 2004;29:103–109

Section IV

Distal Ulna Nonunions

14 Resect Ulnar Styloid Fracture with Repair of Triangular Fibrocartilage Complex

Indications

- Symptomatic nonunion of the ulnar styloid with and without instability of the distal radioulnar joint (DRUJ)
- Patients should be warned of persistent instability of the DRUJ in spite of triangular fibrocartilage complex (TFCC) repair.

Technique

- Zigzag incision along ulnar border of the hand and wrist. The incision begins 1 cm distal to the ulnar styloid and extends to the subcutaneous border of the ulna, palmar to the extensor carpi ulnaris (ECU) tendon sheath (**Fig. 14–1**).

■ Pitfall

Avoid the dorsal cutaneous branch of ulnar nerve that passes obliquely between the ulnar styloid and pisiform.

- Expose with subperiosteal dissection the ulnar aspect of the ulnar head and metaphysis. Do not open the ECU subsheath.
- Open the ulnar aspect of the ulnocarpal joint capsule.
- Expose and resect the nonunited ulnar styloid (**Fig. 14–2**).
- Assess the stability of the DRUJ with the forearm in neutral, supination, and pronation.
- If the styloid fragment is small and DRUJ is stable in all positions close the capsule and skin.

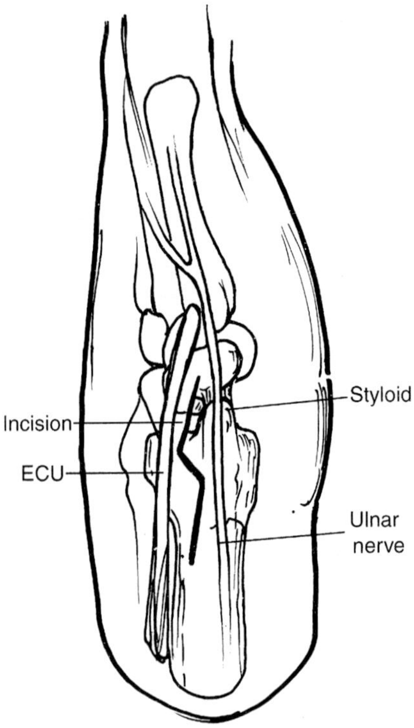

Figure 14–1

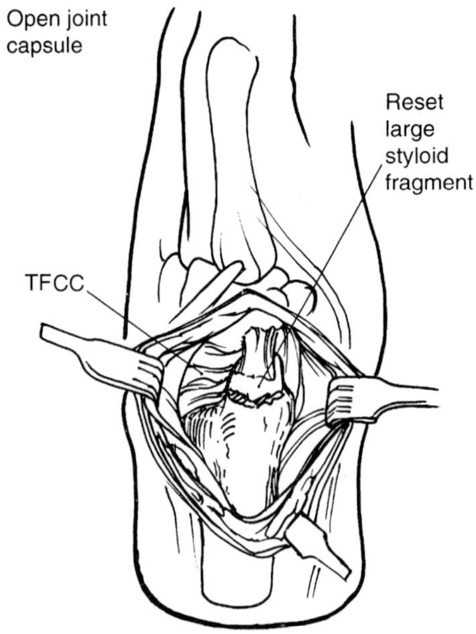

Figure 14–2

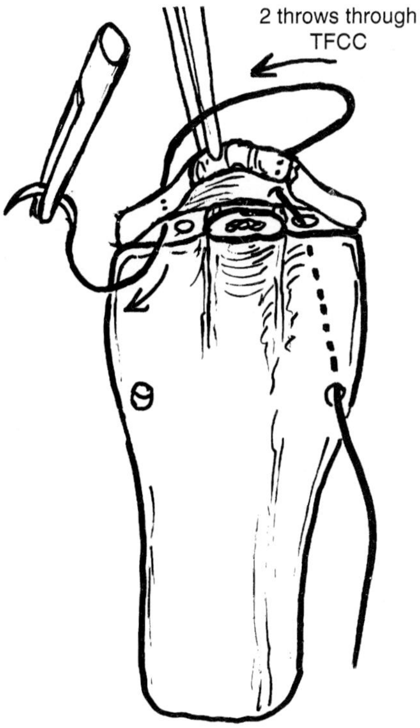

Figure 14–3

- If the styloid fragment is large or if the DRUJ is lax, use a no. 15 blade knife to create a plane between the TFCC and the head and the TFCC and the joint capsule.
- Place two throws with a 2–0 PDS suture on a UCL needle through the ulnar margin of the TFCC (**Fig. 14–3**).
- Remove a 21 gauge needle from its plastic hub and place into a drill chuck. Drill the needle from the ulnar aspect of the ulnar metaphysis into the fovea of the distal ulna (**Fig. 14–4A,B**).
- Pass the suture through the needle and retrieve at the level of the metaphysis (**Fig. 14–4B**).
- Tie the suture ends with the forearm in neutral rotation. Use the same suture to close the joint capsule.
- Close subcutaneous tissue and skin.

Postoperative Care

- Long arm cast with the forearm in neutral rotation for 4 weeks
- Short arm cast for 2 weeks

Alternative Technique

- Ligament weave for instability of the DRUJ
- Sauve-Kapandji procedure for instability with or without associated arthritis of the DRUJ (see Chapter 19)

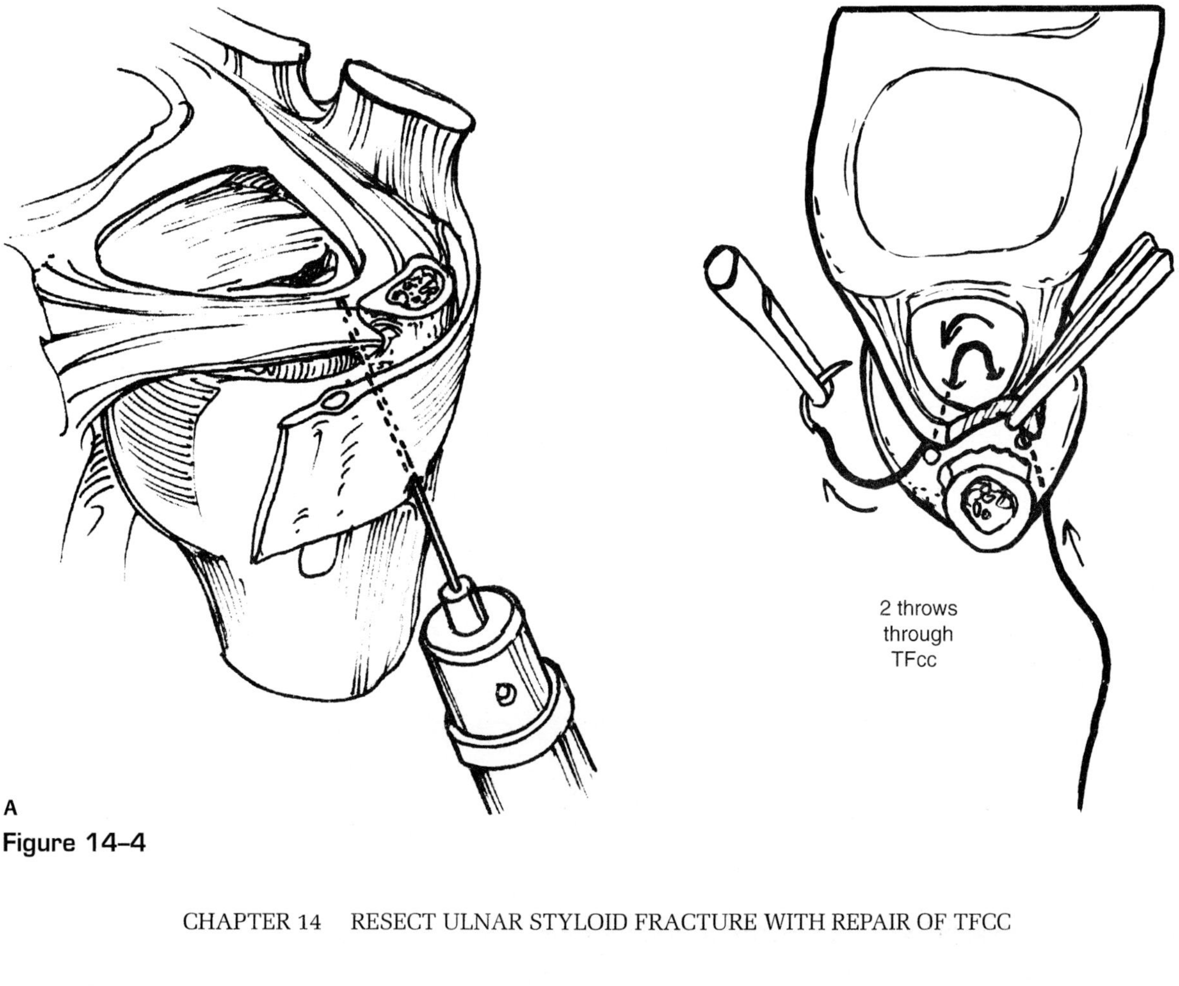

Figure 14–4

Suggested Readings

Faierman E, Jupiter JB. The management of acute fractures involving the distal radioulnar joint and distal ulna. Hand Clin 1998;14:213–229

Hauck CR, Palmer AK. Classification and treatment of ulnar styloid nonunion. J Hand Surg 1996;21A: 418–422

Oskarsson GV, Aaser P, Hjall A. Do we underestimate the predictive value of the ulnar styloid affection in Colles fractures? Arch Orthop Trauma Surg 1997;(116): 341–344

15 Nonunion of an Ulnar Neck Fracture

Indications

- Delayed or nonhealing of a neck fracture following nonoperative treatment
- Failed fixation with nonunion following operative treatment

■ Pitfall

A significant bone defect is typically present after removing the sclerotic margins of the bone and the previously placed hardware. To avoid excessively shortening the ulna it is usually necessary to place intercalary, tricortical iliac crest bone graft.

■ Pearl

To re-create the appropriate ulnar variance take PA projection of the contralateral wrist with the forearm pronated.

Technique

- The distal ulna is exposed through a curvilinear incision extending from the base of the fifth metacarpal to the extensor carpi ulnaris (ECU), ~2 cm proximal to the distal radioulnar joint (DRUJ) (**Fig. 15–1A,B**).
- Expose the dorsal aspect of the ulnar head and neck through the fifth extensor compartment.
- Expose the ulnar aspect of the ulna in the interval between the ECU and flexor carpi ulnaris (FCU). If possible, avoid opening the ECU tendon sheath.
- Remove the sclerotic margin of the nonunion with a micro oscillating or sagittal saw. Irrigate generously to avoid burning the bone.
- Harvest a tricortical iliac crest graft large enough to span the defect.

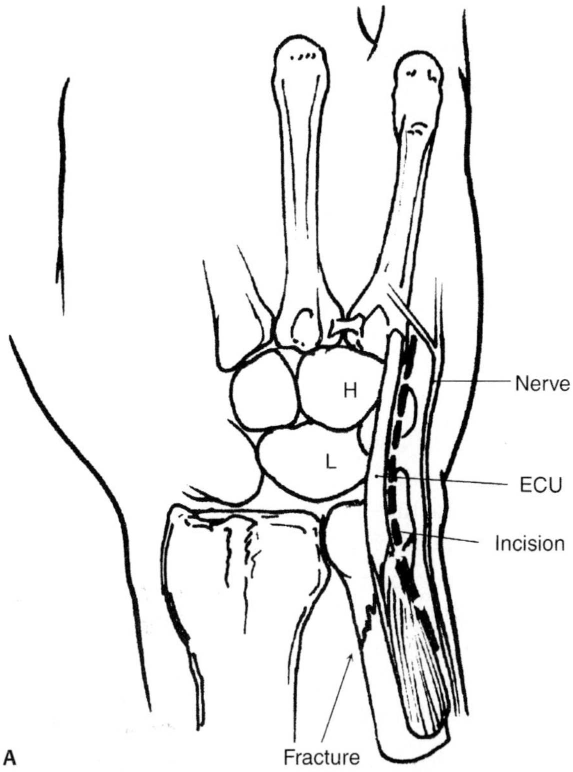

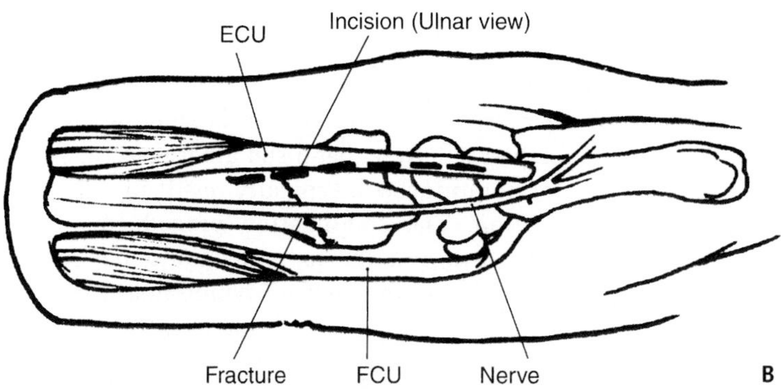

Figure 15–1

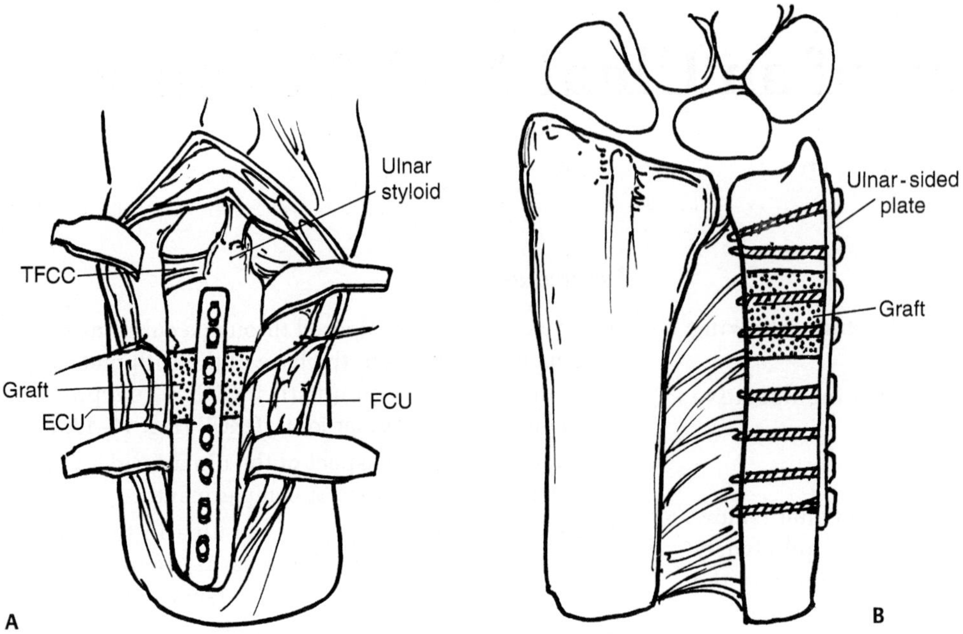

Figure 15–2

■ Pearl

Take a graft several millimeters longer than is expected to be needed. Insert the graft into the defect and provisionally fix with a plate and two or three screws. Check the ulnar variance on a PA projection with the forearm pronated (**Fig. 15–2A,B**).

- Span the graft with two plates placed 90 degrees to each other: one on the dorsal surface of the distal ulna, the other in the interval between the ECU and FCU (**Fig. 15–3**).

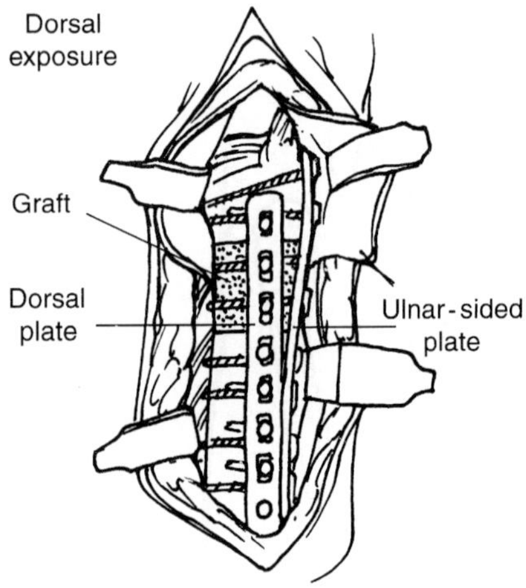

Figure 15–3

■ Pearl

Whenever possible use a mini dynamic compression plate on the dorsal cortex and a T-plate on the ulnar cortex.

■ Pearl

If stable, dual plate fixation is not possible, consider performing a distal ulnar resection with some form of tendon stabilization (see Chapter 22). Note that distal ulnar resection for treatment of nonunion will typically result in a very proximal resection. The stabilization procedure should be done with care and the patient should be warned preoperatively about the risk of symptomatic instability.

- Check the fracture reduction and hardware placement with intraoperative imaging.
- Check forearm rotation. Loss of rotation can result from malreduction of the ulna or a capsular contracture of the DRUJ.
- Close the dorsal retinaculum over the dorsal plate, leaving the EDQ superficial to the retinaculum.

Postoperative Care

- Long arm immobilization for 4 weeks
- Immediate finger motion
- Short arm cast until fracture healed
- Gentle, active, assisted forearm rotation until fracture healed
- Therapy and static, progressive splinting for residual loss of forearm rotation

Alternative Techniques

- Stabilized resection of the distal ulna
- Resection with placement of a distal ulna prosthesis

Suggested Readings

Faierman E, Jupiter JB. The management of acute fractures involving the distal radioulnar joint and distal ulna. Hand Clin 1998;14:213–229

Section V.1

The Distal Radioulnar Joint: Unstable Distal Ulna, Head Intact

16 Open Repair of an Ulnar-Sided Triangular Fibrocartilage Complex Tear

Indications

- A tear of the triangular fibrocartilage complex (TFCC) from the fovea of the ulnar head with or without distal radioulnar joint (DRUJ) instability.

Technique

- Approach the ulnocarpal joint and DRUJ through the fifth extensor compartment (**Fig. 16–1**).
- Open the DRUJ capsule with an L-shaped incision, with one limb along the sigmoid notch and one just proximal to the dorsal radioulnar ligament (**Fig. 16–2**).

■ Pitfall

Avoid cutting the dorsal radioulnar ligament by beginning the capsulotomy at the proximal aspect of the sigmoid notch.

- Open the ulnocarpal joint through an incision just distal to the dorsal radioulnar ligament and extend it distally along the radial margin of the extensor carpi ulnaris (ECU) sheath (**Fig. 16–2**).
- Inspect the TFCC on its proximal and distal surfaces and determine whether it is repairable (**Fig. 16–3**).

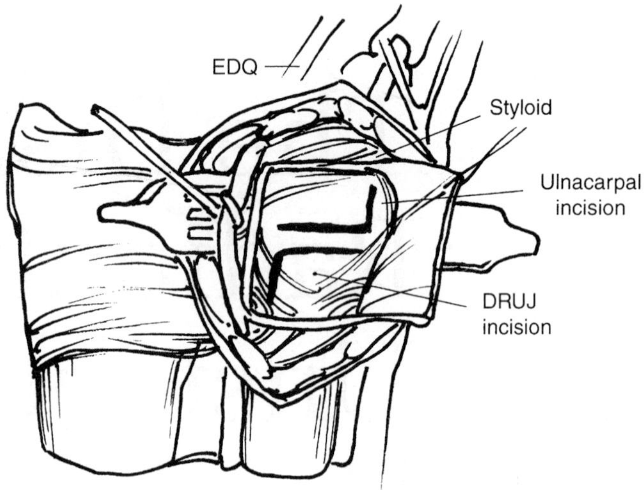

Figure 16–2

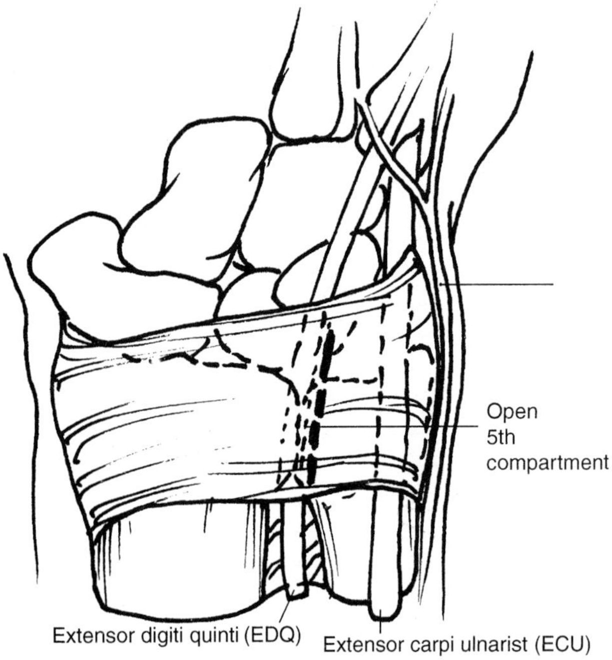

Figure 16–1

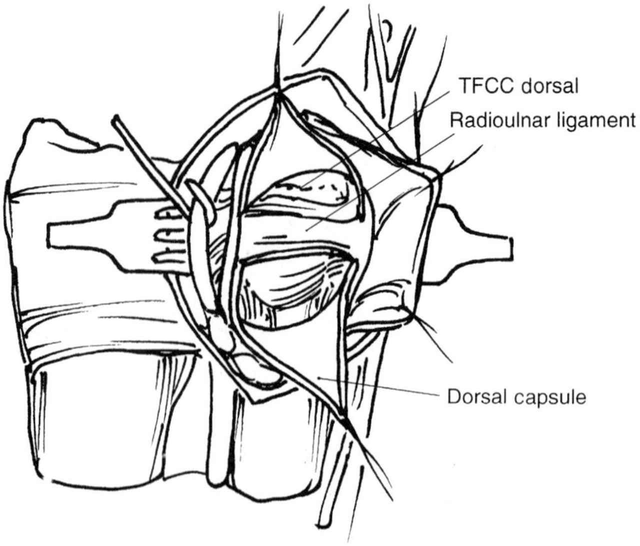

Figure 16–3

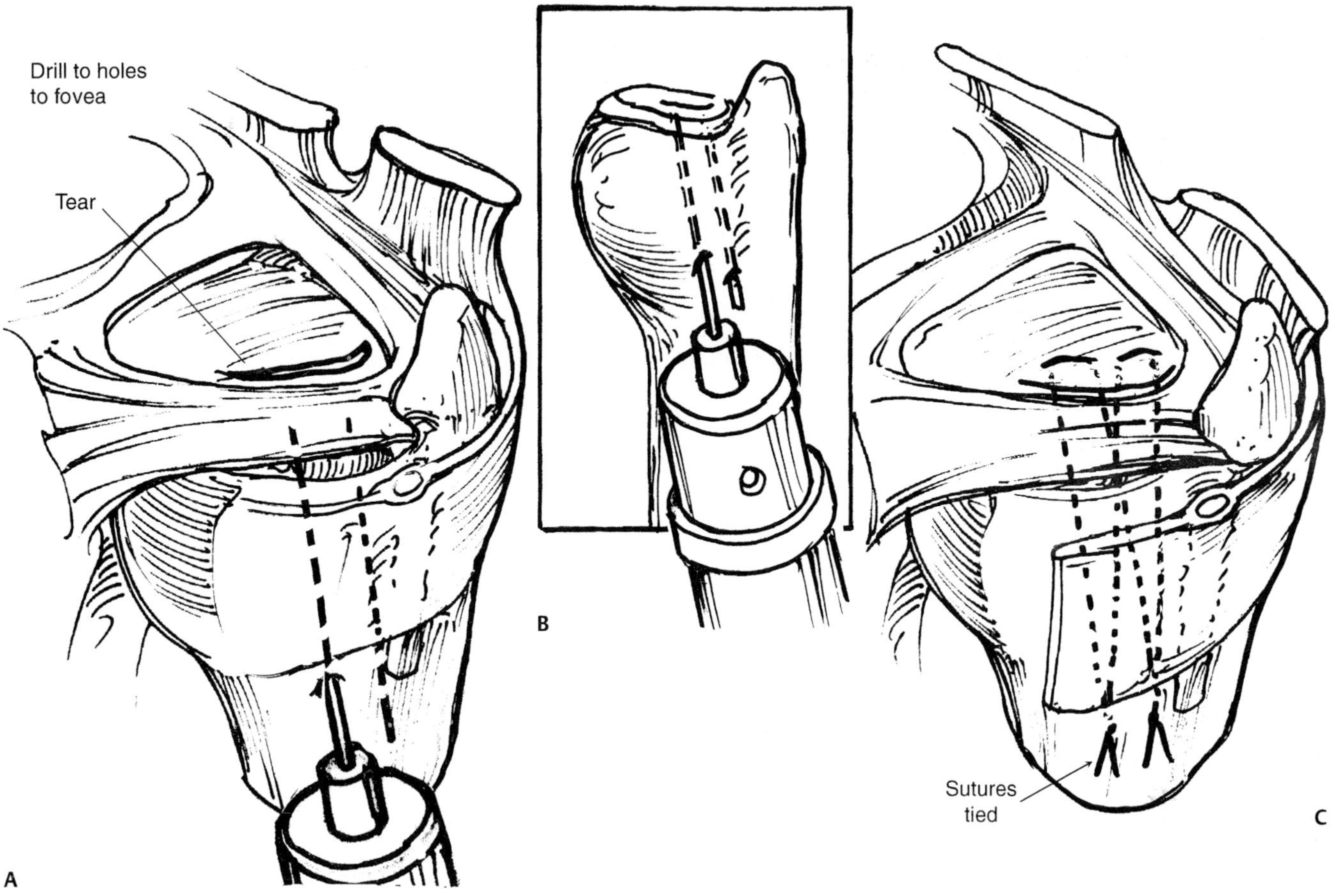

Figure 16–4

- Prepare the fovea by removing granulation tissue and scar.
- Drill two or three holes with a 0.45 in. K-wire from the dorsal aspect of the ulnar neck to the fovea (**Fig. 16–4A,B**).

■ Pearl

Improve the exposure of the fovea by flexing the wrist and retracting the ECU sheath.

- Place two 2–0 monofilament horizontal mattress sutures through the ulnar aspect of the TFCC from distal to proximal.
- Using small Keith needles, pass the sutures through the drill holes.
- Tie the sutures directly against the bone (**Fig. 16–4C**).
- Close the joint capsules, including the dorsal radioulnar ligament in the suturing.

Postoperative Care

- Long arm cast with the forearm in neutral rotation for 3 to 4 weeks
- Well molded short arm cast for 2 weeks
- Splint during strenuous activities for 1 month

Alternative Techniqı'e

Use an arthroscopic technique; however, recognize this may not be effective at restoring DRUJ instability.

Suggested Readings

Cooney WP III. Tears of the triangular fibrocartilage of the wrist. In: Cooney WP III, Linscheid RL, Dobyns JH, eds. The Wrist: Diagnosis and Operative Treatment. St. Louis: Mosby; 1998:710–742

Hermansdorfer JD, Kleinman WB. Management of chronic peripheral tears of the triangular fibrocartilage complex. J Hand Surg [Am] 1991;16A:340–346

17 Peripheral Tear of the Triangular Fibrocartilage Complex from the Ulna: Arthroscopic Repair

Indications

- Peripheral tear of the triangular fibrocartilage complex (TFCC) from its attachments to the ulna or the joint capsule.

■ Pitfall

May not restore stability to the distal radioulnar joint (DRUJ) in cases of advanced or chronic instability

Technique

- The arthroscope is placed in the 3–4 or 4–5 portal depending on the size of the wrist and visualization.
- A probe is inserted through the 6R or 6U portal. Loss of normal TFCC tension under probe pressure, the so-called trampoline test, is a sign of a peripheral tear.

■ Pearl

When making portals, nick the skin and spread the subcutaneous tissue to prevent cutaneous nerve and tendon injury.

- A 1.5 cm skin incision is made just dorsal to the ulnar styloid. The extensor retinaculum and extensor carpi ulnaris (ECU) subsheath are opened 1 cm and the tendon retracted enough to visualize the floor of the sixth compartment.

■ Pitfall

Protect any branches of the dorsal sensory ulnar nerve that pass nearby.

- Using a specialized suture cannula set or 20 gauge needle, pierce the ECU sheath floor and pass through the TFCC just radial to its torn edge.
- A second cannula is inserted through the sheath floor ~5 to 10 mm distal to the first, which will enter the joint capsule distal to the TFCC.
- Second cannula can be placed to create either a horizontal mattress. **(Fig. 17–1)** or simple suture **(Fig. 17–2)** technique.

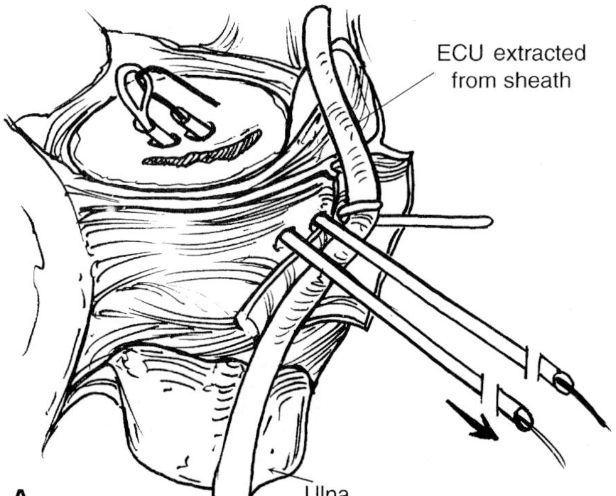

A

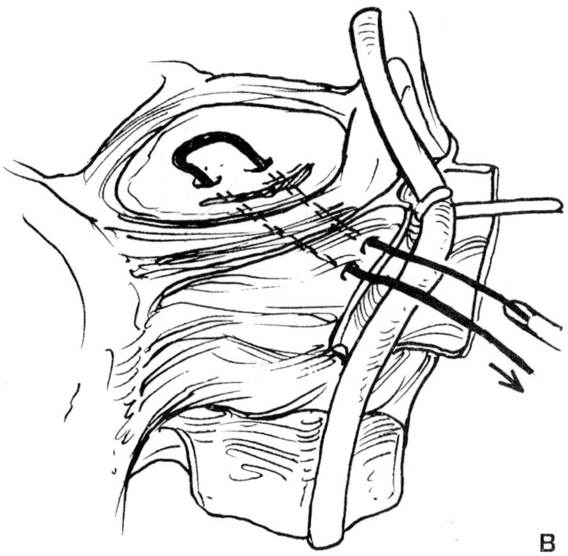

B

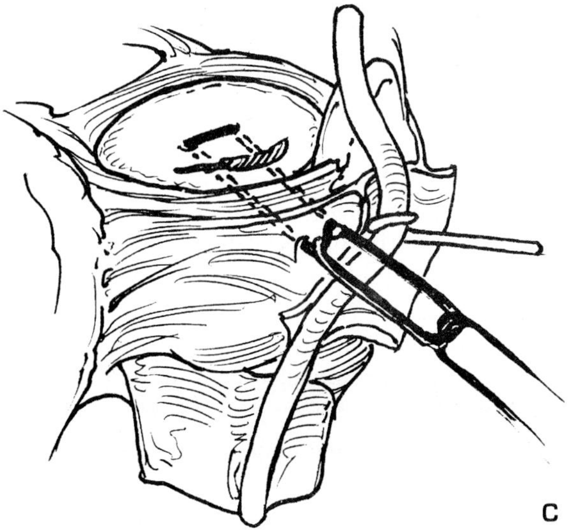

C

Figure 17–1

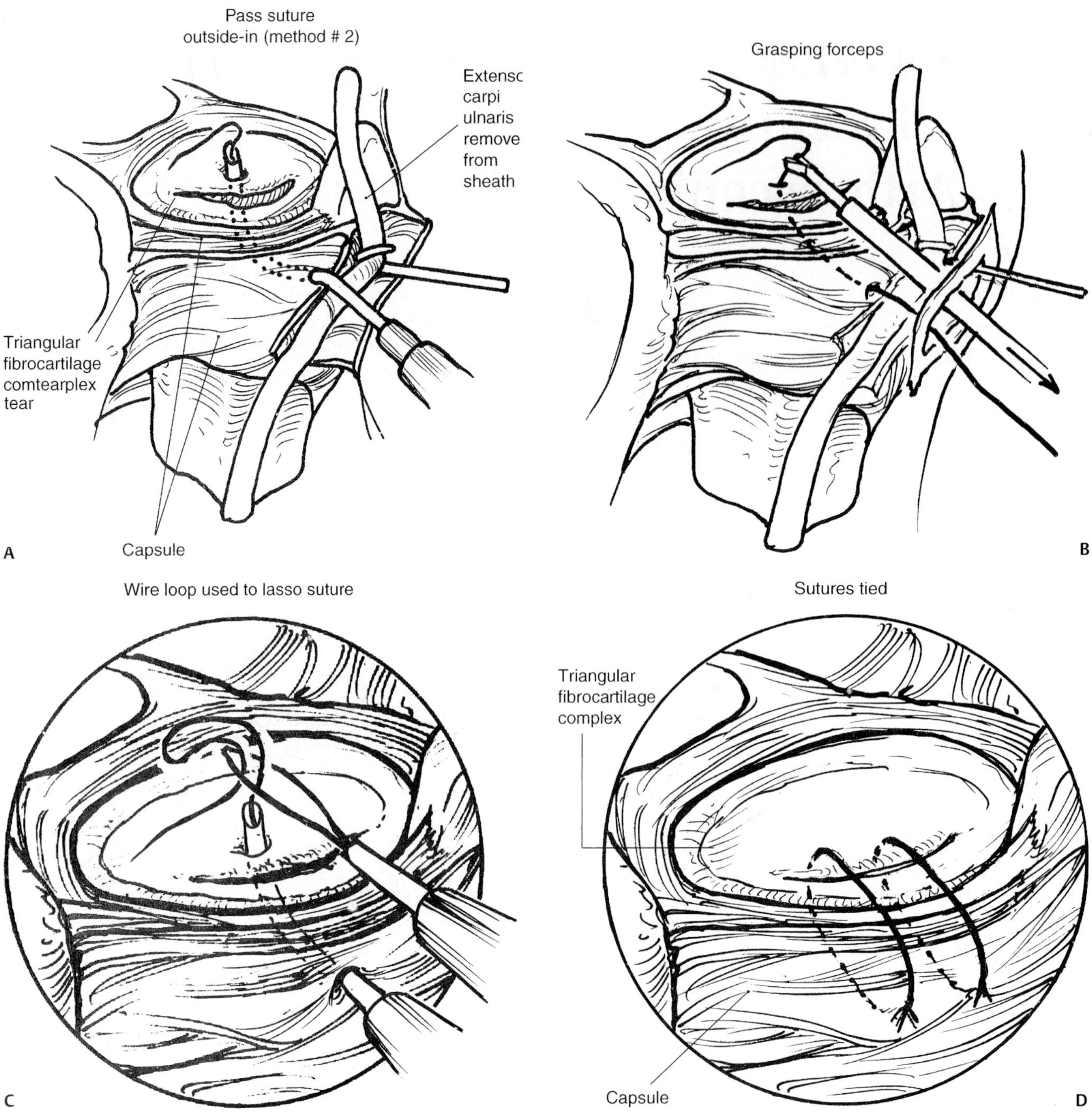

Figure 17–2

- Pass a 2–0 polydioxanone suture through the first cannula and retrieve it through the second using a suture snare. Withdraw the cannulas (**Fig. 17–1A, B,C**).
- In a similar fashion, place one or two additional sutures through the torn edge a few millimeters apart (**Fig. 17–2A,B,C**).
- Tie the sutures over the floor of the subsheath (**Fig. 17–2D**).
- Close the ECU subsheath and retinaculum.

Postoperative Care

- Sugar-tong splint or long arm are cast in 60 degrees of supination for 3 to 4 weeks
- Removable wrist splint for an additional 3 weeks, with gentle wrist motion but avoiding full pronation

Alternative Techniques

- Inside-out technique using Touhy needle (**Fig. 17–3A–E**)
- Open TFCC repair

Inside-out Touhy Technique

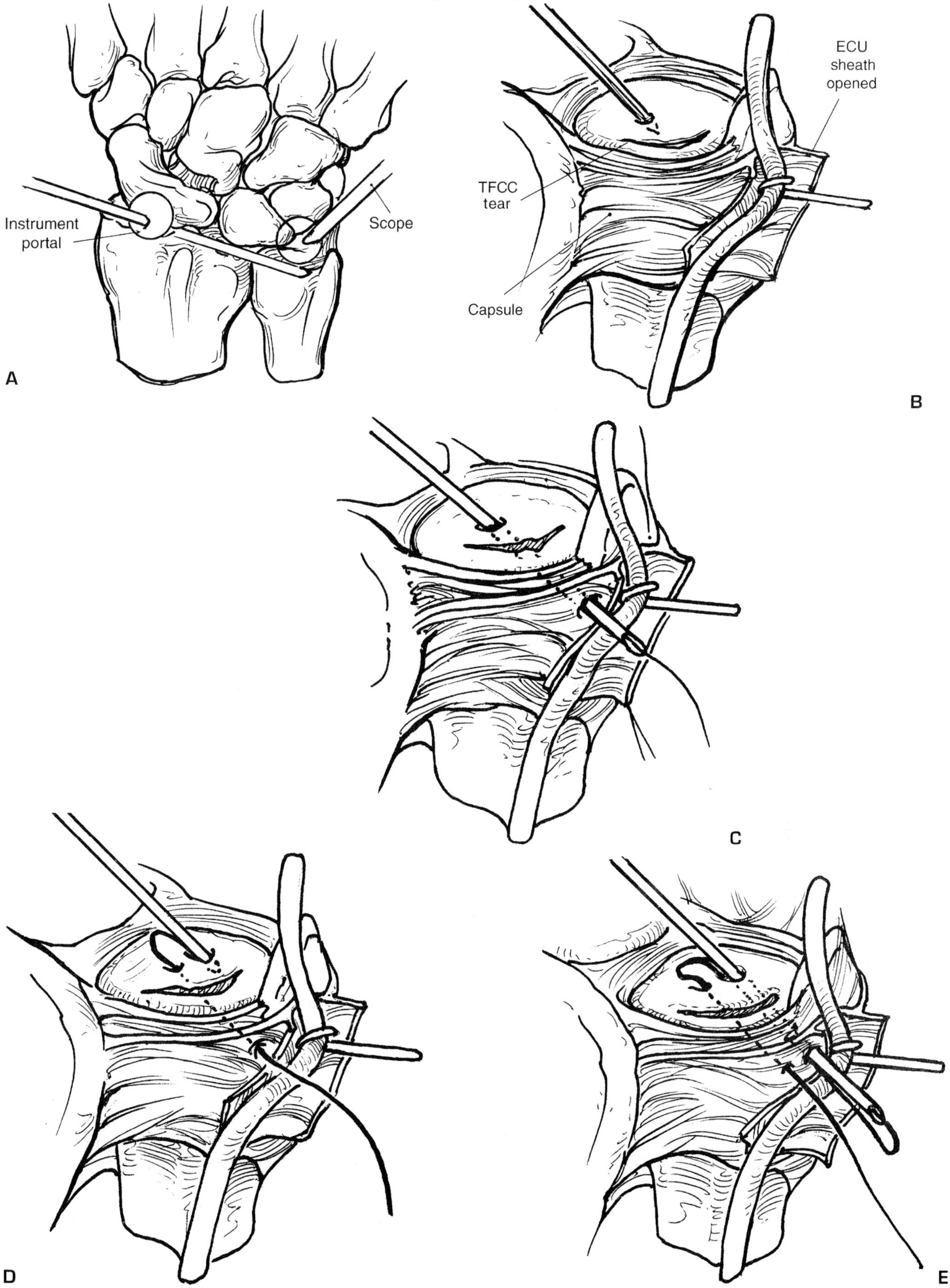

Figure 17–3

Suggested Readings

Ruch DS, Ritter MR. Repair of Peripheral Triangular Fibrocartilage Complex Tears. Atlas of Hand Clinics: New Techniques in Wrist Arthroscopy 2001;6:211–220

Trumble TE, Gilbert M, Vedder N. Isolated tears of the triangular fibrocartilage: management by early arthroscopic repair. J Hand Surg [Am] 1997;22A:57–65

18 Reconstruction of Distal Radioulnar Ligaments

Indications

- Distal radioulnar joint (DRUJ) instability with an irreparable triangular fibrocartilage complex (TFCC) tear and no appreciable arthritis
- Distal radial malunion with DRUJ instability that is not corrected by the osteotomy

Technique

- Approach the DRUJ through fifth extensor compartment, leaving its distal portion intact.
- Reflect the retinaculum ulnarly but do not open the sixth extensor compartment (**Fig. 18–1**).
- Create an L-shaped capsulotomy with one limb just proximal to the dorsal radioulnar ligament and the other along the edge of the sigmoid notch (**Fig. 18–2**).

■ Pitfall

Avoid cutting the triangular fibrocartilage complex (TFCC) remnant by gradually incising the capsule from proximal to distal along the sigmoid notch until the dorsal radioulnar ligament is reached.

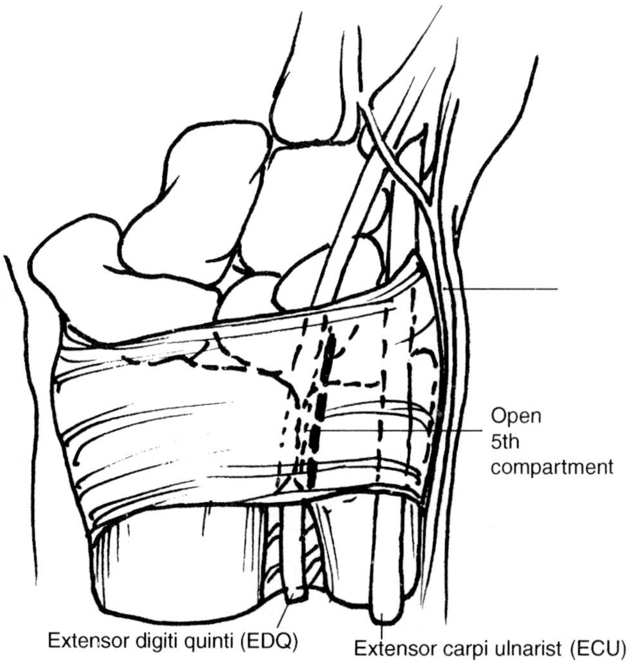

Figure 18–1

- Using a cannulated drill system, create a dorsal to volar tunnel through the distal ulnar corner of the radius (**Fig. 18–3**).

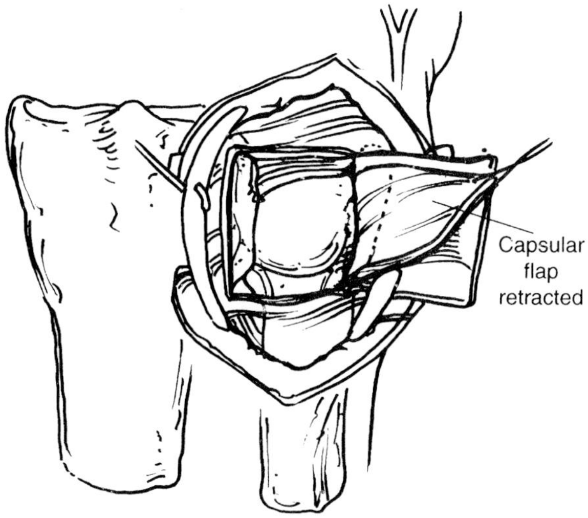

Figure 18–2

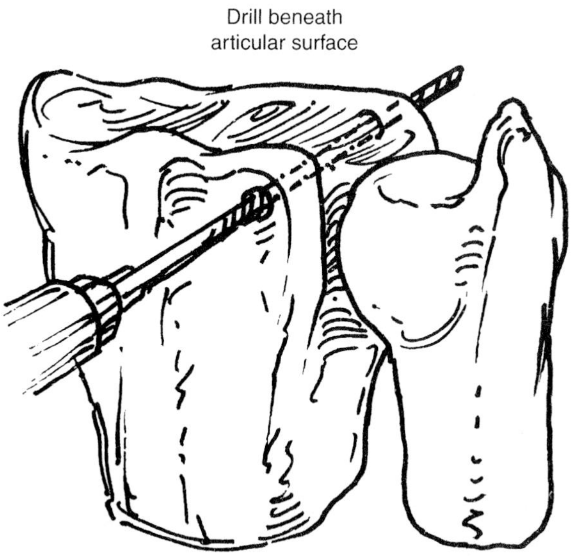

Figure 18–3

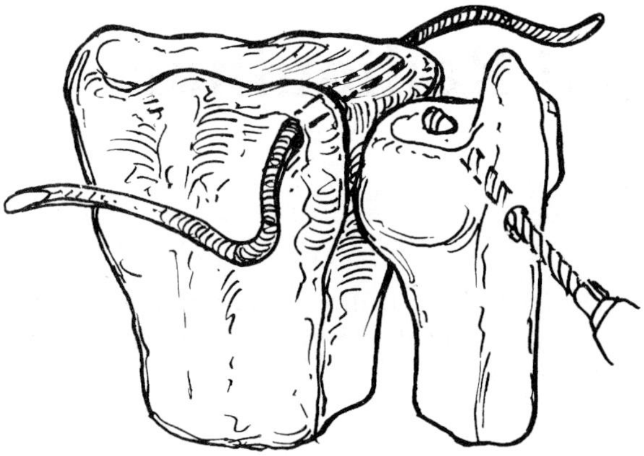

Figure 18–4

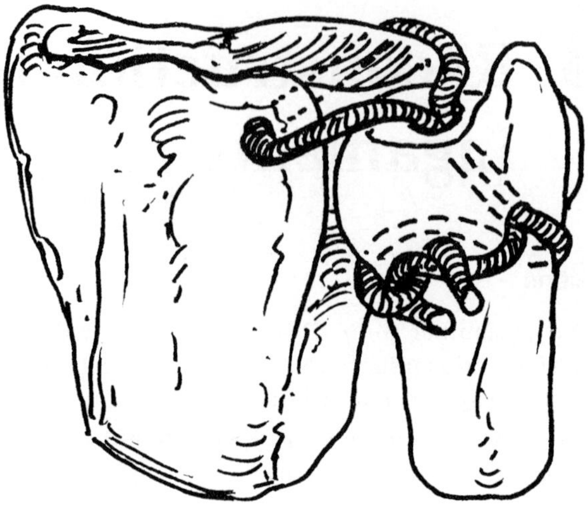

Figure 18–5

■ **Pearl**

Use fluoroscopy to confirm accurate placements of the guide wires.

- Create a tunnel through the ulnar head from the fovea to the ulnar neck using the cannulated drill system (**Fig. 18–4**).

■ **Pearl**

It is easier and more accurate to insert the guide wire distal to proximal but drill over the wire proximal to distal.

- Enlarge the ulnar tunnel slightly with standard drill bits.
- Insert a blunt probe through the radius tunnel to its location volarly and then make an incision at this point.
- Approach the palmar DRUJ capsule between the ulnar neurovascular bundle and the digital flexors.
- Pass a straight hemostat over the ulnar head and penetrate the volar DRUJ capsule.
- Pass one limb of the palmaris longus tendon graft through the radius tunnel using a suture passer (**Fig. 18–4**).
- The other limb is grasped and drawn dorsally through the DRUJ capsule using the previously placed hemostat.
- Pass both limbs of the graft through the ulnar tunnel using the suture passer.
- One limb is passed palmarly around the ulnar neck using a vascular suture passer, and the other limb is passed beneath the extensor carpi ulnaris (ECU) tendon.
- The limbs are pulled taut with the forearm in neutral rotation.
- Make a half-hitch with the graft ends, tighten against the ulnar neck, and secure the limbs to each other with sutures (**Fig. 18–5**).
- Close the dorsal DRUJ capsule but do not overtighten.
- Pinning the ulna to the radius is optional.

Postoperative Care

- Long arm cast for 4 to 6 weeks
- Short arm, well molded cast for 2 to 4 weeks
- Splint for 2 to 4 weeks during strenuous activities.
- Avoid impact loading and forceful forearm rotation for an additional 2 months.

Alternative Technique

Tenodesis procedure using the ECU and flexor carpi ulnaris (FCU) tendons

Suggested Readings

Adams BD, Berger RA. An anatomic reconstruction of the distal radioulnar ligaments for posttraumatic distal radioulnar joint instability. J Hand Surg [Am] 2002;27: 243–251

Scheker LR, Belliappa PP, Acosta R, German DS. Reconstruction of the dorsal ligament of the triangular fibrocartilage complex. J Hand Surg [Br] 1994;19: 310–8

Section V.2

The Distal Radioulnar Joint: Arthritis

19 Sauve-Kapandji Procedure

Indications

- Distal radioulnar joint (DRUJ) arthritis from degenerative joint disease (DJD), inflammatory disease, or trauma

Technique

- Expose the DRUJ through the fifth extensor compartment.

■ Pearl

No need to dissect the sixth extensor compartment from the ulnar head if the extensor carpi ulnaris (ECU) tendon is not subluxated.

- Create an ulnar-based rectangular DRUJ capsular flap (**Fig. 19–1**).
- Insert two parallel guide wires through the ulnar head into the radius across the DRUJ (**Fig. 19–2**).
- Back up the guide pins into the ulnar head.
- Prepare mating surfaces of the ulnar head and sigmoid notch down to cancellous bone (**Fig. 19–3**).

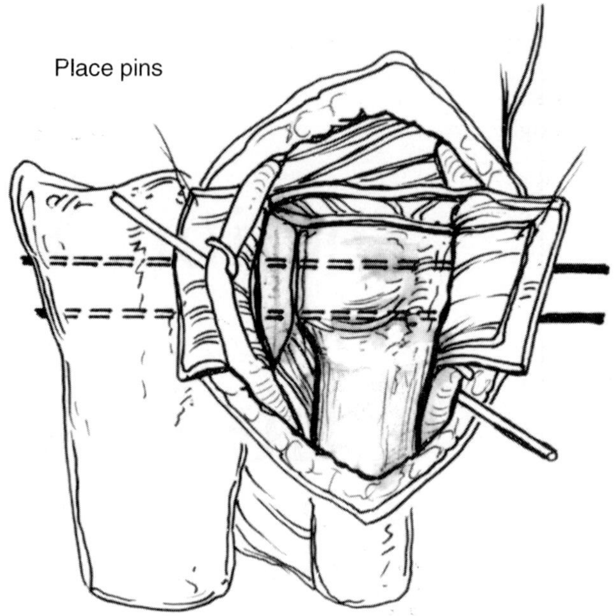

Figure 19–2

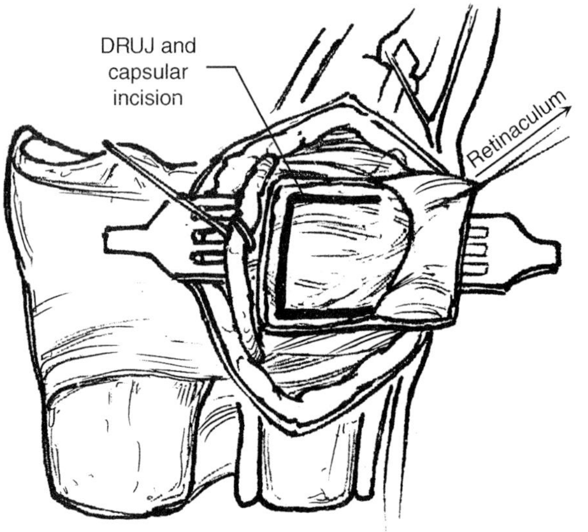

Figure 19–1

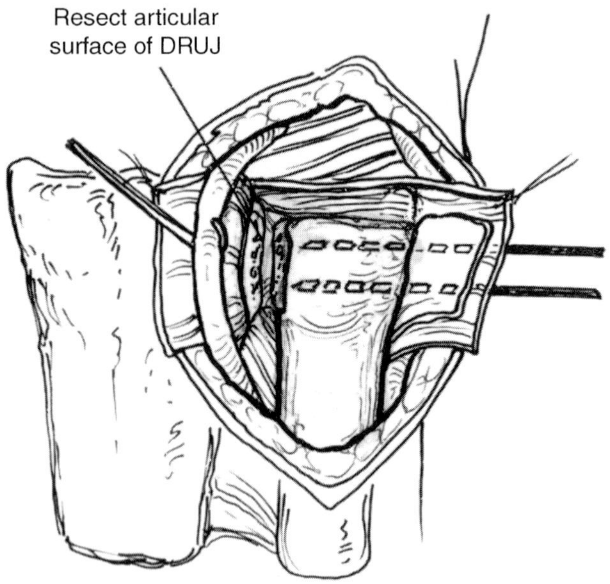

Figure 19–3

■ Pitfall

Although adequate bony preparation is mandatory to attain fusion, over-resection will reduce the ulnocarpal joint space.

- Reinsert the guide wires into the previous holes in the radius while compressing the ulnar head against the radius.
- Drill and insert two 3.0 mm cancellous screws in a lag-compression technique.

■ Pitfall

Overtightening may cause ulnar head fragmentation.

- Resect 1.5 cm of the ulnar neck along with its periosteum (**Fig. 19–4**).
- Close the capsule and retinaculum, leaving the EDQ superficial.
- To improve stability of the ulnar stump, the pronator quadratus can be transferred and interposed in the gap, or a tenodesis using a distally based strip of the flexor carpi ulnaris (FCU) can be used.

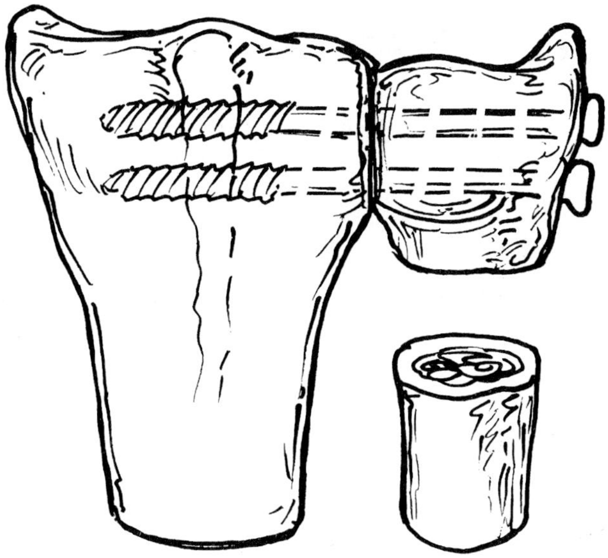

Figure 19–4

Postoperative Care

- Long arm cast for 6 weeks
- Short arm cast until arthrodesis healed

Alternative Techniques

- Hemiresection arthroplasty of the distal ulna
- Darrach procedure

Suggested Readings

Lamey DM, Fernandez DL. Results of the modified Sauve-Kapandji procedure in the treatment of chronic post-traumatic derangement of the distal radioulnar joint. J Bone Joint Surg Am 1998;80:1758–1769

Vincent KA, Szabo RM, Agee JM. The Sauve-Kapandji procedure for reconstruction of the rheumatoid distal radioulnar joint. J Hand Surg [Am] 1993;18A: 978–983

20 Hemiresection Arthroplasty of the Distal Ulna

Indications

- Distal radioulnar joint (DRUJ) arthritis from DJD, inflammatory disease, or trauma

■ Pitfall

Hemiresection arthroplasty will improve arthritic symptoms but will not restore distal ulnar stability.

Technique

- Approach the DRUJ through the fifth extensor compartment, leaving the distal portion intact (**Fig. 20–1**).
- Raise an ulnarly based rectangular capsular flap but do not open the sixth compartment for the extensor carpi ulnaris (**Fig. 20–2**).

■ Pitfall

Avoid cutting the dorsal radioulnar ligament.

- Obliquely resect a portion of the ulnar head, leaving the styloid attached to the triangular fibrocartilage complex (TFCC) (**Fig. 20–3**).

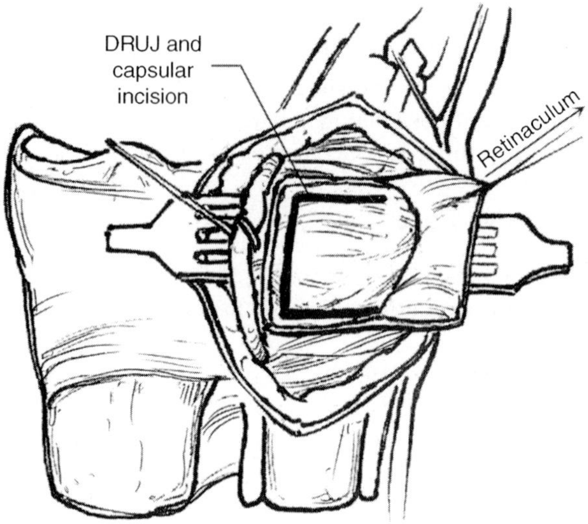

Figure 20–2

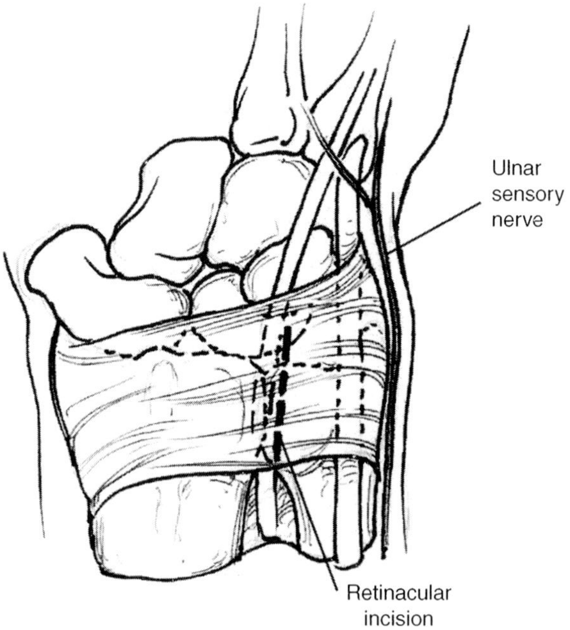

Figure 20–1

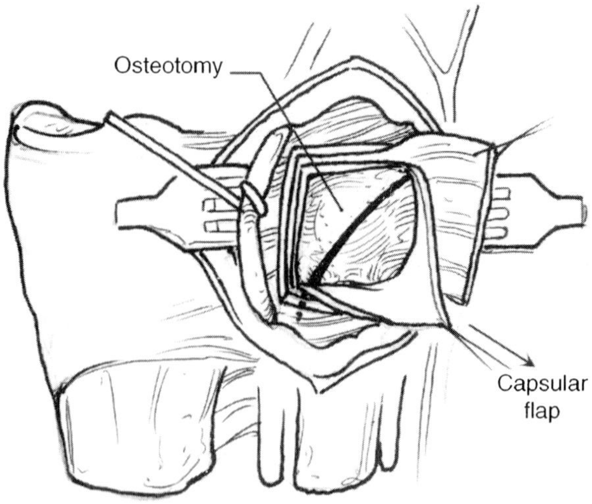

Figure 20–3

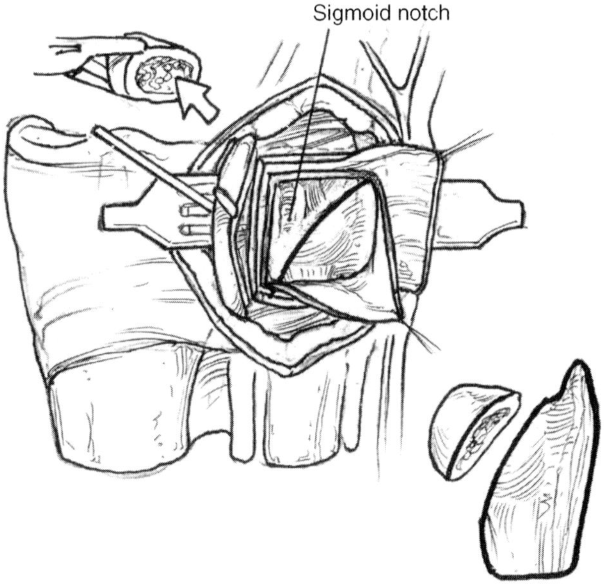

Figure 20–4

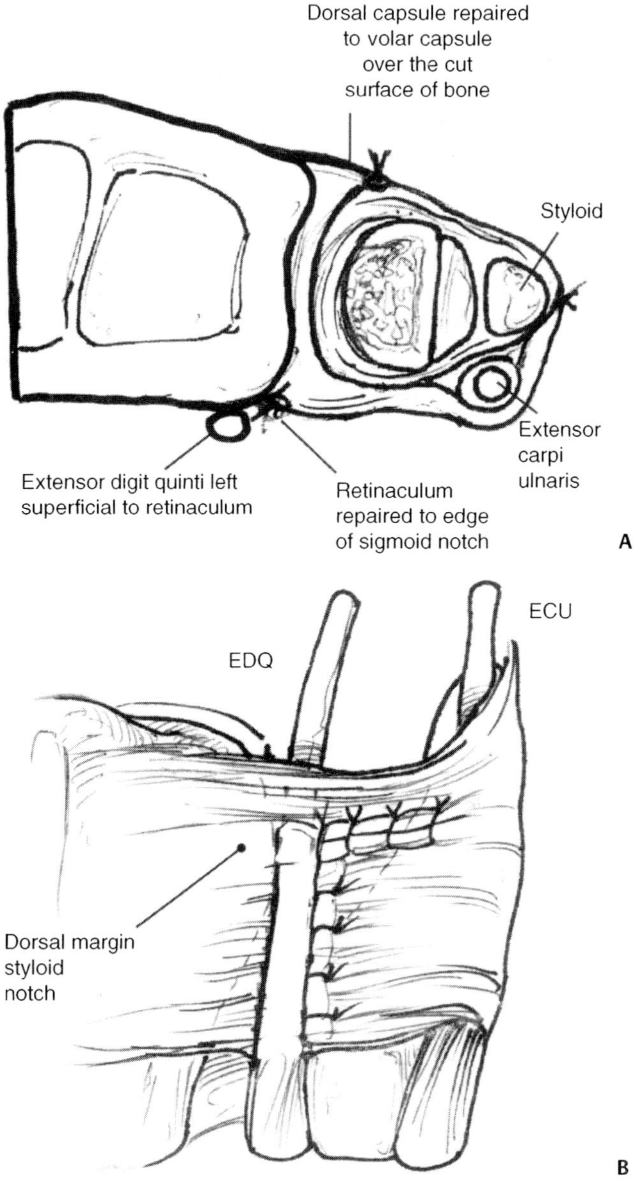

Figure 20–5

- Contour the distal ulna to a hemispherical shape (**Fig. 20–4**).
- Wrap the dorsal capsular flap over the distal ulna and suture to volar DRUJ capsule (**Fig. 20–5A**).
- Extensor retinaculum repaired to dorsal edge of sigmoid notch leaving EDQ superficial to repair (**Fig. 20–5A,B**).

■ Pearl

If the capsule and retinaculum are deficient from previous surgery, the pronator quadratus can be released from the ulna and interposed between the radius and ulna.

Postoperative Care

- Long arm cast with forearm in neutral rotation for 3 weeks
- Wrist splint for comfort and support for 4 weeks

Alternative Techniques

- Darrach resection is appropriate in a lower-demand patient.
- Sauve-Kapandji procedure is preferred by some surgeons.

Suggested Readings

Bowers WH. Distal radioulnar joint arthroplasty: the hemiresection-interposition technique. J Hand Surg [Am] 1985;10A:169–178

Watson HK, Ryu JY, Burgess RC. Matched distal ulnar resection. J Hand Surg [Am] 1986;11A:812–817

21 Darrach Procedure (Distal Ulna Resection)

Indications

- Rheumatoid disease with distal radioulnar joint (DRUJ) arthritis
- Elderly, low-demand patients with DRUJ incongruity or positive ulnar variance (e.g., distal radial malunion)

■ Pitfall

Instability of the ulnar stump may develop resulting in radioulnar impingement. Younger patients may complain of weakness. Ulnar translation of the carpus may occur in rheumatoid patients.

Technique

- Make a dorsal incision between the fifth and sixth extensor compartments.
- Open the sixth dorsal compartment along its palmar edge.
- Reflect the retinaculum radially to the 4–5 extensor compartment septum, and extract the EDQ tendon (**Fig. 21–1**).

■ Pearl

In the nonrheumatoid patient leave the retinaculum intact distal to the ulnar styloid to help maintain EDQ and extensor carpi ulnaris (ECU) stability.

- Create a radially based, rectangular capsular flap with the distal limb just proximal to the dorsal radioulnar ligament, the ulnar limb in the floor of the sixth extensor compartment, and the proximal limb across the ulnar neck (**Fig. 21–2**).
- Osteotomize the ulnar styloid through its base leaving the attachments to the triangular fibrocartilage complex (TFCC) intact.

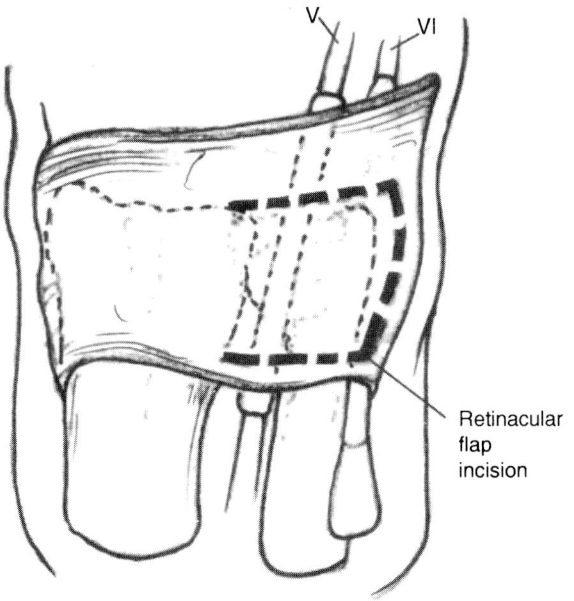

Figure 21–1

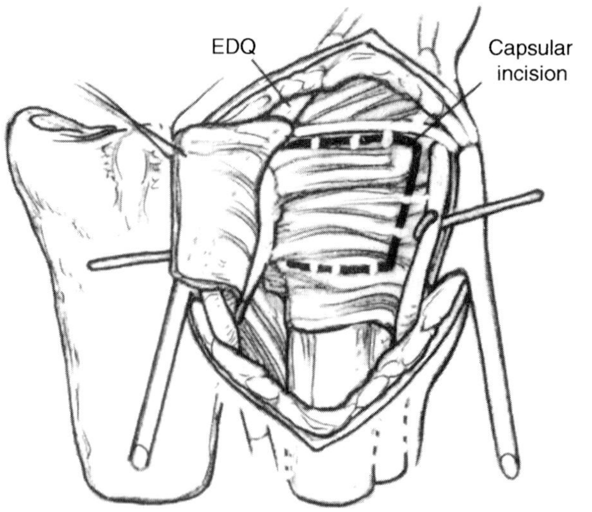

Figure 21–2

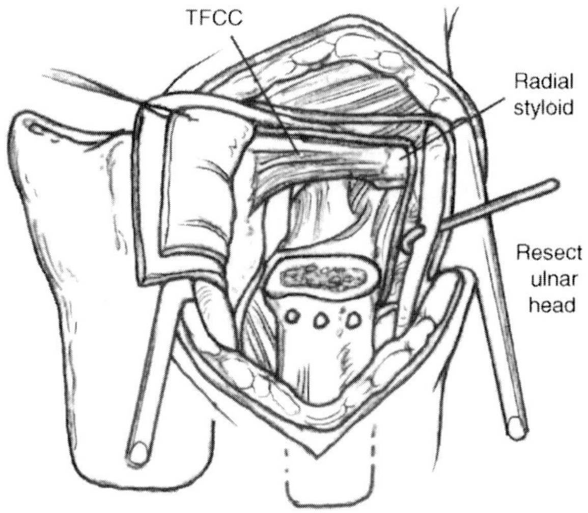

Figure 21–3

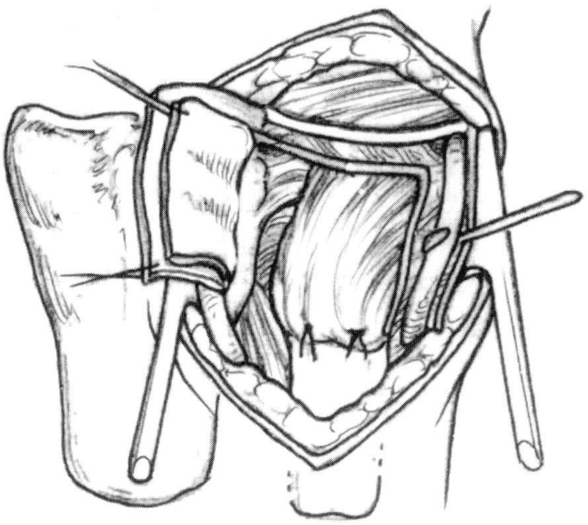

Figure 21–4

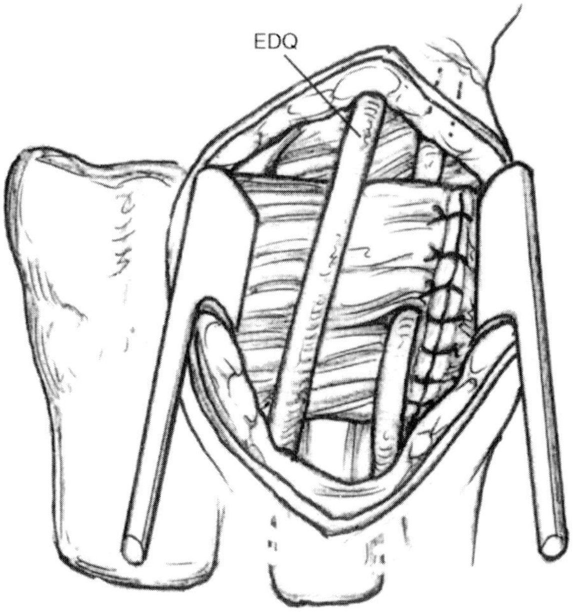

Figure 21–5

- Expose the ulnar head by subperiosteal dissection beginning at the floor of the sixth compartment.
- Resect the ulnar head just proximal to the sigmoid notch (**Fig. 21–3**).
- Create a distally based, rectangular flap of palmar DRUJ capsule and suture it to the dorsal aspect of the distal ulna with sutures placed through bone holes (**Fig. 21–4**).
- Close the remaining DRUJ capsular tissue.
- Transpose the retinaculum beneath the EDQ and ECU tendons (**Fig. 21–5**).

Pitfall

If the distal ulna is unstable, perform a tenodesis stabilization procedure.

- After reapproximating the retinaculum along the ulnar side of the wrist, make an oblique retinacular sling for the ECU to maintain it dorsal to the ulna.

Postoperative Care

- Long arm cast for 3 weeks
- Short arm cast for 2 weeks
- Splint until comfortable

Alternative Techniques

- Hemiresection arthroplasty of the distal ulna
- Sauve-Kapandji procedure (see Chapter 19)

Suggested Readings

Bieber EJ, Linscheid RL, Dobyns JH, Beckenbaugh RD. Failed distal ulna resections. J Hand Surg [Am] 1988;13A:193–200

Tulipan DJ, Eaton RG, Eberhart RE. The Darrach procedure defended: technique redefined and long-term follow-up. J Hand Surg [Am] 1991;16A:438–444

Section V.3

The Distal Radioulnar Joint: Unstable Distal Ulna, Post-Darrach

22 Flexor Carpi Ulnaris Tenodesis Stabilization of the Resected Distal Ulna

Indications

- Unstable distal ulna after a distal ulnar resection (Darrach procedure)
- Performed in conjunction with a distal ulnar resection

Technique

- An incision is made over the flexor carpi ulnaris (FCU) tendon extending to the distal wrist crease.

■ Pitfall

Avoid cutting or placing excess traction on the dorsal cutaneous branch of the ulnar nerve as it passes obliquely over the ulnar border of the wrist.

- Dissect the FCU from the pisiform to its musculotendinous junction (**Fig. 22–1**).
- Split the tendon longitudinally in half and cut one half at its musculotendinous junction, producing a tendon strip ~10 cm long.
- Pass the FCU strip dorsal through a window created in the connective tissue deep to the ulnar artery and nerve.
- A dorsal incision is made to expose the ulnar head or neck.
- Excise the ulnar head if it has not been done previously as described for the Darrach procedure.
- Drill a large oblique hole through the dorsoradial cortex ~1.5 cm from the end of the neck; direct the drill to exit through the open end of the medullary canal (**Fig. 22–2**).

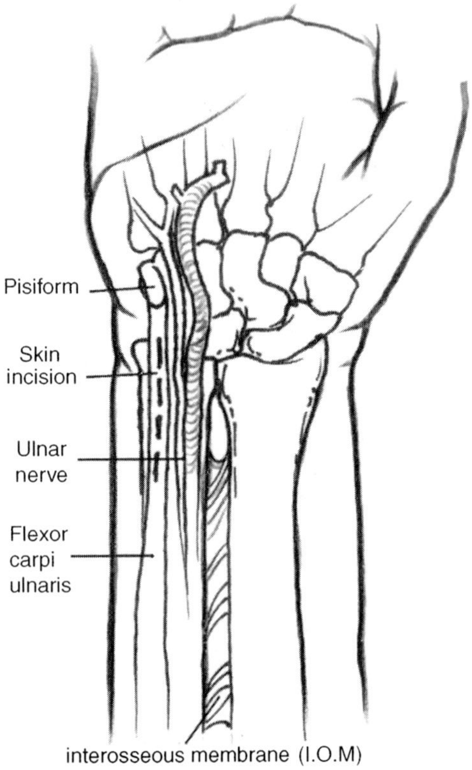

Figure 22–1

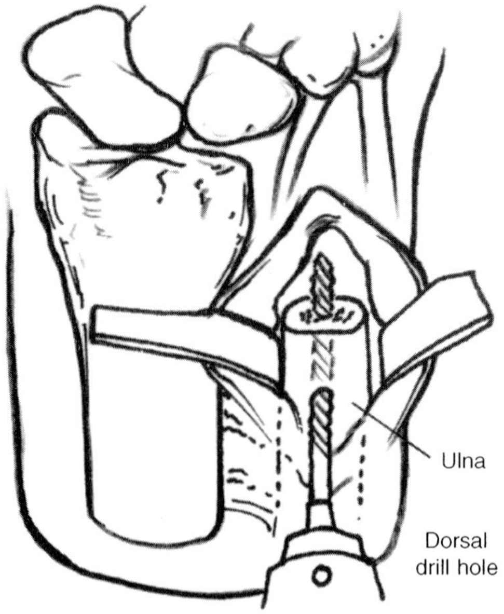

Figure 22–2

Pearl

Enlarge the hole gradually with sequentially larger drill bits to avoid fracture.

- The tendon strip is passed through the open end of the canal and out the drill hole (**Fig. 22–3**).
- Make an incision in the distal part of the interosseous membrane (IM) near the end of the ulna.
- Pass the tendon strip through the incision in IM in a dorsal to palmar direction (**Fig. 22–4**).
- Apply traction to the end of the strip with the forearm supinated and suture it to the IM.
- Loop the tendon around the extensor carpi ulnaris tendon (ECU) and suture it back to itself where it passes through the IM (the loop will prevent the ECU from subluxating over the ulnar stump) (**Fig. 22–5**).

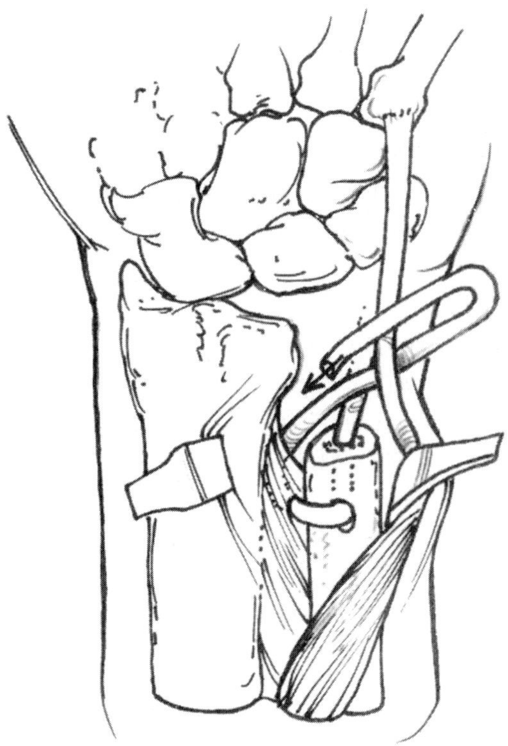

Figure 22–4

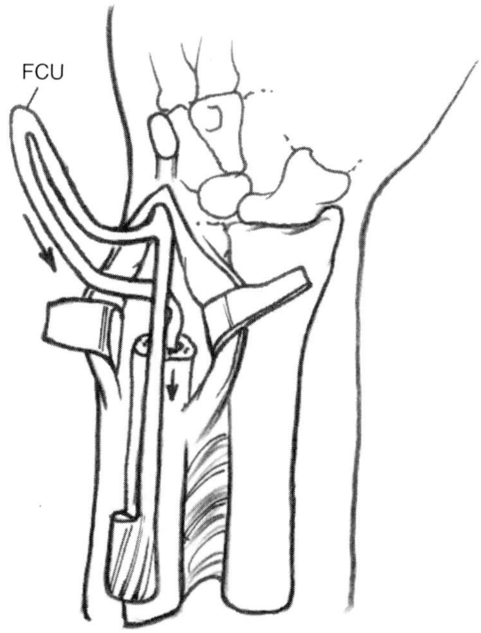

Figure 22–3

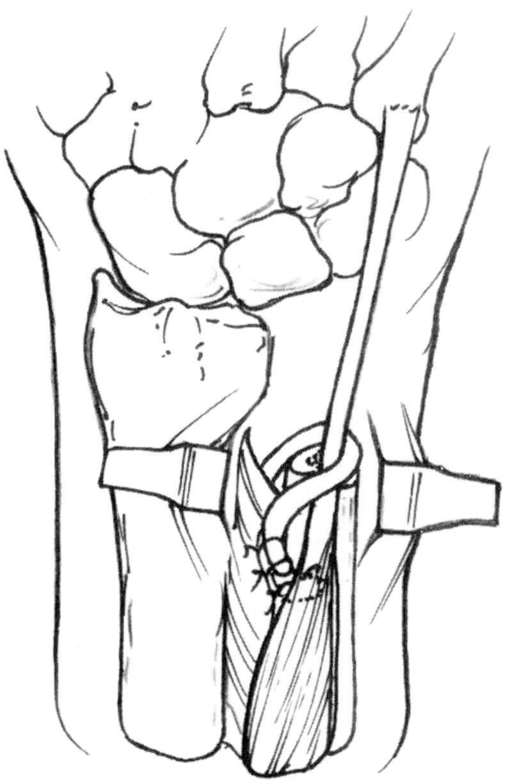

Figure 22–5

■ Pitfall

Do not create a tight loop that will prevent ECU excursion.

Postoperative Care

- Long arm cast with the forearm in supination rotation for 4 weeks
- Short arm cast for 2 weeks with the forearm in neutral
- Splint until comfortable

Alternative Technique

- Several variations of tenodesis and radioulnar tethers using tendon grafts have been described.

Suggested Readings

Breen TF, Jupiter JB. Extensor carpi ulnaris and flexor carpi ulnaris tenodesis of the unstable distal ulna. J Hand Surg [Am] 1989;14A:612–617

Tsai TM, Stilwell JH. Repair of chronic subluxation of the distal radioulnar joint (ulnar dorsal) using flexor carpi ulnaris tendon. J Hand Surg [Br] 1984;9B:289–294

23 Extensor Carpi Ulnaris–Flexor Carpi Ulnaris Tenodesis Stabilization of the Resected Distal Ulna

Indications

- Unstable distal ulna after a distal ulnar resection (Darrach procedure)
- Performed in conjunction with a distal ulnar resection

Technique

- Make an incision along the subcutaneous ulnar border to the level of the distal wrist crease (**Fig. 23–1**).

■ Pitfall

Avoid cutting or traction injury to the dorsal cutaneous branch of the ulnar nerve, which passes obliquely over the ulnar border of the wrist.

- Expose the extensor carpi ulnaris (ECU) and flexor carpi ulnaris (FCU) tendons over the full extent of the incision.
- Split the ECU and FCU tendons in half longitudinally (**Fig. 23–1**).
- Cut one half of the ECU tendon distally and one half of the FCU tendon proximally.
- Resect the ulnar head if not already removed, but retain the ulnar styloid with its triangular fibrocartilage complex (TFCC) attachments.

■ Pearl

Maintain the ECU subsheath in continuity with the TFCC.

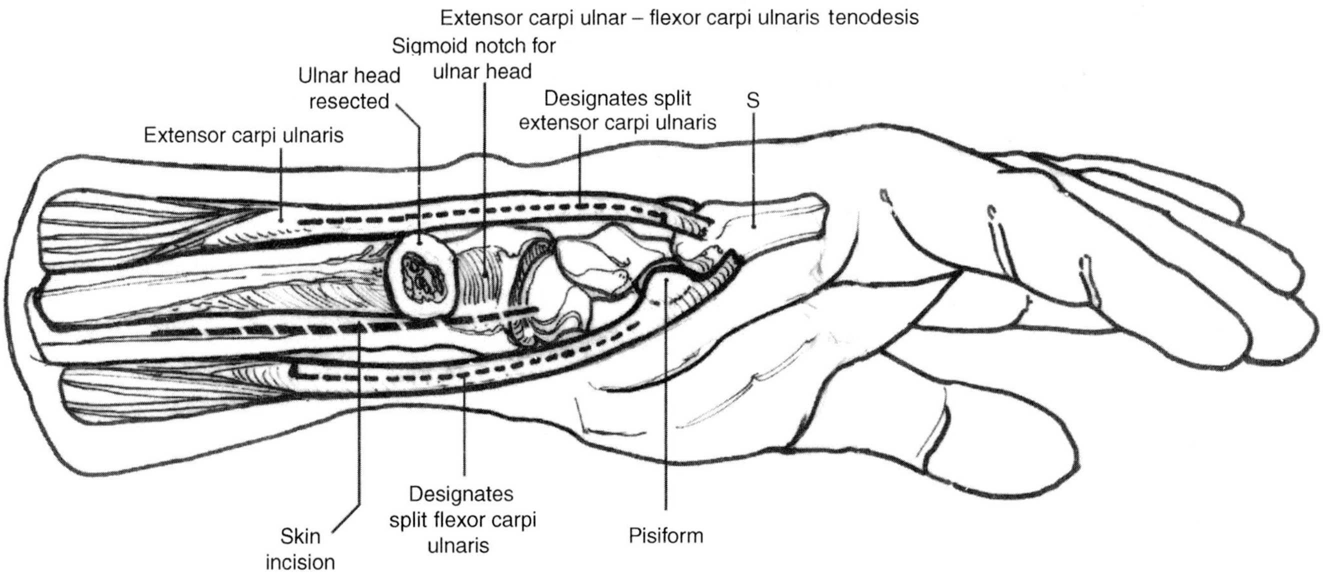

Figure 23–1

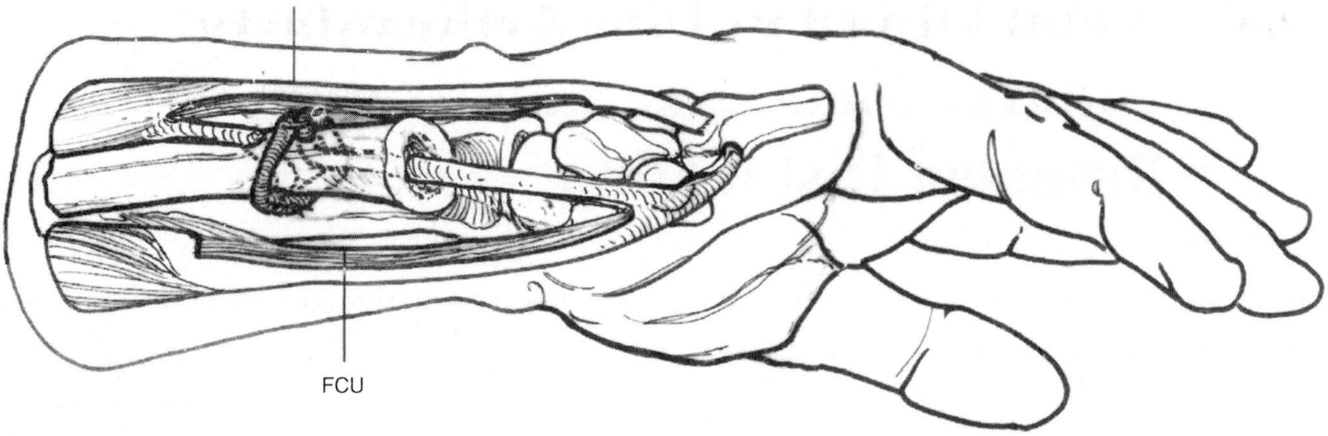

Figure 23–2

- Drill a dorsal to volar tunnel through the ulnar shaft ~2 cm from its end.
- Pass the distally based FCU tendon strip through the medullary canal and out the volar hole (**Fig. 23–2**).
- Direct the proximally based ECU tendon strip completely through the tunnel from dorsal to volar (**Fig. 23–2**).

Pearl

Place the forearm in the position in which the distal ulna is best stabilized by the tenodesis.

- Pass the two ends in opposite directions around the shaft and pull them taut.
- Make a half-hitch with the ends, tighten them against the shaft, and secure with sutures (**Fig. 23–2**).
- Close the skin but not the fascia.

Postoperative Care

- Long arm cast with the forearm in neutral rotation for 3 weeks
- Short arm cast for 2 weeks
- Splint until comfortable

Alternative Technique

Several variations of tenodesis and radioulnar tethers using tendon grafts have been described.

Suggested Readings

Breen TF, Jupiter JB. Extensor carpi ulnaris and flexor carpi ulnaris tenodesis of the unstable distal ulna. J Hand Surg [Am] 1989;14A:612–617

Tsai TM, Stilwell JH. Repair of chronic subluxation of the distal radioulnar joint (ulnar dorsal) using flexor carpi ulnaris tendon. J Hand Surg [Br] 1984;9B:289–294

24 Distal Ulna Implant Arthroplasty

Indications

- Chronic instability of the distal ulna after Darrach resection (see Chapter 21)
- Osteoarthritis or posttraumatic arthritis in patients with low activity demands

■ Pitfall

Implant stability may be difficult to achieve in cases with preoperative radioulnar divergence.

Technique

- The skin is incised along the subcutaneous border of the ulna, extending 6 to 8 cm proximally from the triquetrum (**Fig. 24–1**).
- Identify and protect the dorsal sensory branch of the ulnar nerve.
- The extensor retinaculum is incised between the extensor carpi ulnaris (ECU) and flexor carpi ulnaris (FCU).
- Elevate the ECU sheath subperiosteally from the distal ulna along with the triangular fibrocartilage complex (TFCC) and other soft tissues (**Fig. 24–2**).

■ Pearl

A dorsal approach is particularly useful when there is a preexisting dorsal incision or if joint inspection is required to decide optimal treatment.

- Use radiographs and templates to choose the proper head size.

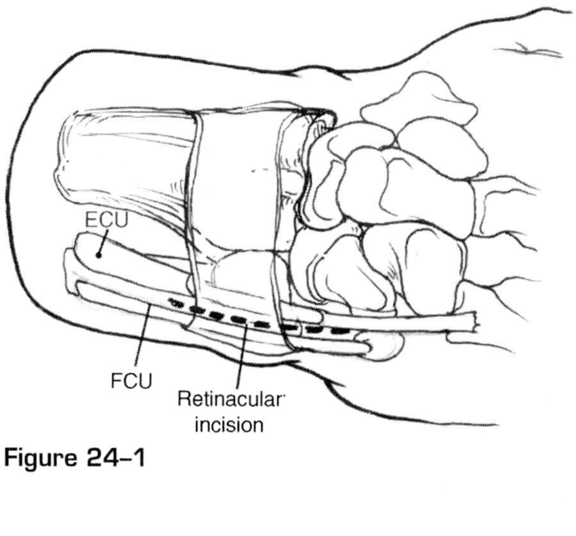

Figure 24–1

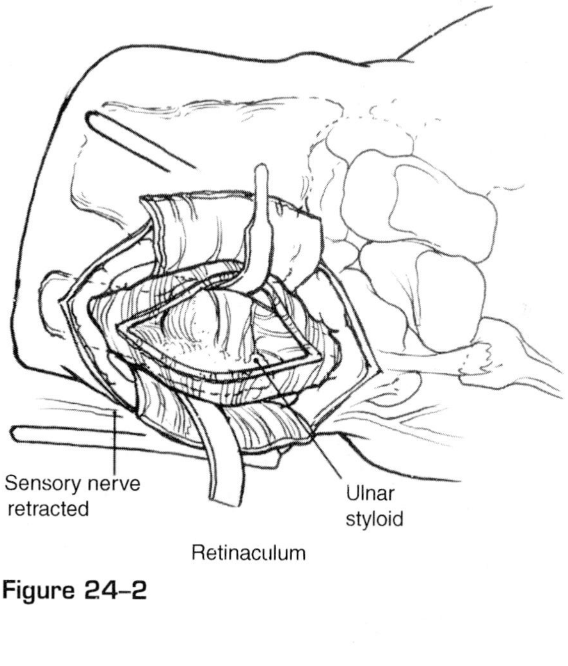

Figure 24–2

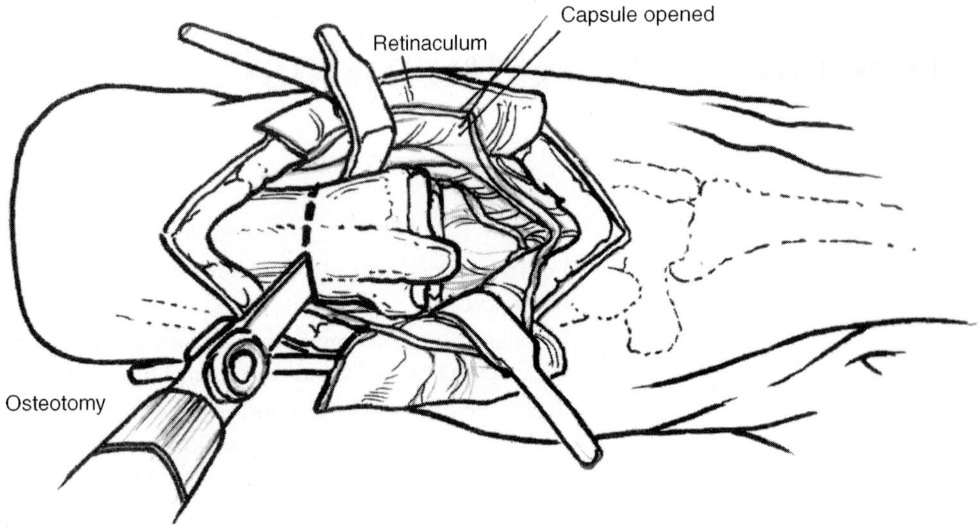

Figure 24–3

- A resection guide is used to determine the osteotomy level through the ulnar neck.
- The distal ulna is removed, preserving all soft tissues, which will form a pocket for the prosthetic head (**Fig. 24–3**).

Pearl

A stem with an extended collar may be required when there has been a previous ulnar resection.

- Inspect the sigmoid notch for osteophytes and incongruity.
- Use fluoroscopy to confirm proper length of the distal ulna, and revise the osteotomy if necessary.
- The medullary canal is prepared using a broach, and a trial stem and head are inserted (**Fig. 24–4**).
- Test the implant through a full range of pronation and supination for smooth joint motion and stability.
- Try different head sizes to achieve optimum stability and motion.

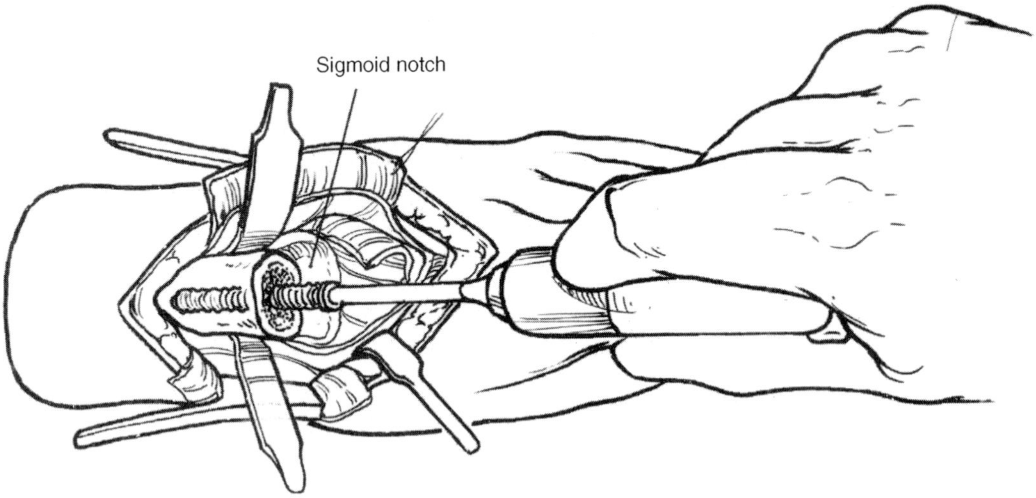

Figure 24–4

■ Pitfall

The sigmoid notch must have a smooth contour and sufficient depth for proper implant stability and motion.

- Place sutures in the most ulnar remnants of the TFCC and the ECU sheath and through the existing holes in the implant head (**Fig. 24–5A,B**).
- Seat the ulnar head on the stem and tie the previously placed sutures with the forearm in midrotation (**Fig. 24–6**).
- Close the remaining soft tissues over the implant head and reapproximate the extensor retinaculum (**Fig. 24–7**).

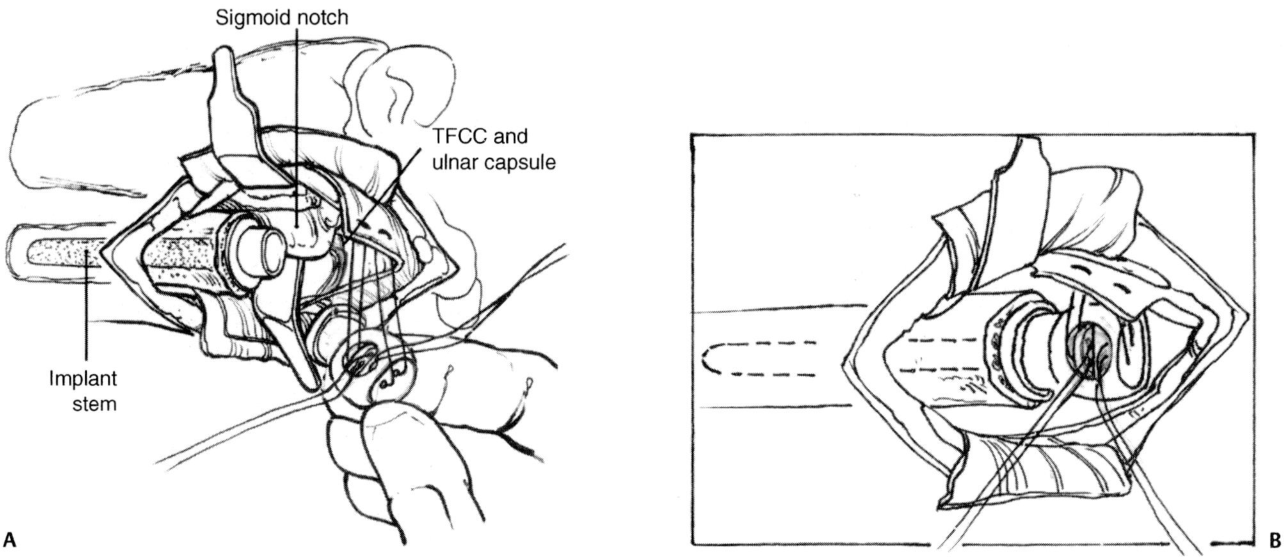

Figure 24–5

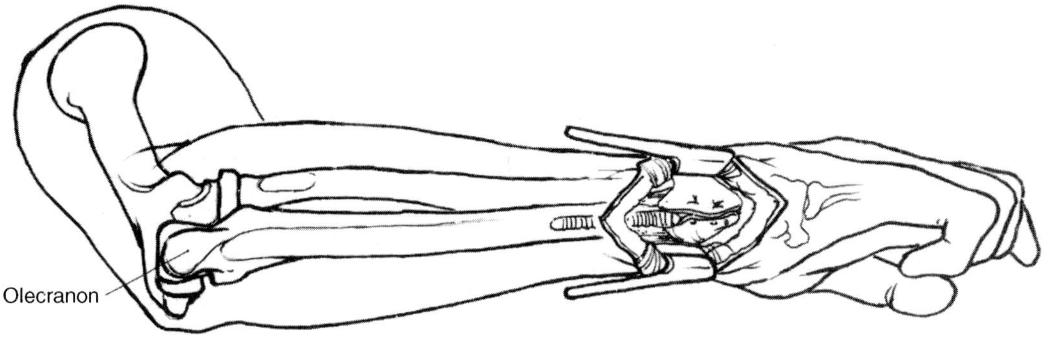

Figure 24–6

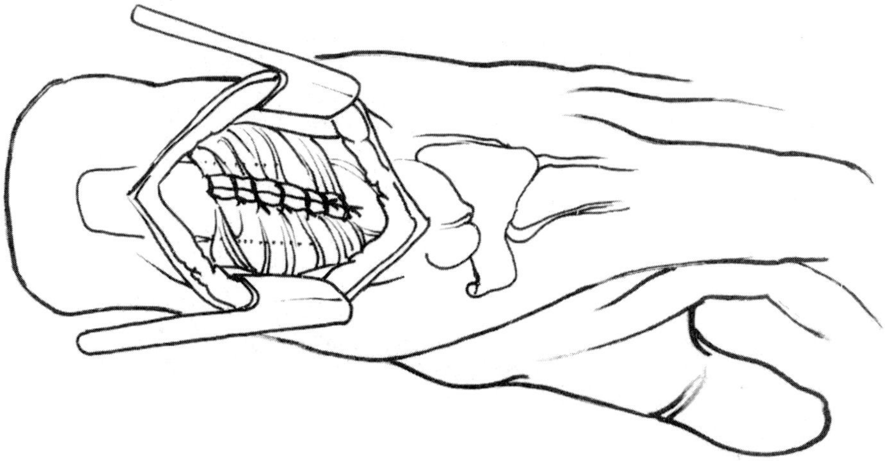

Figure 24–7

Postoperative Care

- Wrist and forearm are immobilized with the forearm in midrotation using a long arm or Muenster-type cast for 3 weeks.
- A well-molded short arm split is used for an additional 3 weeks, with intermittent gentle wrist motion.

Alternative Techniques

- Complete wrist arthrodesis
- Total wrist prosthetic replacement

Suggested Readings

Sauerbier M, Hahn ME, Fujita M, Neale PG, Berglund LJ, Berger RA. Analysis of dynamic distal radioulnar convergence after ulnar head resection and endoprosthesis implantation. J Hand Surg [Am] 2002;27A: 425–434

Scheker LR, Babb BA, Killion PE. Distal ulnar prosthetic replacement. Orthop Clin North [Am] 2001;32:365–376

van Schoonhoven J, Fernandez DL, Bowers WH, Herbert TJ. Salvage of failed resection arthroplasties of the distal radioulnar joint using a new ulnar head prosthesis. J Hand Surg [Am] 2000;25A: 438–446

Section V.4

The Distal Radioulnar Joint: Ulnocarpal Abutment

25 Arthroscopic "Wafer" Procedure

Indications

- Ulnar impaction syndrome

■ Pitfall

Cannot be used if positive ulnar variance is greater than 4 mm or when there is arthritis of the distal radioulnar joint (DRUJ)

Technique

- Standard wrist arthroscopy setup is used.
- Use the 3–4 and 4–5 or 6R portals to inspect the joint, specifically evaluating the triangular fibrocartilage complex (TFCC), lunotriquetral interosseous ligament, lunate, triquetrum, and ulnar head for tears and chondromalacia (**Fig. 25–1**).

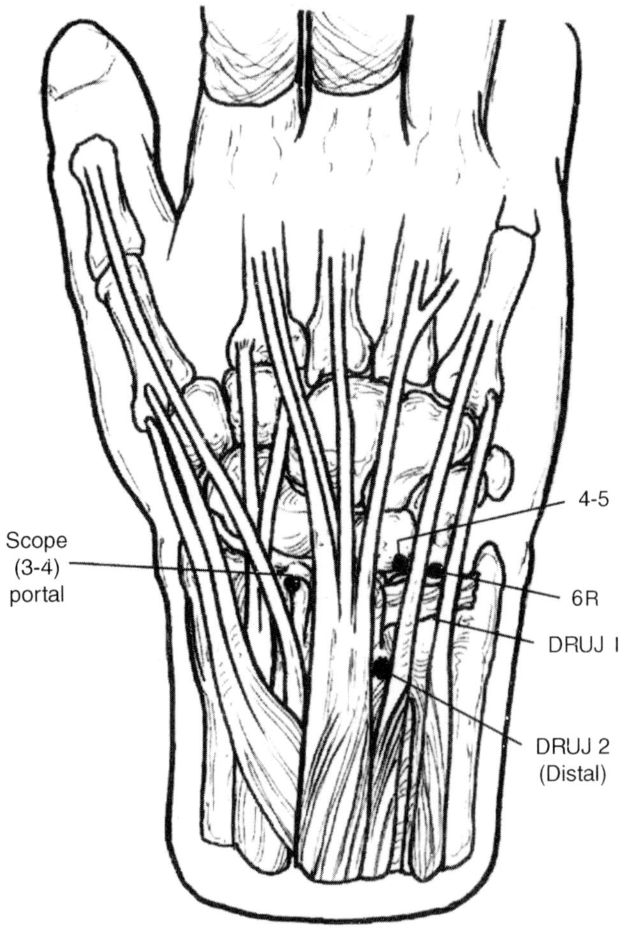

Figure 25–1

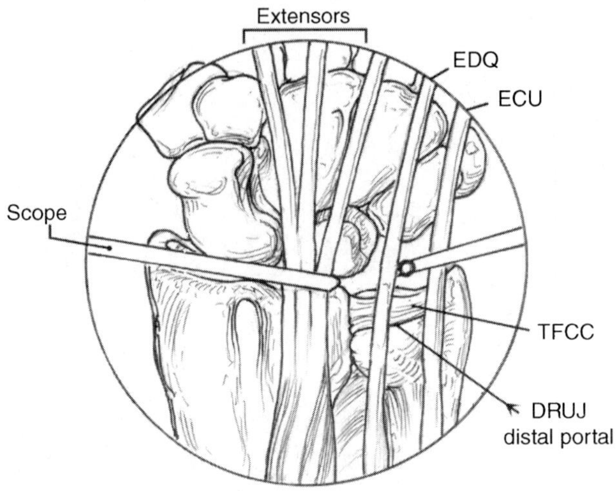

Figure 25–2

- Debride the central two thirds of the TFCC using a shaver, punch, or radiofrequency device in the 4–5 or 6R portal (**Fig. 25–2**).

■ Pitfall

Do not violate the peripheral 2 mm of the articular disk to avoid creating DRUJ instability.

- Using a motorized bur in the 4–5 or 6R portal, remove the central portion of the ulnar head dome through the hole in the TFCC to create 2 mm ulnar negative variance (**Fig. 25–3A,B**).
- A distal DRUJ portal is made 3 mm ulnar to the sigmoid notch and just proximal to the TFCC.

■ Pearl

To make the DRUJ portal, position the forearm in slight pronation and spread a hemostat horizontally between the ulnar head and TFCC.

- Place the bur in the DRUJ portal and remove the periphery of the dome to complete the resection (**Fig. 25–4**).
- Pronate and supinate the forearm to reach the entire periphery of the dome.

■ Pitfall

Do not violate the fovea of the ulnar head where the deep fibers of the radioulnar ligaments attach.

- With wrist traction reduced, confirm a complete and adequate level of resection with fluoroscopy.

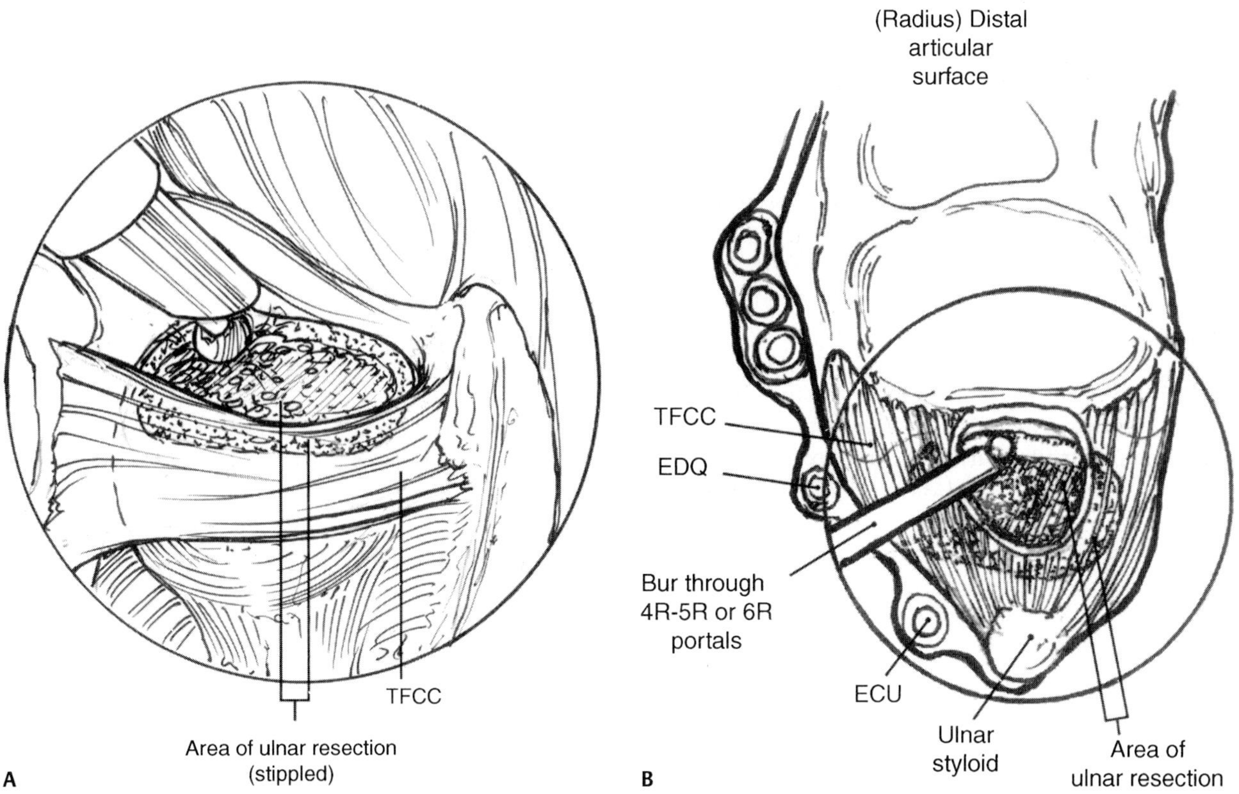

Figure 25–3

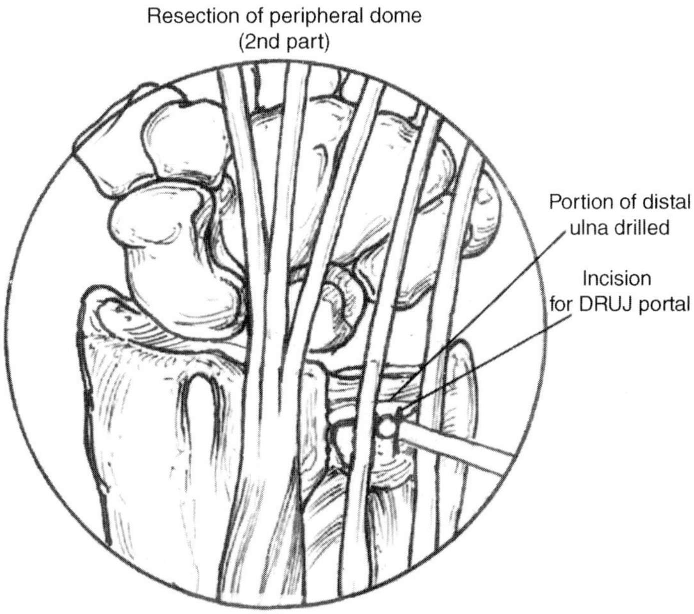

Figure 25–4

- Modify the resection level if necessary and remove any remaining sharp bony edges.

Postoperative Care

- Apply a dressing and plaster wrist splint.
- Convert to a removable wrist splint at the first postoperative visit and begin gentle wrist motion.

■ Pearl

It may take up to several months for recovery and resolution of symptoms.

Alternative Technique

- Open wafer procedure (see Chapter 26)
- Ulnar shortening by shaft osteotomy

Suggested Readings

Tomaino MM, Weiser RW. Combined arthroscopic TFCC debridement and wafer resection of the distal ulna in wrists with triangular fibrocartilage complex tears and positive ulnar variance. J Hand Surg [Am] 2001;26A: 1047–1052

Verheyden JR, Short WH. Arthroscopic Wafer Procedure. Atlas of Hand Clinics: New Techniques in Wrist Arthroscopy 6:241–252, 2001

26 Open "Wafer" Procedure

Indications

- Ulnar impaction syndrome
- In conjunction with repair of a traumatic triangular fibrocartilage complex (TFCC) peripheral tear

■ Pitfall

Cannot be used if positive ulnar variance is greater than 4 mm or when there is arthritis of the distal radioulnar joint (DRUJ).

Technique

- A 5 cm longitudinal dorsal skin incision is made centered over the ulnar head.
- Approach the DRUJ through the fifth extensor compartment, leaving the distal portion of the retinaculum intact.
- Reflect the retinaculum ulnarly but do not open the sixth extensor compartment.
- Create an L-shaped capsulotomy with one limb just proximal to the dorsal radioulnar ligament and the other along the edge of the sigmoid notch (**Fig. 26–1**).

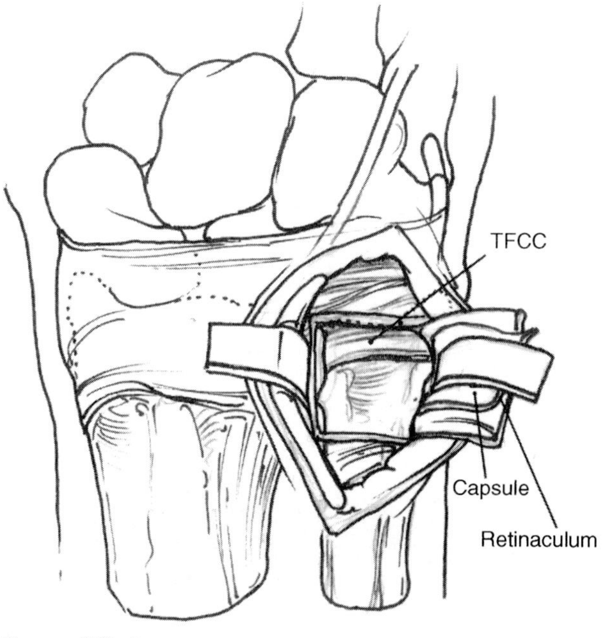

Figure 26–1

■ Pitfall

Avoid cutting the dorsal radioulnar ligament by incising the capsule gradually from proximal to distal.

- Resect 2 to 4 mm of the dome of the ulnar head (**Fig. 26–2A,B**).
- Confirm that the resection is sufficient using fluoroscopy.
- Trim torn edges of the TFCC articular disk.

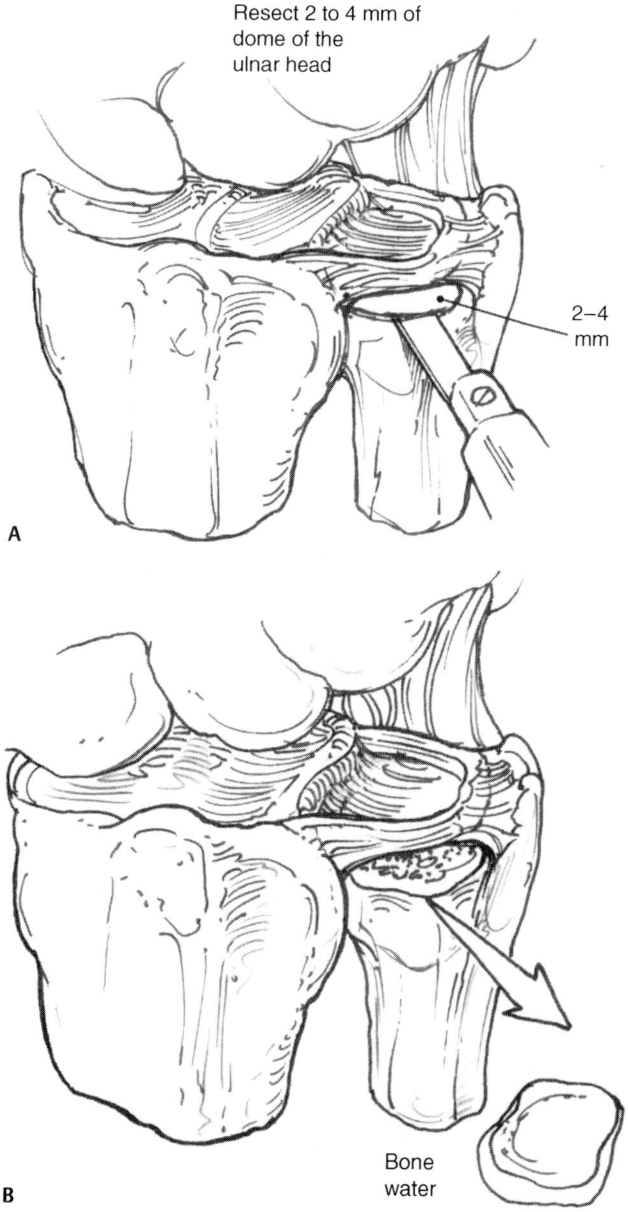

Figure 26–2

■ Pearl

Identify the fovea to avoid injury to the attachments of the radioulnar ligaments.

- Close the capsule and retinaculum in layers leaving the extensor digiti minimi tendon superficial to the retinaculum over the DRUJ.

Postoperative Care

- Apply a dressing and plaster wrist splint.
- Convert to a removable wrist splint and begin gentle wrist motion at 2 weeks.
- Avoid impact loading and power grip for 3 months.

■ Pearl

Recovery and improvement in symptoms may take several months.

Alternative Technique

- Arthroscopic technique for wafer procedure
- Ulnar shortening by shaft osteotomy

Suggested Readings

Bilos ZJ, Chamberland D. Distal ulnar head shortening for treatment of triangular fibrocartilage complex tears with ulna positive variance. J Hand Surg [Am] 1991; 16A:1115–1119

Feldon P, Terrono AL, Belsky MR. Wafer distal ulna resection for triangular fibrocartilage tears and/or ulna impaction syndrome. J Hand Surg [Am] 1992;17A: 731–737

27 Ulnar Shaft Shortening Osteotomy

Indications

- Ulnar impaction syndrome
- Positive ulnar variance from radius malunion (e.g., distal radius fracture)
- Traumatic lunotriquetral interosseous ligament tear with positive or neutral ulnar variance

Preoperative Evaluation

- Measure ulnar variance with shoulder abducted 90 degrees, elbow flexed 90 degrees, and forearm and wrist in neutral positions.

Technique

- Incise along subcutaneous border of ulna, extending to ulnar neck (**Fig. 27–1**).
- Incise periosteum longitudinally and reflect the extensor carpi ulnaris (ECU) muscle (**Fig. 27–2**).

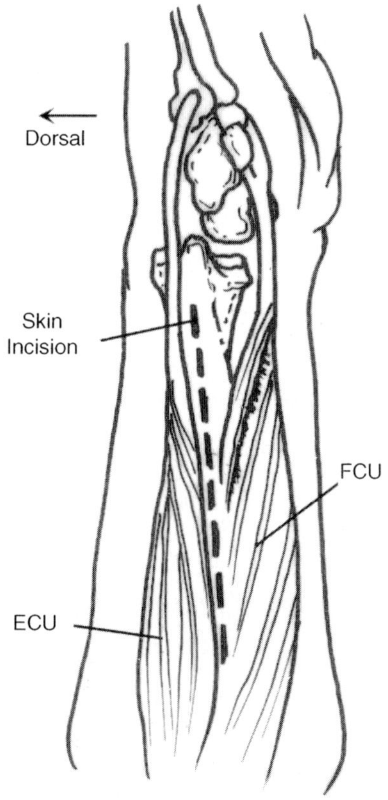

Figure 27–1

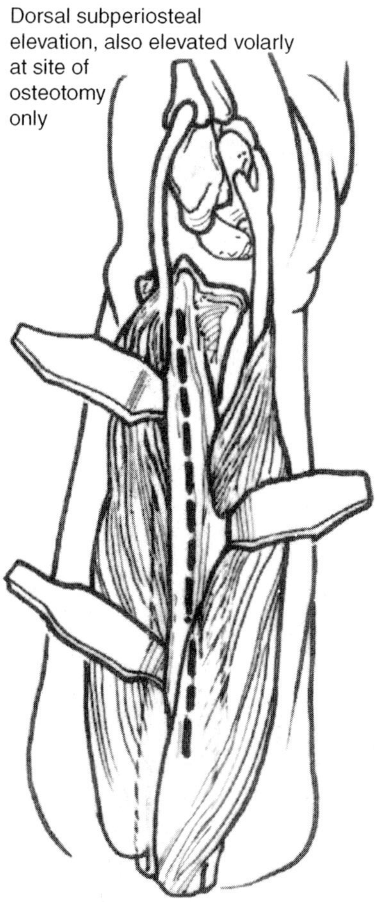

Figure 27–2

Pearl

To improve bone healing, do not strip the flexor carpi ulnaris (FCU) except at the osteotomy site and for applying plate clamps.

- Apply a six- or seven-hole 3.5 mm dynamic compression plate dorsally and insert the middle of the distal three screws (**Fig. 27–3**).

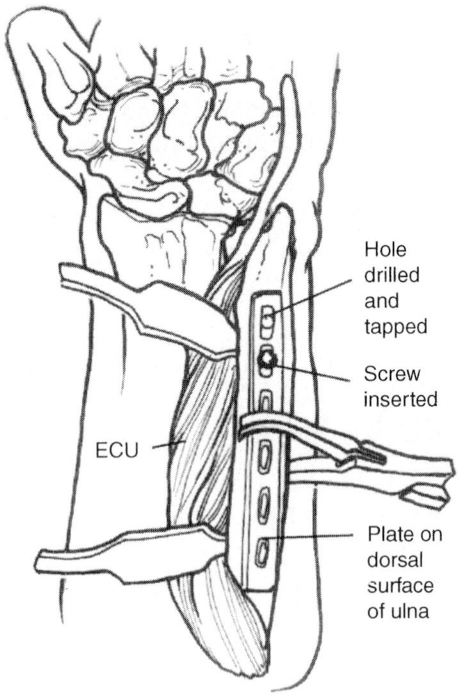

Figure 27–3

- With the screw slightly loose, rotate the plate to access the ulnar shaft.
- Make a distal oblique osteotomy ~45 degrees to the plane of the plate from proximal ulnar to distal dorsal and locate it under the third or fourth plate hole (**Fig. 27–4A,B**).

Pearl

Make a distal cut only partway through the ulna to maintain shaft stability during the second cut.

- Mark and make the complete second cut parallel to the first.
- Reposition the plate and compress the osteotomy.
- Clamp the plate to the shaft proximally and tighten the first screw.
- Insert the fourth and fifth screws sequentially in compression mode.
- Insert the sixth screw in neutral mode.
- Insert the third or fourth screw in lag mode through the plate and across the osteotomy.
- Check screw lengths and osteotomy compression via fluoroscopy (**Fig. 27–5**).
- Close the subcutaneous tissue and skin but not the fascia.

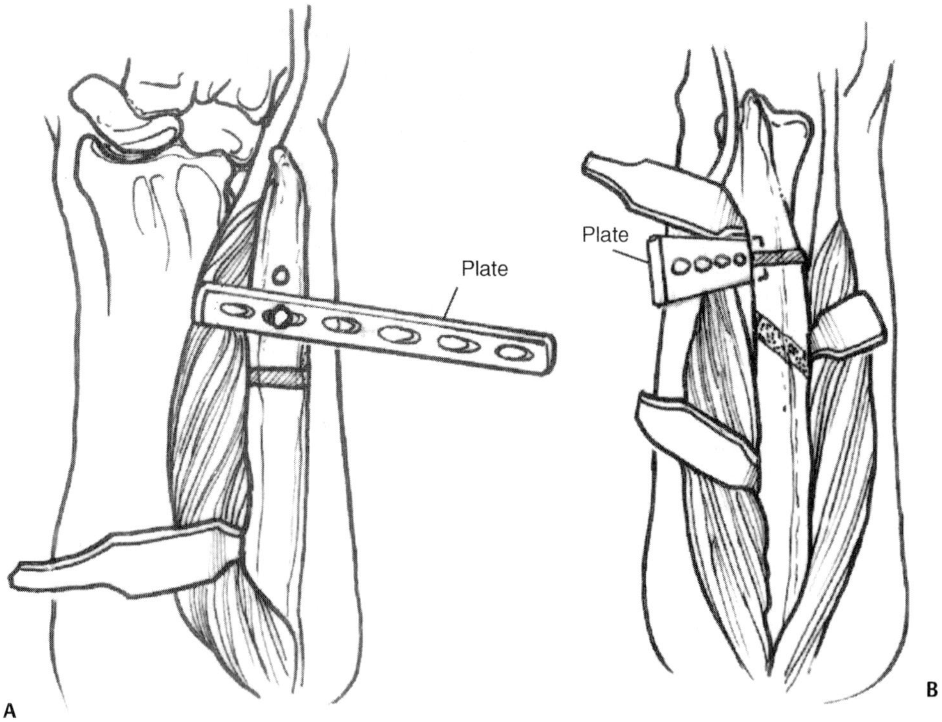

A B

Figure 27–4

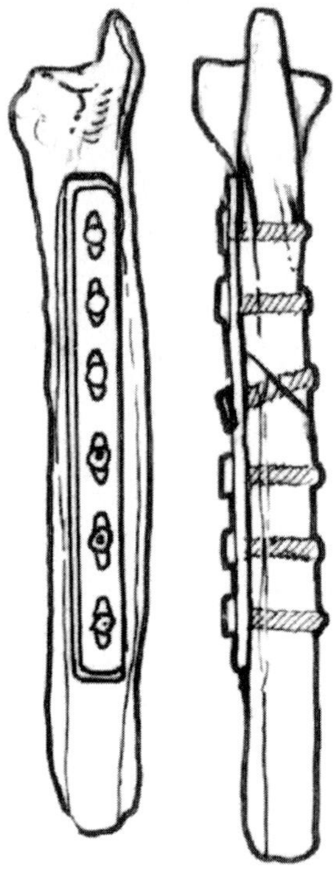

Figure 27–5

Postoperative Care

- Short arm plaster splint is used for 2 weeks.
- Short arm splint extending to near the elbow for strenuous activities is used until the osteotomy is healed.
- Plate removal is optional.

Alternative Techniques

- Use a specialized instrument/plating system for ulnar osteotomy.
- Arthroscopic or open resection (Wafer procedure) of the distal ulna (see Chapter 25)
- Hemiresection arthroplasty of the distal ulna

Suggested Readings

Chun S, Palmar AK. The ulnar impaction syndrome: follow-up of ulnar shortening osteotomy. J Hand Surg [Am] 1993;18A:46–53

Rayhack JM, Gasser SI, Latta LL, Ouellette EA, Milne EL. Precision oblique osteotomy for shortening of the ulna. J Hand Surg [Am] 1993;18A:908–918

Section VI.1

The Wrist Joint: Scaphoid Fractures

28 Percutaneous Screw Fixation of Scaphoid Fractures

Indications

- Acute nondisplaced and displaced fractures of the scaphoid
- Fractures in competitive athletes or laborers or other individuals who wish to avoid prolonged periods of immobilization and a faster return to activity
- Fractures with delayed treatment

Technique

- The patient is positioned supine with the arm extended and the elbow flexed 90 degrees.
- The forearm is pronated and the wrist is flexed ~45 degrees of flexion placing the scaphoid in 90 degrees of flexion (**Fig. 28–1**).
- The guide wire is inserted into the proximal pole from the dorsal aspect of the wrist. The wire is advanced across the fracture and into the proximal pole. The centered position of the wire is confirmed using anteroposterior, lateral, and oblique projections with intraoperative imaging.
- For displaced fractures of the scaphoid, two Kirschner wires can be used as joysticks to reduce the fragments. One of the wires can be advanced to capture the reduction (**Fig. 28–2**).

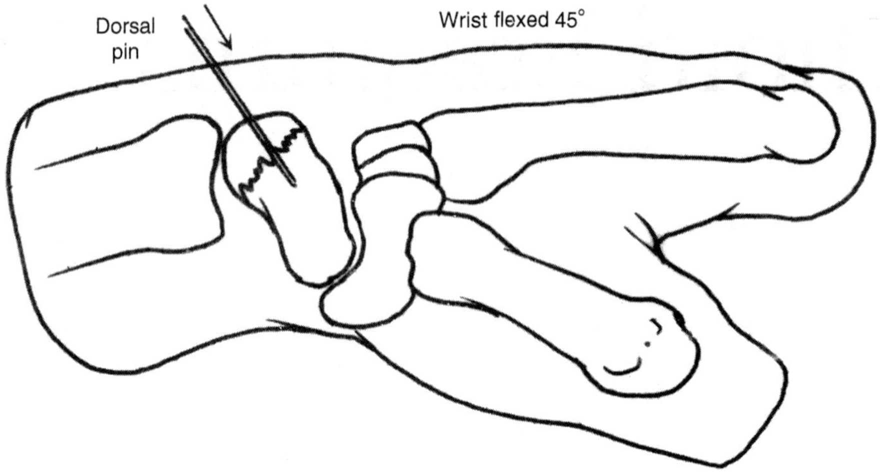

Figure 28–1

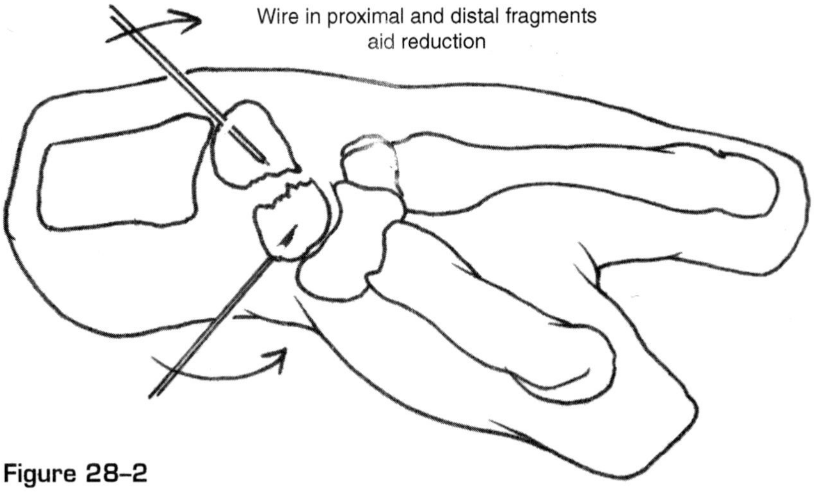

Figure 28–2

- Fluoroscopy or arthroscopy can be utilized to confirm acceptable reduction.

Dorsal Screw Placement (Proximal Pole and Waist Fractures)

- The dorsal entry site over the guide wire can be enlarged with a small longitudinal skin incision and blunt dissection down to the capsule to avoid injury to the extensor tendons.
- The scaphoid is prepared with a hand reamer, reaming no more than 2 mm from the distal cortex.
- A headless, cannulated screw 4 mm shorter than the length of the scaphoid is advanced over the guide wire from proximal to distal.
- The wire is removed and the reduction and screw position is confirmed with fluoroscopy.

Palmar Screw Placement (Distal Third Fractures)

- The guide wire is placed as above.
- A palmar incision is made over the palmar site of wire penetration.
- The scaphoid is prepared with the hand reamer, which is advanced through the palmar edge of the trapezium and then into the scaphoid no more than 2 mm from the proximal cortex.
- A headless, cannulated screw 4 mm shorter than the length of the scaphoid is advanced over the guide wire from distal to proximal (**Fig. 28–3**).
- The wire is removed and the reduction and screw position are confirmed with fluoroscopy.

■ Pearls

Accurate determination of scaphoid length using parallel guide wires and downsizing the screw by 4 mm avoids the complications of oversized screws, including distraction of the fragments and screw penetration of the cortex.

For the palmar approach, reaming the edge of the trapezium and then the scaphoid ensures a starting point that will achieve center–center screw placement.

■ Pitfall

Reaming into the opposite cortex compromises the compressive capacity of the screw.

Alternative Techniques

- Arthroscopically assisted percutaneous screw fixation
- Open reduction and internal fixation through either a dorsal or a palmar approach

Postoperative Care

- A bulky hand dressing and splint are applied. These will be exchanged with a customized, removable palmar splint.
- The patient may remove the splint for gentle motion and strengthening.
- Postoperative radiographs are taken every 2 weeks to assess fracture healing.
- Athletes and laborers are restricted until union is confirmed.

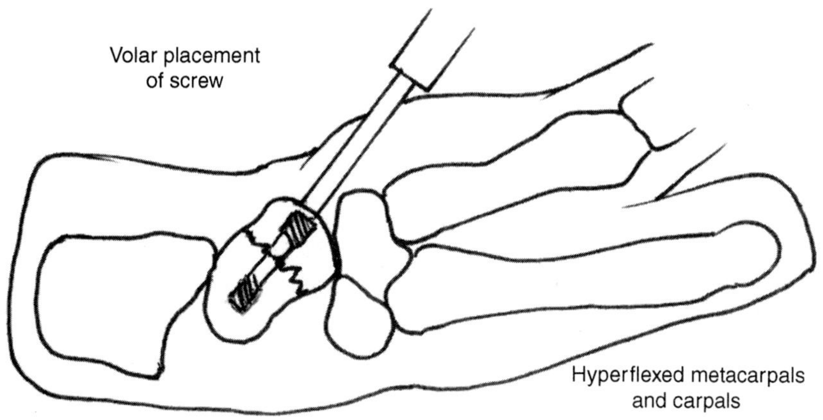

Figure 28–3

Suggested Readings

Adolfson L, Lindau T, Arner M. Acutrak screw fixation versus cast immobilisation for undisplaced scaphoid waist fractures. J Hand Surg [Br] 2001;26B: 192–195

Bond CD, Shin AY, McBride MT, Dao KD. Percutaneous screw fixation or cast immobilization for nondisplaced scaphoid fractures. J Bone Joint Surg Am 2001;83-A: 483–488

McCallister WV, Knight J, Kaliappan R, Trumble TE. Central placement of the screw in simulated fractures of the scaphoid waist: a biomechanical study. J Bone Joint Surg Am. 2003;85-A:72–77

Slade JF, Grauer JN, Mahoney JD. Arthroscopic reduction and percutaneous fixation of scaphoid fractures with a novel dorsal technique. Orthop Clin North Am 2001;32: 247–261

29 Open Reduction and Internal Fixation of Displaced Scaphoid Fractures via Dorsal Approach

Indications

- Acute unstable fractures

  Displacement greater than 1 mm
  Lateral intrascaphoid angulation greater than 35 degrees
  Significant bone loss
  Significant comminution
  Concomitant ligamentous injuries
  Fractures not amenable to closed reduction and cast treatment

- Relative indications

  Multiple upper extremity injuries
  Delayed union—4 to 6 months
  Nonunion
  Early return to sport/occupation

Technique

- 4 cm longitudinal incision ~4 cm on the ulnar border of Lister's tubercle through the third compartment (**Fig. 29–1**)
- Identify extensor pollicis longus (EPL).
- Open overlying extensor retinaculum and elevate subperiosteally.
- Retract radial wrist extensors ulnarly, EPL radially.
- Expose dorsal wrist capsule and incise longitudinally, providing adequate exposure while preserving dorsal intercarpal ligament (**Fig. 29–2**).
- Reduce fragments using joystick K-wires and assess alignment with mini image intensifier.

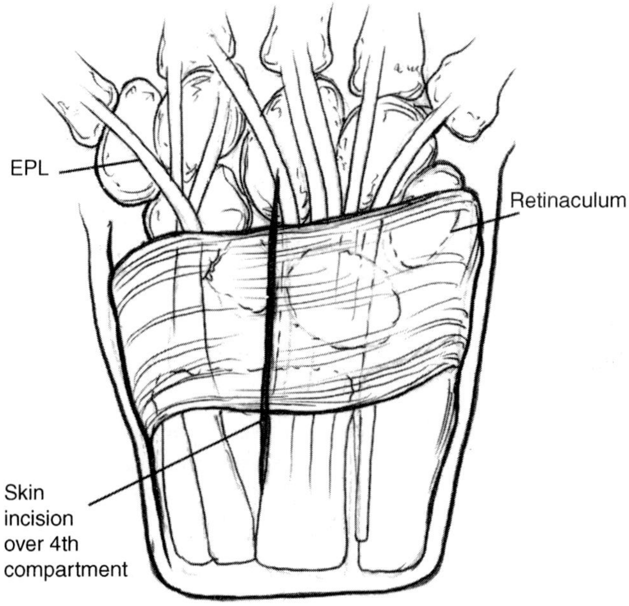

Figure 29–1

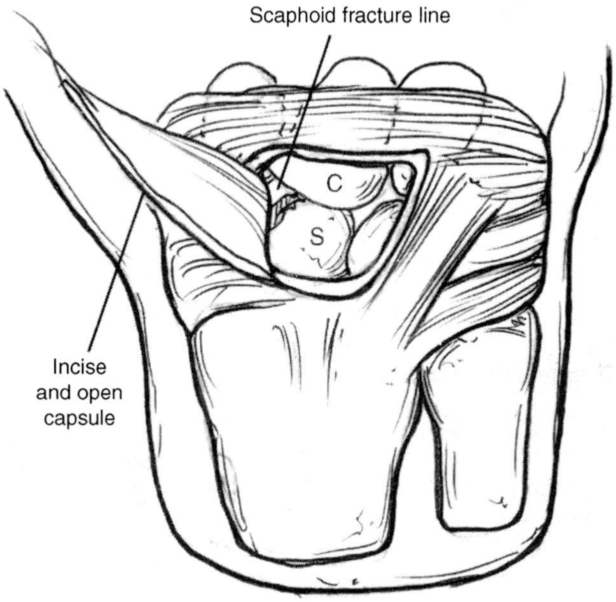

Figure 29–2

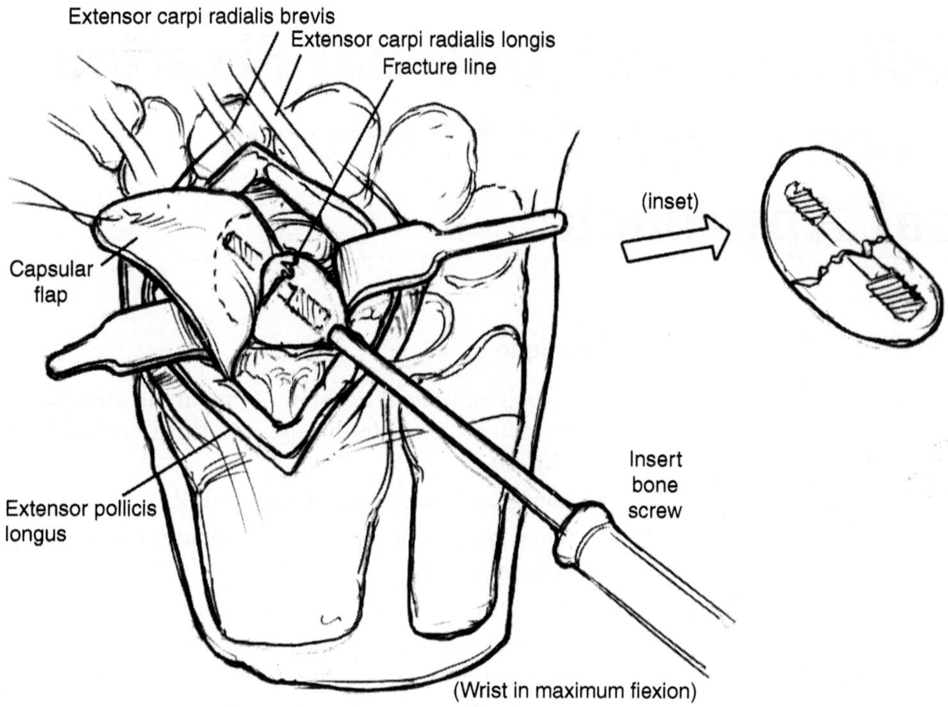

Figure 29–3

- Place stable fixation with cannulated headless screw from proximal to distal over guide wire (**Fig. 29–3**).
- May use additional percutaneous K-wires for more rotational control.
- Close capsule without imbrication.
- Volar thumb gauntlet splint

Postoperative Care

- Remove sutures at 7 to 10 days.
- Continue splinting with custom Orthoplast (Johnson & Johnson, New Brunswick, NJ).
- Plain films every 2 weeks to assess healing; scaphoid view at 6 to 8 weeks to assess union
- If union uncertain, order CT scan—sagittal views in plane of scaphoid (45 degrees to long axis).

■ Pearl

Preserve the dorsal intercarpal ligament.

- Close the capsule without imbrication.

■ Pitfall

- Use multiple views with fluoroscopy to ensure that the guide wire is positioned in the central third of the long axis of the scaphoid.

Suggested Readings

McCallister WV, Knight J, Kaliappan R, Trumble TE. Central placement of the screw in simulated fractures of the scaphoid waist: a biomechanical study. J Bone Joint Surg Am. 2003;85-A:72–77

Rettig ME, Koznl SH, Cooney WP. Open reduction and internal fixation of acute displaced scaphoid waist fractures. J Hand Surg [Am] 2001;26A:271–276

Section VI.2

The Wrist Joint: Scaphoid Nonunions

30 Open Reduction and Internal Fixation of Scaphoid Nonunion via Palmar Approach with Distal Radial Bone Graft

Indications

Scaphoid fails to heal after 3 months. Radiographs show resorption of bone with sclerosis along the edges of the fracture.

■ Pearl

If, on a lateral view, the scaphoid has collapsed into a "humpback deformity" (**Fig. 30–1**), consider correcting this deformity with a wedge of iliac crest or distal radius bone graft.

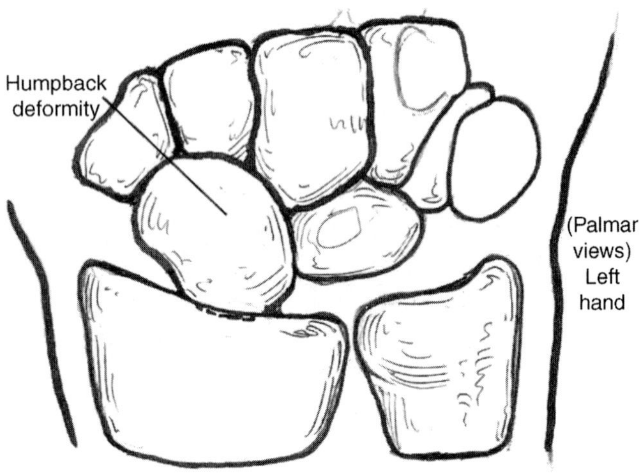

Figure 30–1

Technique

- Brunner incision along the radial aspect of the flexor carpi radialis (FCR) tendon (**Fig. 30–2**).

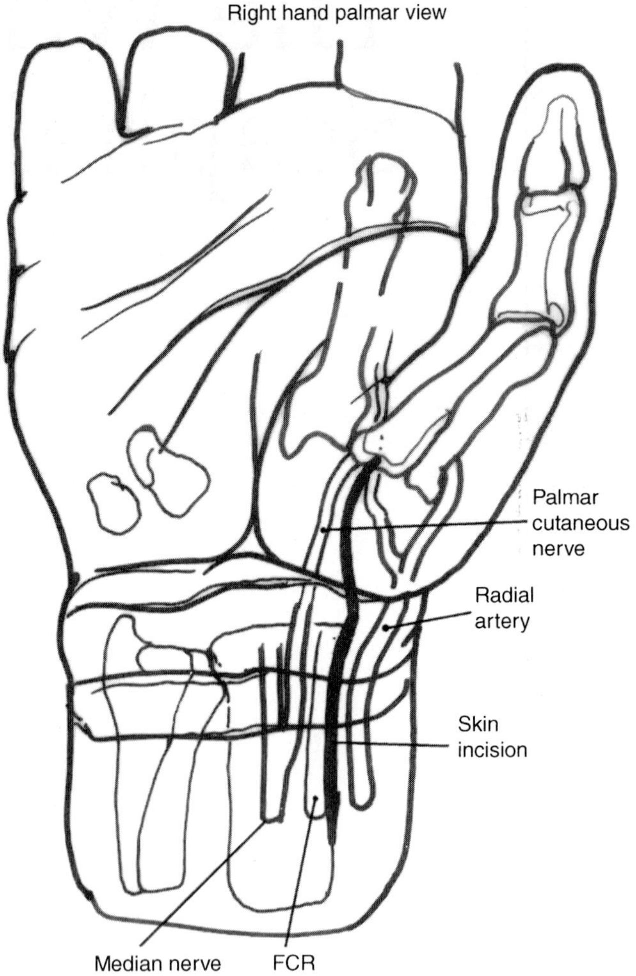

Figure 30–2

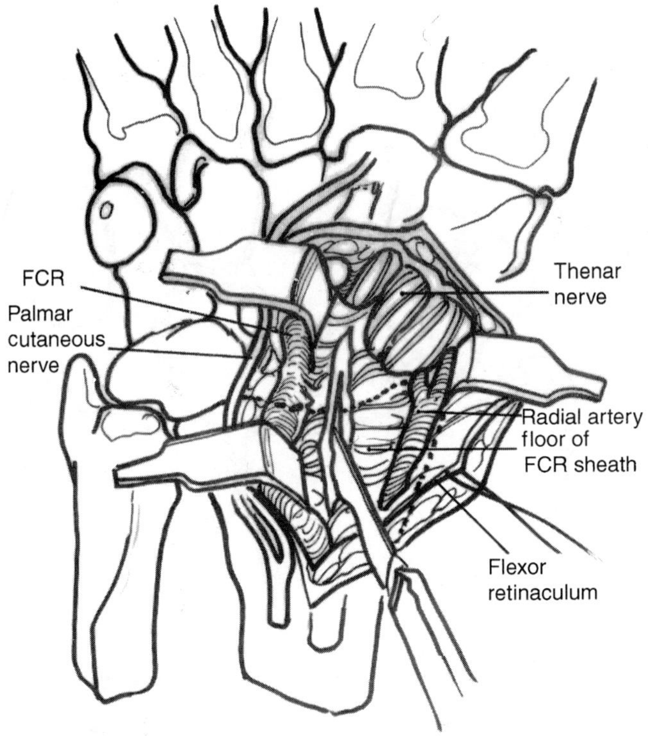

Figure 30–3

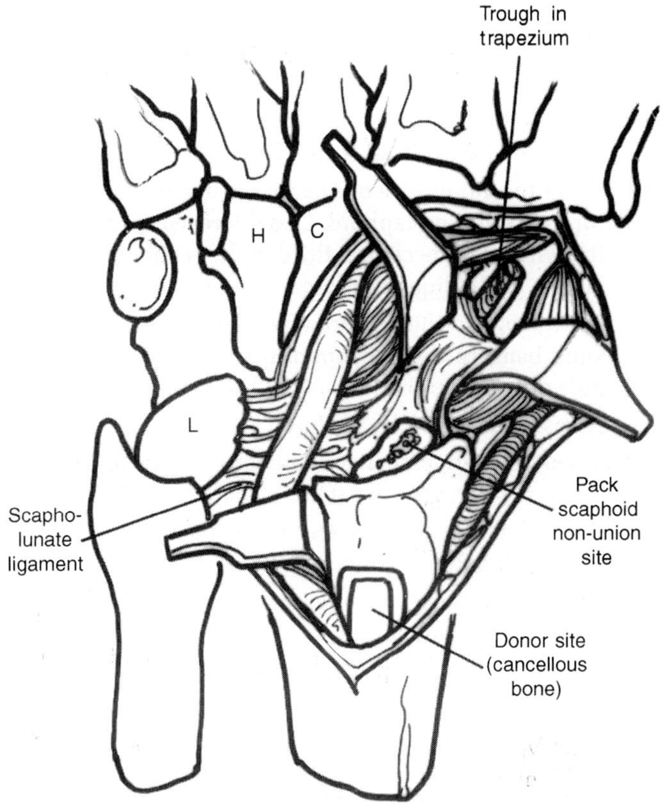

Figure 30–4

- Retract the FCR tendon ulnarly and incise the floor of the FCR sheath (**Fig. 30–3**).

■ Pitfall

The palmar cutaneous branch of the median nerve runs along the ulnar aspect of the FCR tendon. The nerve is at risk if the dissection strays ulnar to the FCR tendon.

- Directly beneath the sheath are the joint capsule and distal radius.
- Elevate the capsule off the scaphoid and the periosteum off the radius via a longitudinal incision. Extend the exposure to the scaphotrapezial joint by splitting the fibers of the thenar musculature (**Fig. 30–4**).
- Debride the nonunion site with a curette and small rongeur.
- Use a small osteotome to wedge open the nonunion site and restore the scaphoid to its normal length (**Fig. 30–5**).
- Measure the dimensions of the defect.
- Expose the palmar aspect of the distal radius.
- Use a sagittal saw to harvest a piece of corticocancellous graft to match the defect in the scaphoid.

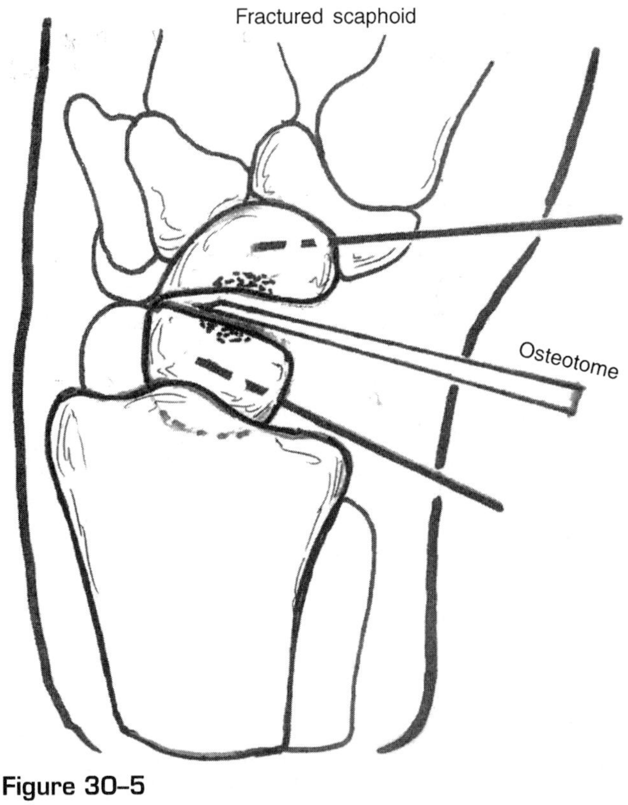

Figure 30–5

- Harvest cancellous bone and pack in the defects within either pole of the scaphoid.
- Trim and inset the corticocancellous graft.
- Create a trough in the palmar aspect of the trapezium for access to the distal scaphoid.
- Insert the guide wire of a cannulated screw down the long axis of the scaphoid. Use fluoroscopy to ensure the wire is in the central third of the scaphoid on PA, lateral, and oblique fluoroscopic projections.
- Drill, tap, and then insert a headless screw, countersunk beneath the subchondral surface of the distal pole of the scaphoid (**Fig. 30–6**).
- Assess stability of the fracture.
- Check the radiocarpal and midcarpal joints to ensure that screw threads have not violated either joint.
- Check fracture position and screw position on three views using fluoroscopy.
- Irrigate and close capsule and skin. Place in bulky dressing with thumb spica splint.

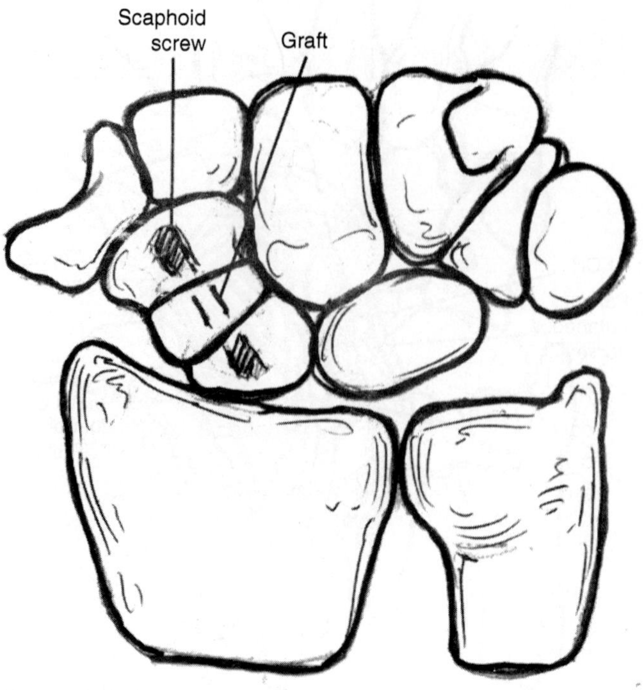

Figure 30–6

Postoperative Care

- Remove stitches after 10 to 14 days and place in short arm–thumb spica cast.
- Recheck every 3 to 4 weeks with exam and radiograph. Convert to thumb spica splint when union appears imminent.
- Questions about healing can usually be resolved by imaging with a CT scan taken in the plane of the scaphoid.

■ Pearl

Repeat surgery for persistent scaphoid nonunion has a high failure rate. Your first chance is your best chance. Don't cut corners on technique or postoperative immobilization. Make sure your patient doesn't smoke.

Suggested Readings

Eggli S, Fernandez DL, Beck T. Unstable scaphoid fracture nonunion: a medium-term study of anterior wedge grafting procedures. J Hand Surg [Br] 2002;27:36–41

Merrell GA, Wolfe SW, Slade JF III. Treatment of scaphoid nonunions: quantitative meta-analysis of the literature. J Hand Surg [Am] 2002;27:685–691

31 Open Reduction and Internal Fixation of Scaphoid Nonunion with Vascularized Bone Graft

Indications

- Proximal pole scaphoid nonunion, especially in cases of an avascular proximal pole and after failed open reduction and, internal fixation (ORIF) with autogenous nonvascularized graft.

Technique

- Loosely wrap the arm with an elastic wrap prior to elevating the tourniquet. This will leave the vessels partially filled and easier to identify.
- Use a dorsal approach to expose the wrist and distal radius.
- Identify the supraretinacular artery between the first and second extensor compartments (**Fig. 31–1**).
- Harvest a block of corticocancellous bone from the dorsum of the distal radius along with periosteum and the vascular pedicle (**Fig. 31–2**).

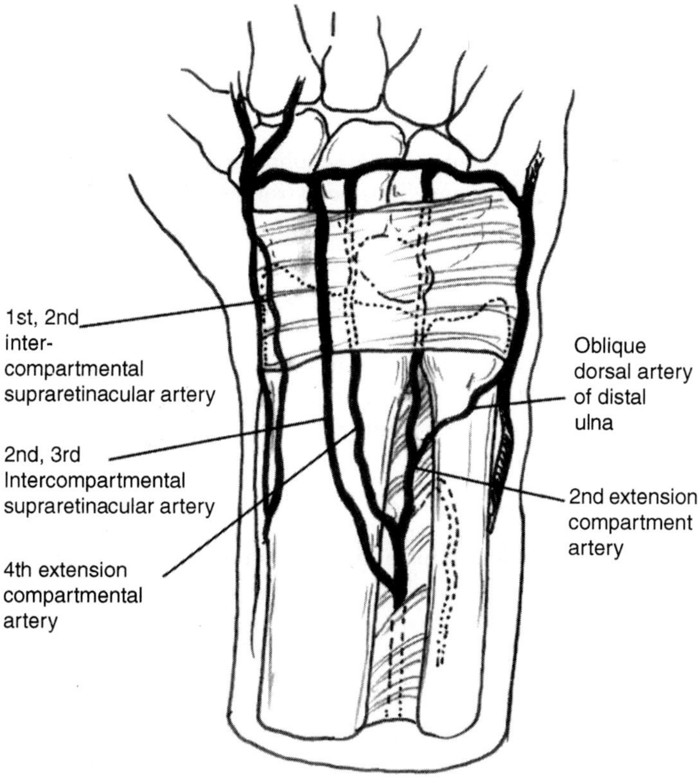

Figure 31–1

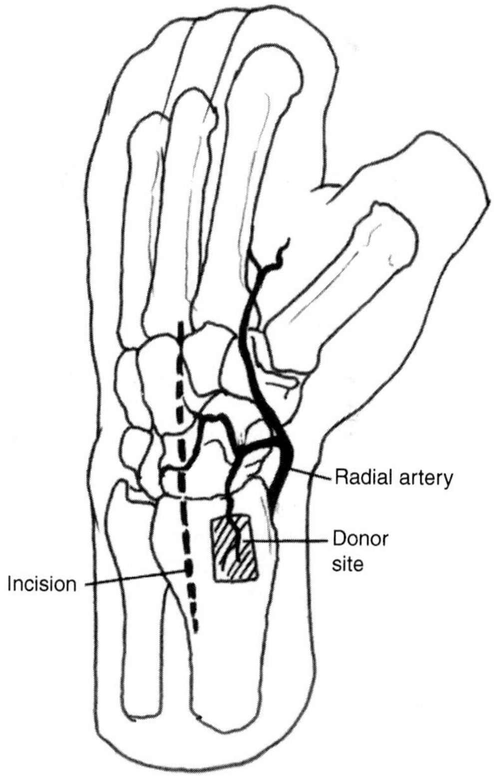

Figure 31–2

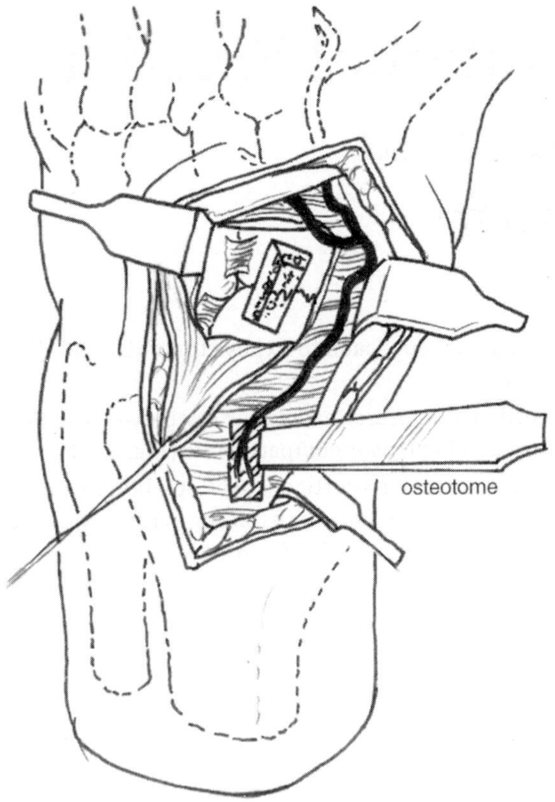

Figure 31–3

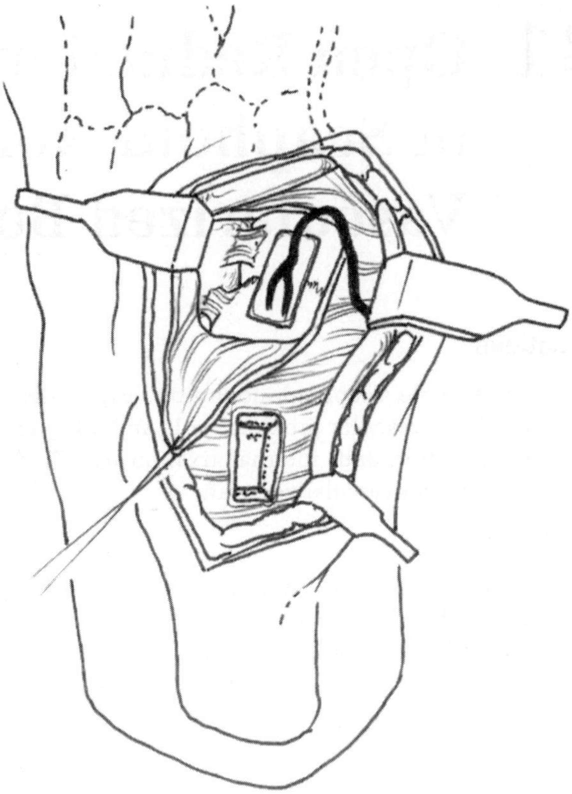

Figure 31–4

- Mobilize the pedicle you have chosen by elevating the artery and its vein(s) along with a cuff of adjacent tissue (**Fig. 31–3**).
- Debride the site of the scaphoid nonunion, creating an oval-shaped defect in the nonarticular surface of the dorsal cortex.
- Contour the vascularized bone to fit the shape of the defect.
- Press fit the vascularized graft into the defect in the scaphoid (**Fig. 31–4**).
- Choose a form of scaphoid fixation. In most instances the scaphoid can be fixed with a screw and the graft secured as the two poles of the scaphoid are compressed. If the proximal pole is too small to accept a screw, place one or two 0.045 in. pins through the scaphoid and graft directed from proximal to distal. The pins will exit the skin superficial to the scaphoid tubercle and can be withdrawn to ensure that the tips of the pins are contained within the proximal pole.
- Fill gaps between the scaphoid and the vascularized graft with cancellous bone from the distal radius.
- Close the capsule and extensor retinaculum over the extensor digitorum communis (EDC) tendons. Leave the extensor pollicis longus (EPL) free in the subcutaneous tissues.
- Release the tourniquet and cauterize bleeding vessels. Close skin after irrigation with interrupted sutures. Apply a bulky dressing with a palmar splint.

Postoperative Care

- Remove sutures and apply short arm thumb–spica cast.
- Check radiographs until union imminent, then switch to thumb-spica splint.
- If there is any uncertainty about healing by 3 months postsurgery examine the fracture with either a tomogram or a CT scan.

Suggested Readings

Shin AY, Bishop AT. Pedicled vascularized bone grafts for disorders of the carpus: scaphoid nonunion and Kienböck's disease. J Am Acad Orthop Surg 2002; 10:210–216

Waters PM, Stewart SL. Surgical treatment of nonunion and avascular necrosis of the proximal part of the scaphoid in adolescents. J Bone Joint Surg Am 2002;84-A: 915–920

Section VI.3

The Wrist Joint: Nonunion Hook of Hamate

32 Excision Hook of Hamate for Nonunion

Indications

- Palmar pain and tenderness directly over hook of hamate
- Weak grip
- Ulnar nerve paresthesia
- Small finger flexor digitorum sublimis (FDS) rupture

Preoperative Evaluation

Nonunion may be visible on carpal tunnel view; if not, it should be easily visualized on CT scan.

Technique

- Local anesthesia with sedation; forearm tourniquet
- Palmar approach, radial aspect of hypothenar eminence. In patients with thick palms exposure may be facilitated by extending incision across wrist crease (**Fig. 32–1**).
- Split muscles of the hypothenar region longitudinally.
- Identify and mobilize the ulnar nerve, particularly the motor branch as it sweeps around the ulnar aspect of the hamate hook (**Fig. 32–2**).
- Peel periosteum off of hamate hook.

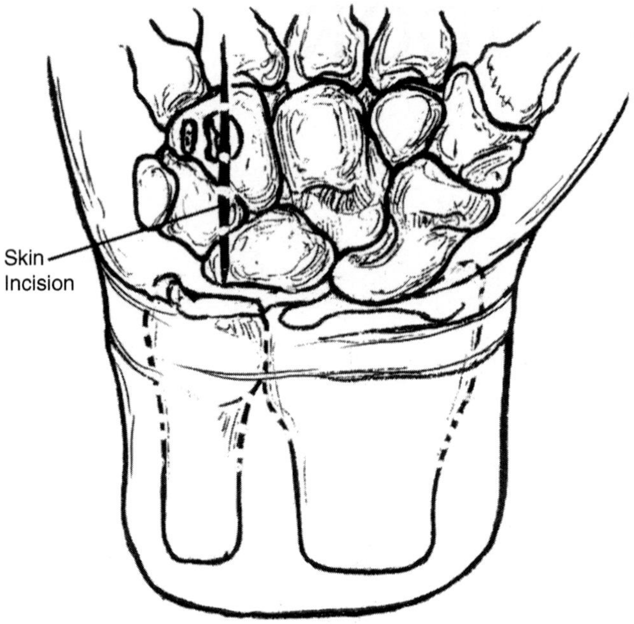

Figure 32–1

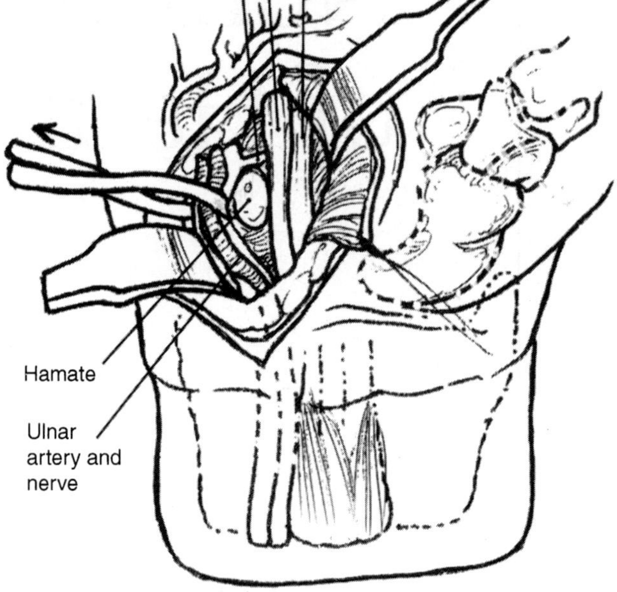

Figure 32–2

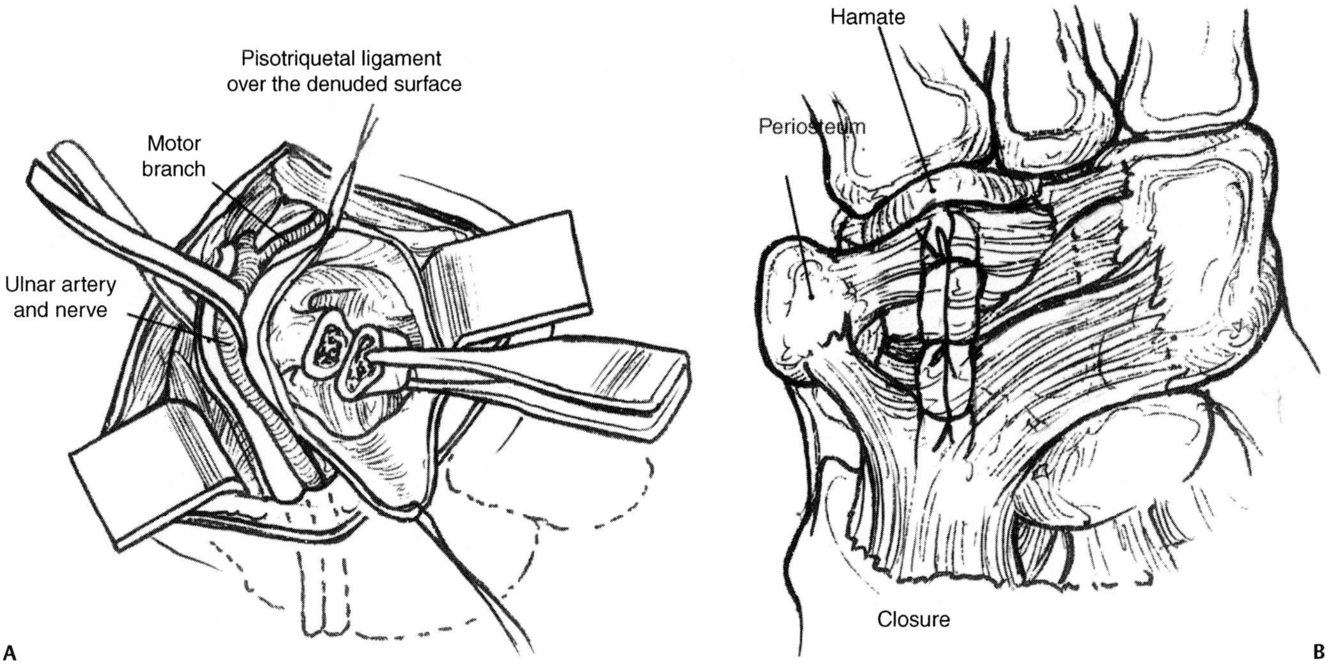

Figure 32–3

- Excise hook and repair periosteum over exposed bone (**Fig. 32–3A,B**).

■ Pearls

Don't hesitate to extend the incision to identify the ulnar nerve and artery in Guyon's canal.

- During subperiosteal exposure of the hamate hook protect the motor branch of the ulnar nerve with a small curved retractor around on the motor branch of the ulnar nerve.
- Grasping the hamate hook with a bone tenaculum facilitates hook excision.

■ Pitfalls

In some cases the fibrous union is stable enough that the site of nonunion is not immediately apparent. Continue the dissection toward the base; the hook is often larger than expected.

- Attritional fraying of flexor tendons from tendons rubbing against the irregular surface created by the nonunion. Make sure to inspect the flexors and repair or reconstruct as necessary.

Postoperative Care

- Soft dressing until sutures out in 10 to 14 days
- Finger motion immediately
- Grip exercises in 3 to 4 weeks
- Silicone patch as necessary for scar sensitivity

Suggested Readings

Bishop AT, Beckenbaugh RD. Fractures of the hamate hook. J Hand Surg [Am] 1988;13A:135–139

Parker RD, Berkowitz MS, Brahms MA, Bohl WR. Hook of hamate fractures in athletes. Am J Sports Med 1986;14: 517–523

Section VI.4

The Wrist Joint: Scapholunate Ligament Injuries

Arthroscopy and Percutaneous Pin Fixation of Scapholunate Ligament Injuries

Indications

- Acute (< 3 months) partial tear or stretch injury of the scapholunate (SL) ligament where dynamic instability is present
- < 3 mm SL interval
- No dorsiflexion of the lunate on a lateral projection

Technique

- Index and long fingers in finger trap traction with 10 lb of distraction via traction tower
- Evaluate SL ligament through radiocarpal and midcarpal portals (**Fig. 33–1A,B**).
- The view through the midcarpal portal allows the surgeon to quantify the diastasis at the SL joint using a 2 mm probe and the Geissler "drive through" test (**Table 33–1**).
- Debridement alone is indicated for SL tears with minimal evidence of SL joint instability (Geissler 1 or 2) (**Fig. 33–2A,B**).
- Percutaneous pinning is considered when a probe can be passed between the scaphoid and the lunate and there is a step-off at the SL joint when examined through a midcarpal portal (Geissler 3).
- Reduce the SL joint with percutaneously placed joysticks into the scaphoid and lunate (see Chapter 38).

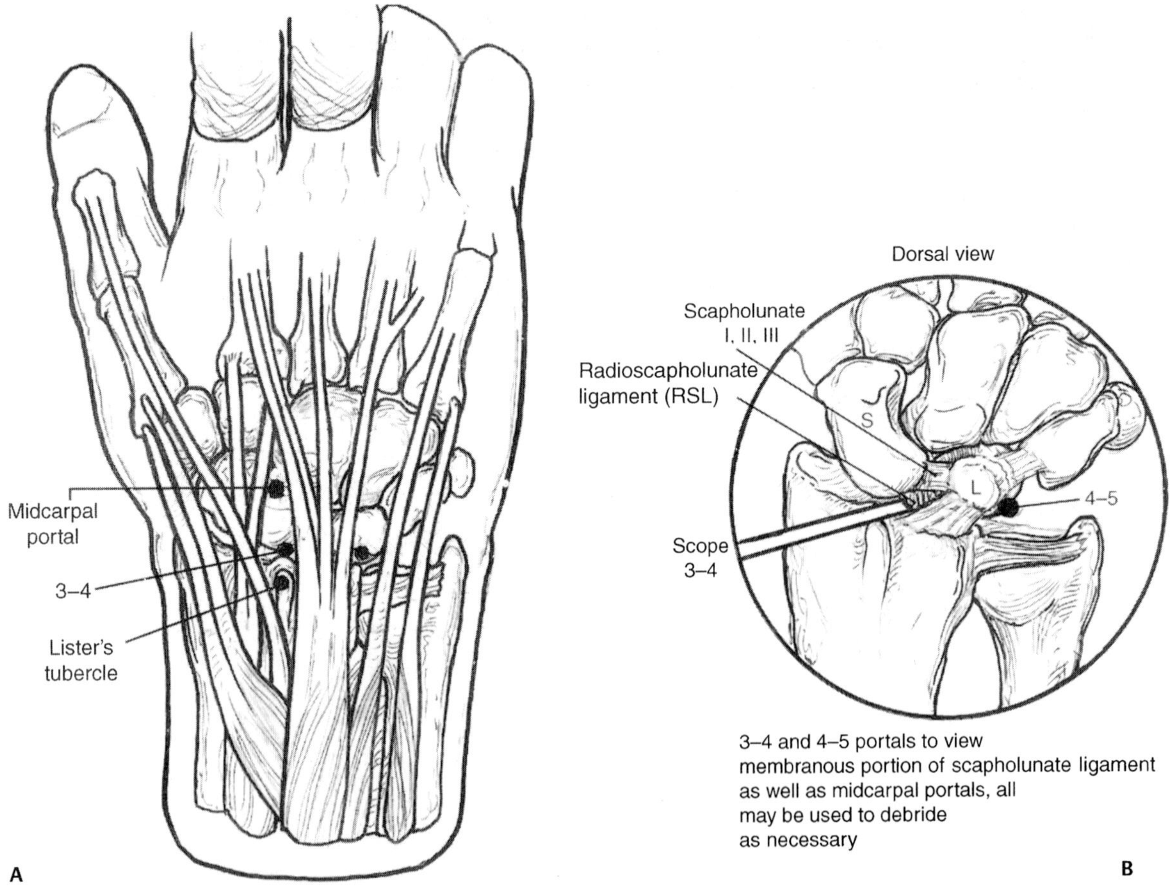

Figure 33–1

Table 33–1 Geissler's "Drive Through" Classification of Scapholunate Ligament Injury

Grade	Findings
1	Attenuation or hemorrhage, no incongruency
2	Incongruency or step-off of carpal space; slight gap less than width of probe
3	Incongruency or step-off of carpal space; probe passed between scaphoid and lunate
4	Incongruency or step-off of carpal space; scope (2.7 mm) passed through gap between scaphoid and lunate

- Extend the scaphoid and flex the lunate. Confirm the reduction through the midcarpal portal.
- Maintain the reduction with multiple 0.045 in. wires placed across the SL and scaphocapitate joints.
- Use fluoroscopy to confirm reduction and placement of wires (**Fig. 33–3**).

Postoperative Care

- The wrist is immobilized in a short–arm thumb spica cast for 8 weeks.
- The pins are removed at 8 weeks and a removable splint is used for 4 weeks.
- Occupational therapy is begun at 12 weeks.

■ Pearl

Multiple pins are necessary to adequately stabilize the SL and scaphocapitate ligament.

■ Pitfall

Complete SL ligament tears should be treated with open reduction of the joint and SL ligament repair or reconstruction.

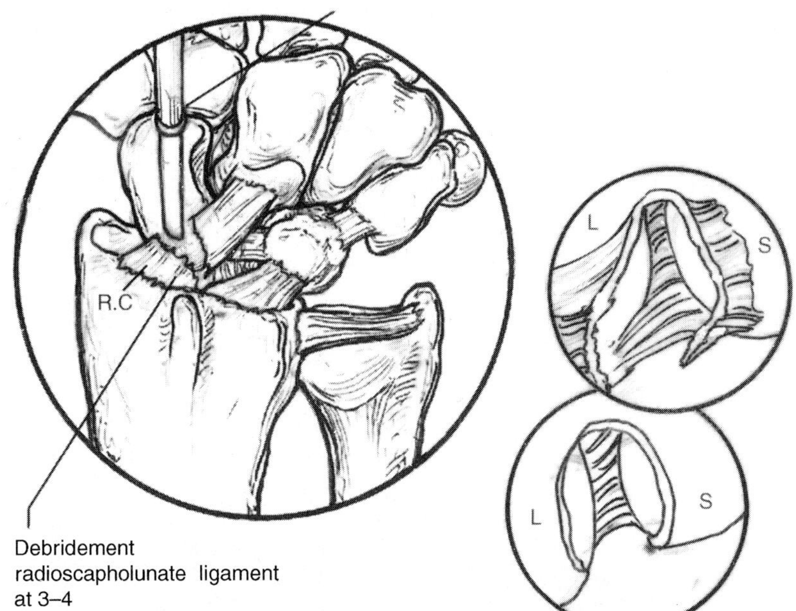

Figure 33–2

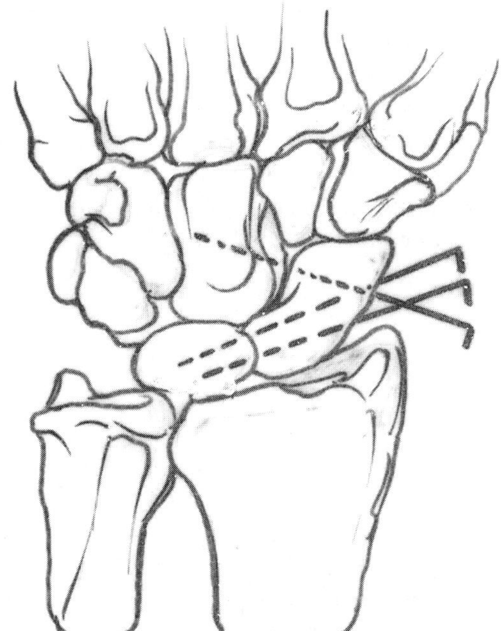

Figure 33–3

Suggested Readings

Ruch DS, Smith BP. Arthroscopic and open management of dynamic scaphoid instability. Orthop Clin North Am 2001;30:233–240

Weiss AP, Sachar K, Glowacki KA. Arthroscopic debridement alone for intercarpal ligament tears. J Hand Surg [Am] 1997;22A:344–349

34 Open Scapholunate Ligament Repair

Indications

- Wide scapholunate (SL) joint (> 3 mm) and a dorsiflexed lunate
- Repairable remnant of SL ligament (can be present up to 3 months postinjury)
- Reducible scaphoid
- No radioscaphoid or capitolunate arthritis

Technique

- Dorsal longitudinal incision
- Incise the third dorsal compartment and retract the extensor pollicis longus radially (**Fig. 34–1**).
- Incise the radial wall of the fourth compartment and retract the extensor digitorum communis tendons ulnarly.
- The dorsal capsule is incised with a radial-based triangular flap to preserve the dorsal intercarpal ligament and dorsal radiocarpal ligaments (**Fig. 34–2A,B**).
- The SL ligament is inspected; typically it has avulsed from the lunate.

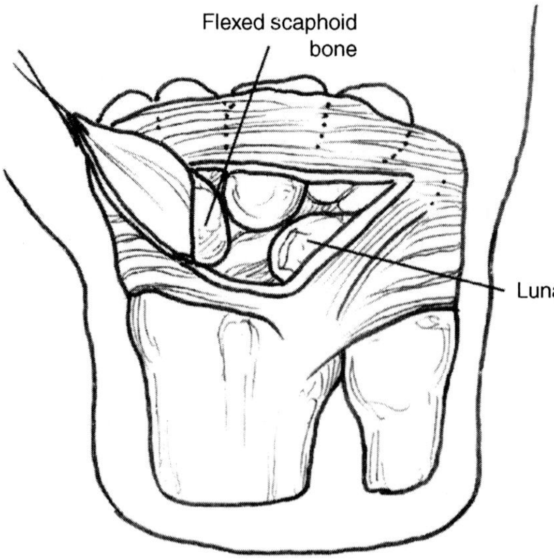

Figure 34–1

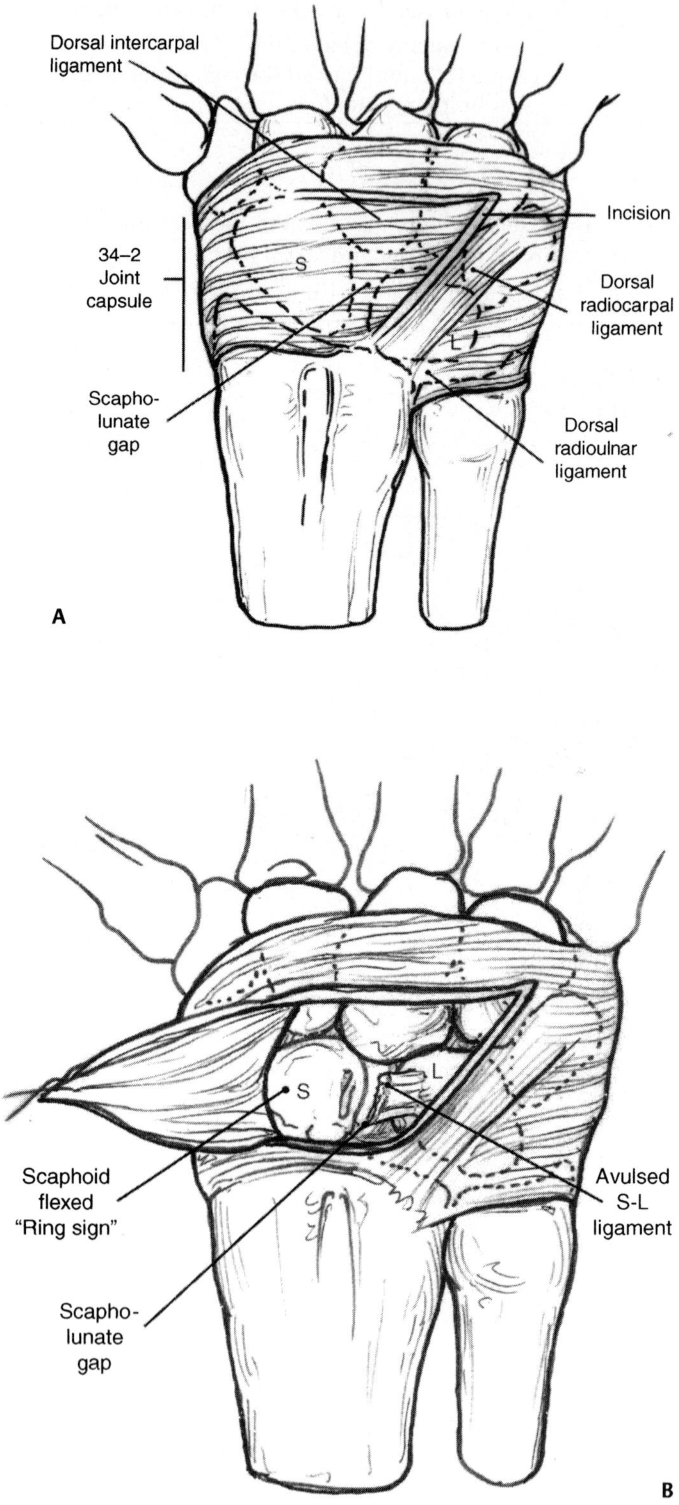

Figure 34–2

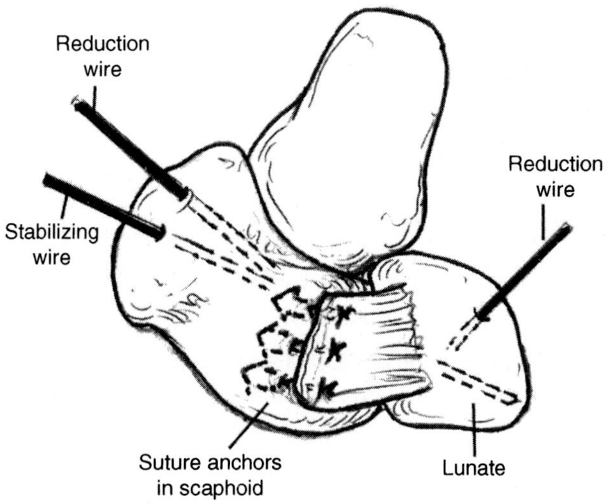

Figure 34–3

■ **Pearl**

If there is insufficient ligament to repair, consider a soft tissue reconstruction as described in Chapters 35, 36, and 37, or a RASL procedure as described in Chapter 38.

- Two 0.045 in. wires are drilled into the scaphoid and lunate and are used as joysticks to reduce the SL joint, which is then pinned with two 0.045 in. wires (**Fig. 34–3**).

■ **Pearl**

If the scaphoid is not reducible consider a reconstructive procedure, such as a proximal row carpectomy or scaphoid excision and CLTH fusion.

- A third 0.045 in. wire is use to pin the scaphoid to the capitate.
- Fluoroscopy confirms reduction as well as appropriate pin placement.
- Pins are cut so that the ends lie beneath the skin.
- Suture anchors are placed into dorsal scaphoid at the previous insertion site of the dorsal fibers of the SL ligament.
- Use the suture anchors to reapproximate the SL ligament to bone.
- Additional suture anchors can be used to repair the dorsal intercarpal ligament to either or both the scaphoid and the lunate.
- The dorsal capsule is repaired utilizing nonabsorbable, braided suture and the retinaculum is closed.

■ **Pitfall**

Avoid imbricating the capsule during closure because it is likely to compromise wrist flexion.

- The extensor pollicis longus tendon is left transposed.
- The wound is closed and the wrist is immobilized in a short arm, thumb spica splint.

Postoperative Care

- Postoperative splint and sutures are removed after 10 to 14 days.
- The patient is placed in a short arm, thumb spica cast for 6 weeks followed by a short arm, Orthoplast (Johnson & Johnson, New Brunswick, NJ) splint for 4 weeks.
- Wires are maintained for as long as possible or a maximum of 12 weeks.
- From week 8 to week 12 gentle wrist motion is permitted out of the splint.

■ **Pearl**

Obtain frequent postoperative radiographs to catch failures early.

Suggested Readings

Wyrick JD, Youse BD, Kiefhaber TR. Scapholunate ligament repair and capsulodesis for the treatment of static scapholunate dissociation. J Hand Surg [Br] 1998;23B: 776–780

35 Scapholunate Reconstruction with Dorsal Capsular Flap (Blatt Procedure)

Indications

- Acute or chronic, static or dynamic scapholunate (SL) instability
- No arthritis at radioscaphoid or capitolunate joint
- Reducible scaphoid

Technique

- Dorsal midline incision
- Release extensor pollicis longus (EPL) and retract radially; open and retract the fourth extensor compartment in an ulnar direction.
- Design and mobilize proximally based capsular flap with distal margin at the STT joint. The width of the flap is 10 to 15 mm (**Fig. 35–1**).
- If dorsal portion of SL ligament is substantial enough to repair, place suture anchors at site of ligament avulsion. If the ligament is not repairable, debride the remnants.
- Place a 1 to 2 cm, V-shaped incision on the radial aspect of the wrist (**Fig. 35–2**).
- Identify and protect branches of the radial sensory nerve.
- Place two 0.045 in. pins into the radial aspect of the scaphoid, one directed toward the SL joint, the second toward the scaphocapitate (SC) joint.
- Place two additional 0.045 in. pins in the dorsal aspect of the scaphoid and lunate to use as joysticks.

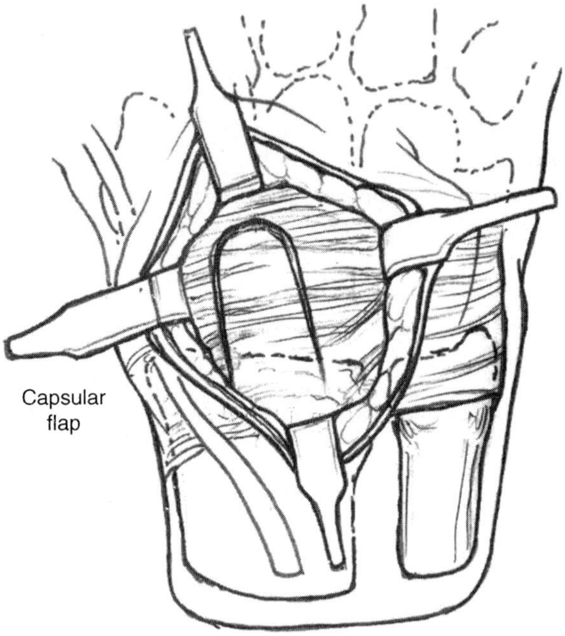

Figure 35–1

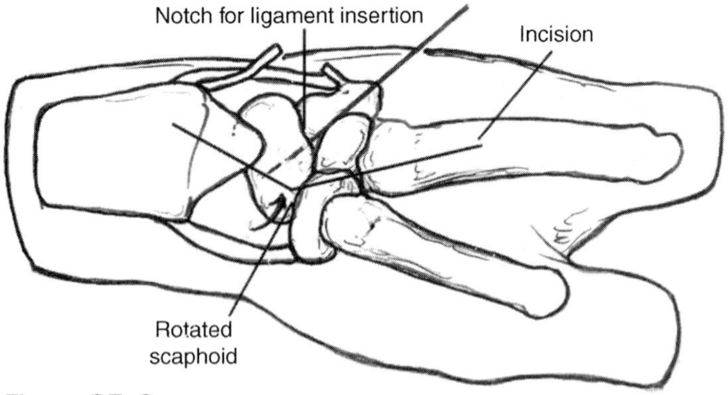

Figure 35–2

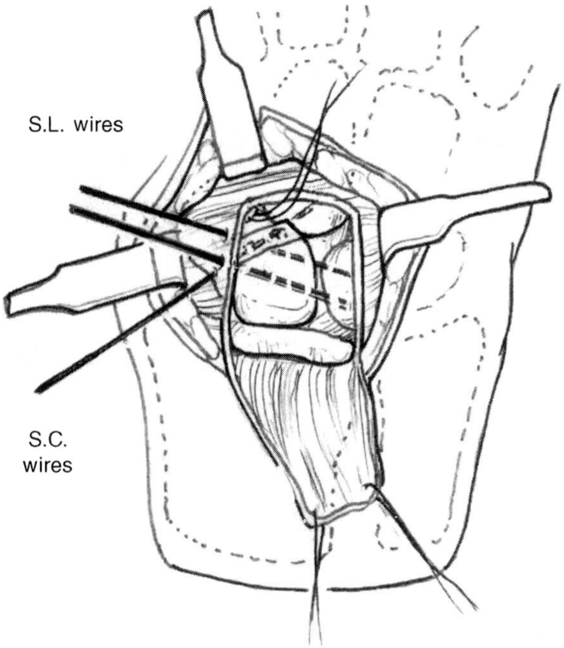

Figure 35–3

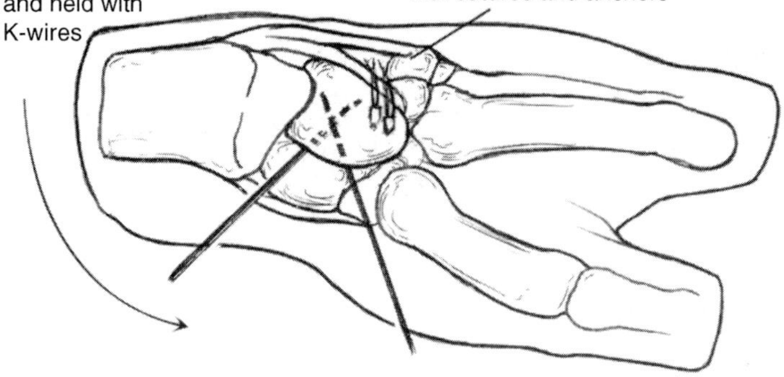

Figure 35–4

- Reduce the SL joint under fluoroscopy and advance the SL and SC pins (**Fig. 35–3**).
- Remove joystick pins.
- Create trough on dorsal aspect of distal pole of scaphoid, distal to dorsal ridge.
- Place suture anchors in trough.
- Suture capsule to trough with wrist in slight extension (**Fig. 35–4**).
- Close capsule.
- Leave EPL free in subcutaneous tissues. Repair fourth compartment and close skin.
- Cut pins beneath skin.

Postoperative Care

- Splint wrist for 10 to 14 days.
- Finger motion immediately
- Cast for 6 weeks
- Convert to removable splint at 8 weeks; allow intermittent wrist motion.
- Pins removed in 12 weeks
- Occupational therapy as necessary

■ Pearl

The width of the capsular flap should be as wide as the distal pole of the scaphoid.

■ Pitfalls

Beware the PA radiograph with an apparent SL diastasis and a lateral radiograph with a normal radiolunate angle (i.e., a lunate that is not dorsiflexed).

- The capitate head may appear triangular. This can be seen in patients with a congenital diastasis.
- Check the contralateral wrist. The findings are often bilateral and the symptoms can be managed nonoperatively.

Suggested Readings

Blatt G. Capsulodesis in reconstructive hand surgery: dorsal capsulodesis for the unstable scaphoid and volar capsulodesis following excision of the distal ulna. Hand Clin 1987;3:81–102

Wintman BI, Gelberman RH, Katz JN. Dynamic scapholunate instability: results of operative treatment with dorsal capsulodesis. J Hand Surg [Am] 1995;20A: 971–979

Wyrick JD, Youse BD, Kiefhaber TR. Scapholunate ligament repair and capsulodesis for the treatment of static scapholunate dissociation. J Hand Surg [Br] 1998;23B: 776–780

36 Flexor Carpi Radialis Tendon Stabilization of the Scapholunate Joint (Brunelli Procedure)

Indications

- Patients with symptomatic static scapholunate dissociation without arthritis at the radioscaphoid or scaphotrapeziotrapezoidal joints

Technique

- Dorsal longitudinal incision
- Incise the third dorsal compartment and retract the extensor pollicis longus radially.
- Incise the radial wall of the fourth compartment and retract the extensor digitorum communis tendons ulnarly.
- The dorsal capsule is incised with a radially based triangular flap to preserve the dorsal intercarpal ligament and dorsal radiocarpal ligaments (**Fig. 36–1**).
- The scar tissue between the scaphoid and lunate is removed.
- More distally, the Scaphotrapezial-trapezoida (STT) joint is exposed and any interarticular scar that formed in the dorsal angle created by the scaphoid flexion is removed.
- A second volar incision is made over the flexor carpi radialis (FCR) tendon (**Fig. 36–2**).
- The fibrous sheath of the FCR tendon is incised to the level of the trapezium and trapezoid. The deep portion of the sheath is preserved.
- The FCR tendon is split longitudinally and a 7 cm tendon slip is prepared, preserving its distal attachment to the base of the second metacarpal.

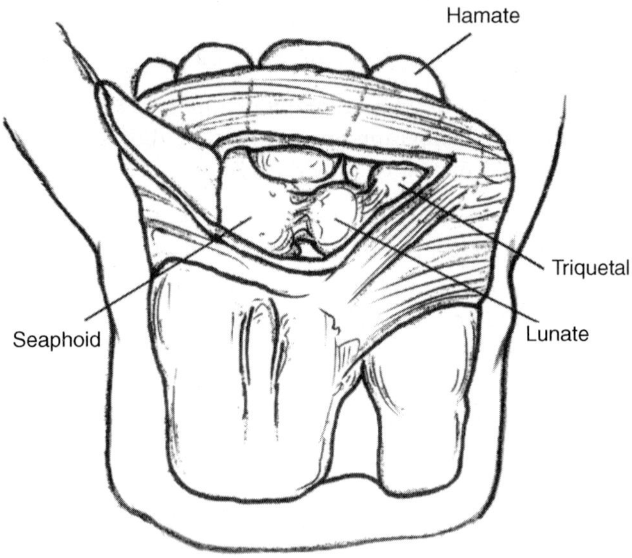

Figure 36–1

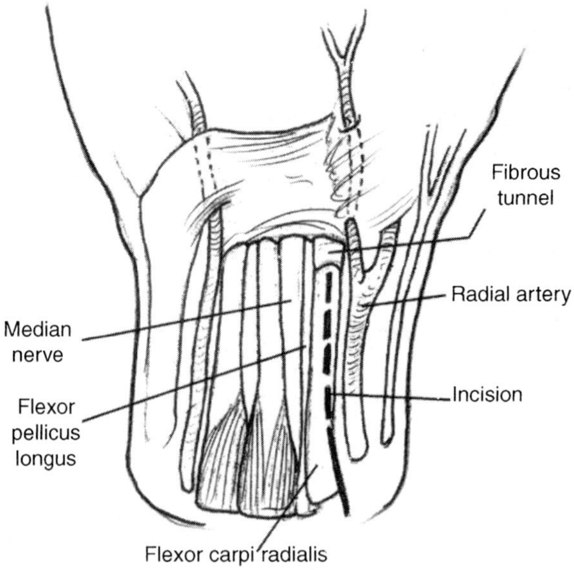

Figure 36–2

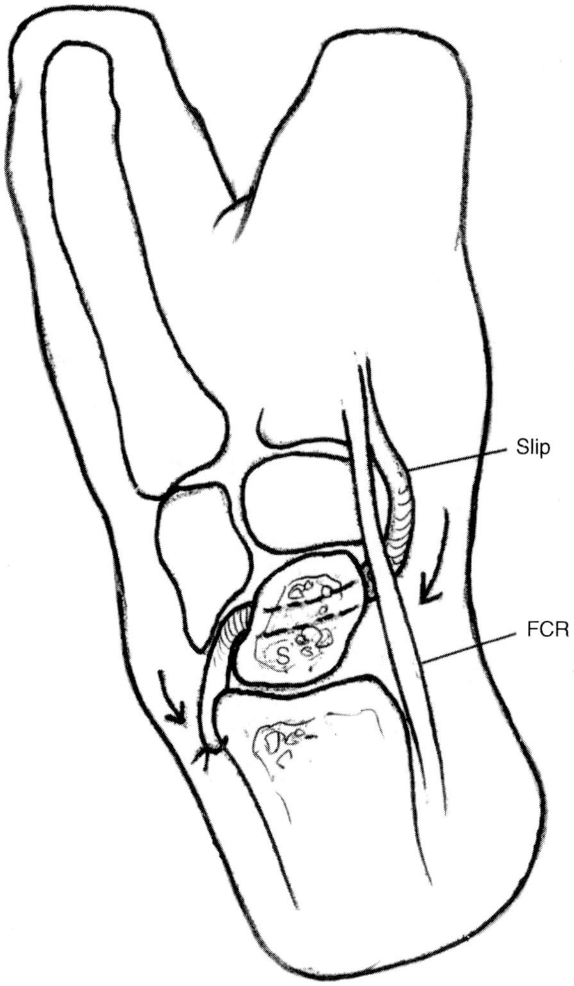

Figure 36–3

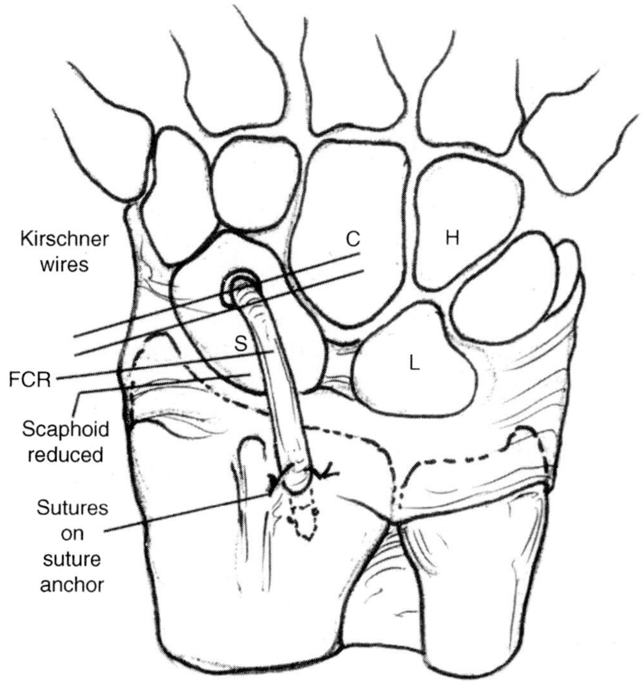

Figure 36–4

- The tendon slip is passed from volar to dorsal through a 2.5 mm diameter tunnel drilled in the distal pole of the scaphoid parallel to its distal articular surface (**Fig. 36–3**).
- The scaphoid is reduced by pulling the tendon slip dorsally.
- The reduced scaphoid is fixed with a Kirschner wire that crosses the distal part of the scaphoid and capitate.
- The tendon slip is sutured to the fibrous remains of the lunate ligament and to the fibrous tissue of the dorsoulnar edge of the radius (**Fig. 36–4**).
- The wounds are closed in standard fashion and a sterile dressing and plaster splint are applied.

Postoperative Care

- The dressing, splint, and sutures are removed after 10 days.
- Long arm cast immobilization continues for 4 weeks.
- The Kirschner wire is removed after 4 weeks.
- Physical therapy begins 8 weeks after surgery.

■ Pitfall

Tendon graft does not have the same "material properties" as the SL ligament. The tendon may stretch, leading to loss of reduction with resulting instability and pain.

■ Pearls

When opening the fibrous sheath of the FCR tendon during the volar approach, care must be taken to preserve the deep portion of the tendon.

- When removing scar tissue from around the carpus take care to spare the cartilage surfaces.

Suggested Readings

Brunelli GA, Brunelli GR. A new technique to correct carpal instability with scaphoid rotary subluxation: a preliminary report. J Hand Surg [Am] 1995;20A: S82–S85

37 Bone Graft–Bone Autograft Reconstruction

Indications

- Patients with symptomatic dynamic scapholunate (SL) dissociation without arthritis at the radioscaphoid or scaphotrapeziotrapezoidal joints

Technique

- Dorsal longitudinal incision
- Incise the third dorsal compartment and retract the extensor pollicis longus (EPL) radially (**Fig. 37–1**).
- Incise the radial wall of the fourth compartment and retract the extensor digitorum communis tendons ulnarly.
- The dorsal capsule is incised with a radially based triangular flap that spares half the dorsal intercarpal ligament and half the dorsal radiocarpal ligaments.
- The area over Lister's tubercle is marked to harvest a 20 × 8 × 8 mm block of bone.
- Using an osteotome, the bone is harvested with the overlying periosteum and retinaculum attached.
- An osteotome and curette are used to fashion troughs in both the dorsal proximal scaphoid and the radial lunate to receive the autograft (**Fig. 37–2**).
- Kirschner wires are drilled into the scaphoid (S) and lunate (L) and are used as joysticks to reduce the SL joint, which is then pinned with two 0.045 in. wires (**Fig. 37–3**).
- A third Kirschner wire is passed from the scaphoid into the capitate (C) for additional fixation.
- Using a fine rongeur, the middle 2 to 3 mm of the cortical and cancellous bone of the autograft bone block is carefully removed, preserving the overlying periosteum and retinaculum.

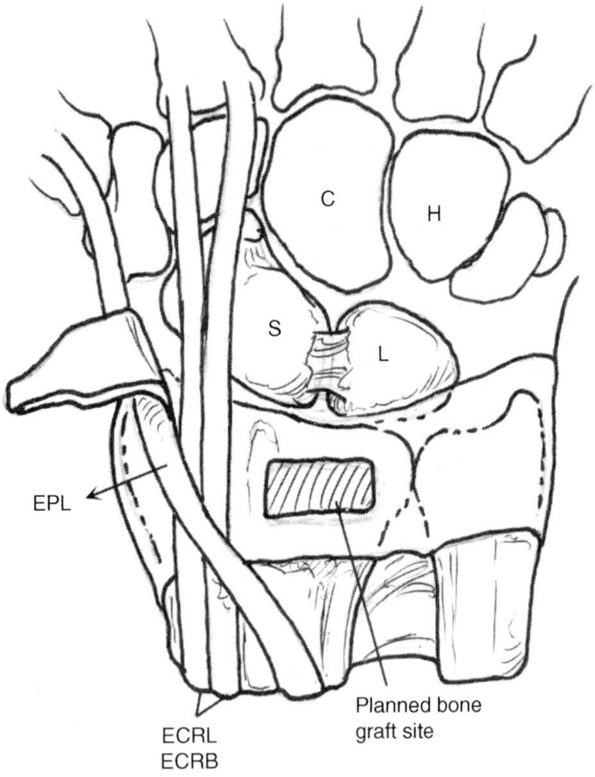

Figure 37–1

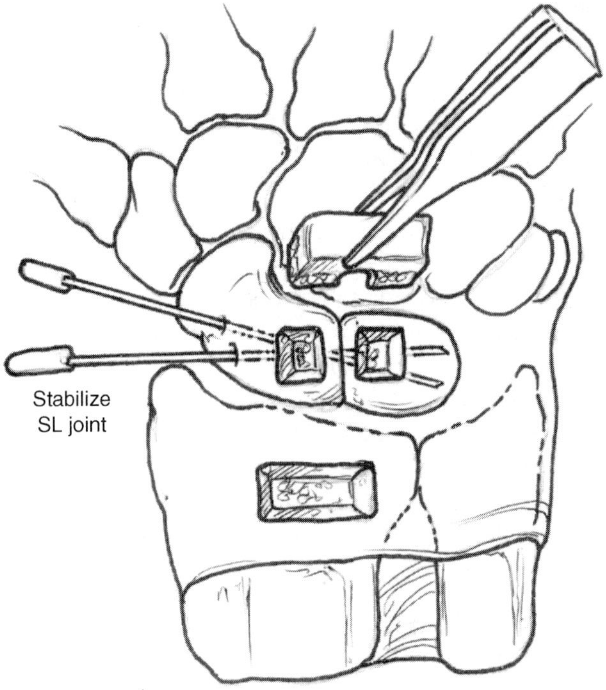

Figure 37–2

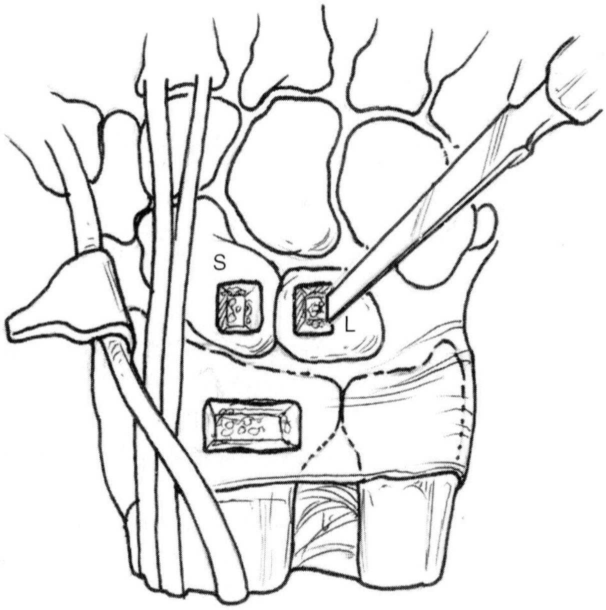

Figure 37–3

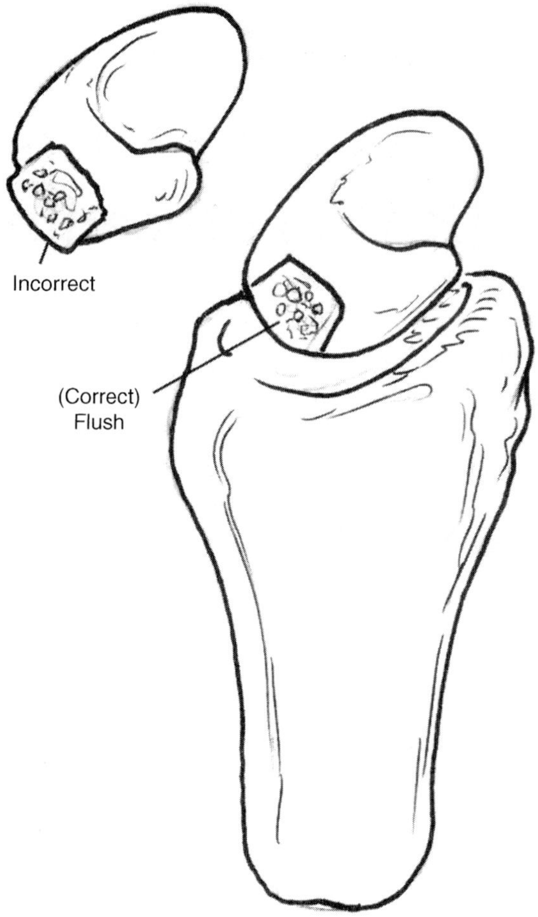

Figure 37–4

- The autograft is placed into the prepared trough and once seated should allow full radiocarpal motion in flexion and extension (**Fig. 37–4**).

■ Pearl

The troughs created in the dorsal scaphoid and lunate to receive the autograft should be slightly undersized to create a snug fit. If the graft is not stable in the troughs it can be stabilized with temporary Kirschner wire fixation or mini screws.

- The dorsal capsule is repaired and imbricated, creating a tight closure to support the graft.
- The extensor retinaculum is closed with the EPL tendon transposed.
- The wound is closed in standard fashion and a sterile dressing and plaster splint are applied with the wrist extended 30 degrees to protect the graft.

Postoperative Management

- Splint for 10 to 14 days
- Short arm cast for 6 to 8 weeks
- After 8 weeks the cast and Kirschner wires are removed.

■ Pitfalls

Patients with static scalo lunate dissociation (SLD) do not appear to do as well. This may be due to tension on the graft as a result of the significant soft tissue and bony changes that occur in patients with long-standing SLD. Studies indicate that the bone–retinaculum–bone autograft from the distal radius may be significantly weaker and less stiff than the SL ligament. Cadaveric studies indicate carpometacarpal and navicular-first cuneiform ligaments may have biomechanical characteristics more similar to the SL ligament.

Suggested Readings

Davis CA, Culp RW, Hume EL, Osterman AL. Reconstruction of the scapholunate ligament in a cadaver model using a bone–ligament–bone autograft from the foot. J Hand Surg [Am] 1998;23A: 884–892

Harvey EJ, Hanel D, Knight JB, Tencer AF. Autograft replacements for the scapholunate ligament: a biomechanical comparison of hand-based autografts. J Hand Surg [Am] 1999;24A:963–967

Shin SS, Moore DC, McGovern RD, Weiss AP. Scapholunate ligament reconstruction using a bone– retinaculum–bone autograft: a biomechanic and histologic study. J Hand Surg [Am] 1998;23A:216–220

Weiss AC. Scapholunate ligament reconstruction using a bone–retinaculum–bone autograft. J Hand Surg [Am] 1998;23A:205–215

38 Screw Fixation: Reduction and Association of the Scapholunate (RASL) Procedure

Indications

- Subacute to chronic scapholunate (SL) dissociation
- Static or dynamic SL instability
- Irreparable scapholunate interosseous ligament (SLIL)
- No SL advanced collapse wrist or advanced osteoarthritis of the radiocarpal joint
- Focal radial styloid–scaphoid arthritis is not a contraindication.

Technique

- 6 cm longitudinal dorsal incision just ulnar to Lister's tubercle
- Oblique retinaculum incision between third and fourth dorsal compartment, retract extensor pollicis longus (EPL) radially, retract extensor indicis proprius (EIP) and extensor digitorum communis (EDC) ulnarly.
- Longitudinal incision in capsule, retract to visualize scaphoid and lunate
- Insert two 0.062 in. Kirschner wires into the scaphoid and lunate to use as joysticks for reduction. The Kirschner wire in the scaphoid is placed distal and directed proximally in the palmar-flexed scaphoid. The Kirschner wire is placed as proximal as possible and directed distally in the dorsiflexed lunate. Placement of the Kirschner wires is planned to allow the Herbert screw fixation after SL reduction (**Fig. 38–1A,B**).
- Use the joysticks to spread the SL joint and allow dechondrification of the contacting surfaces (**Fig. 38–2**).

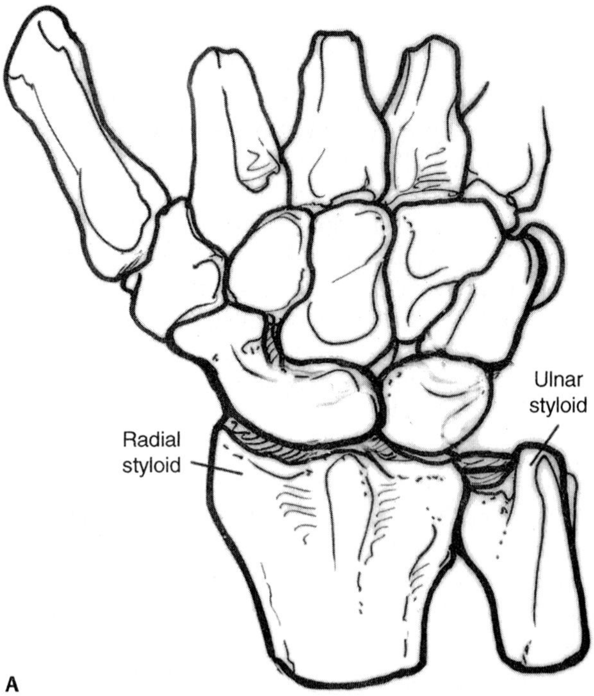

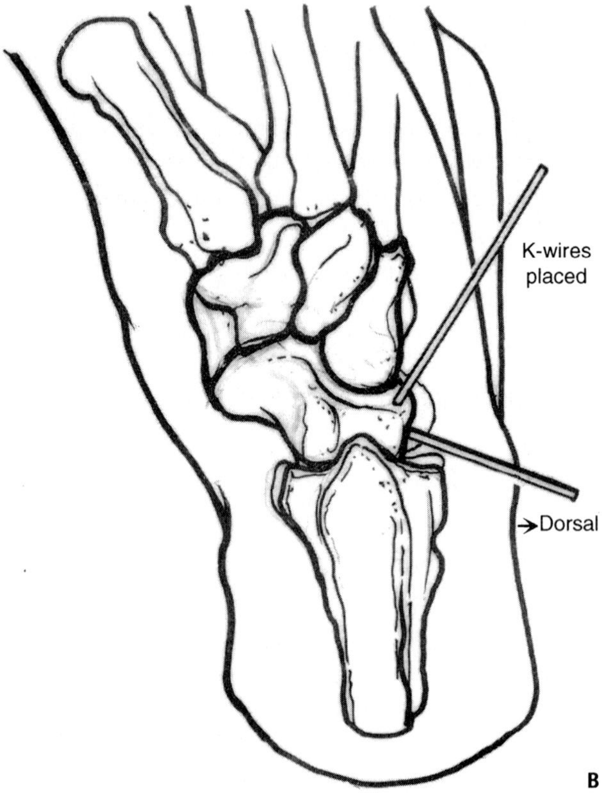

Figure 38–1

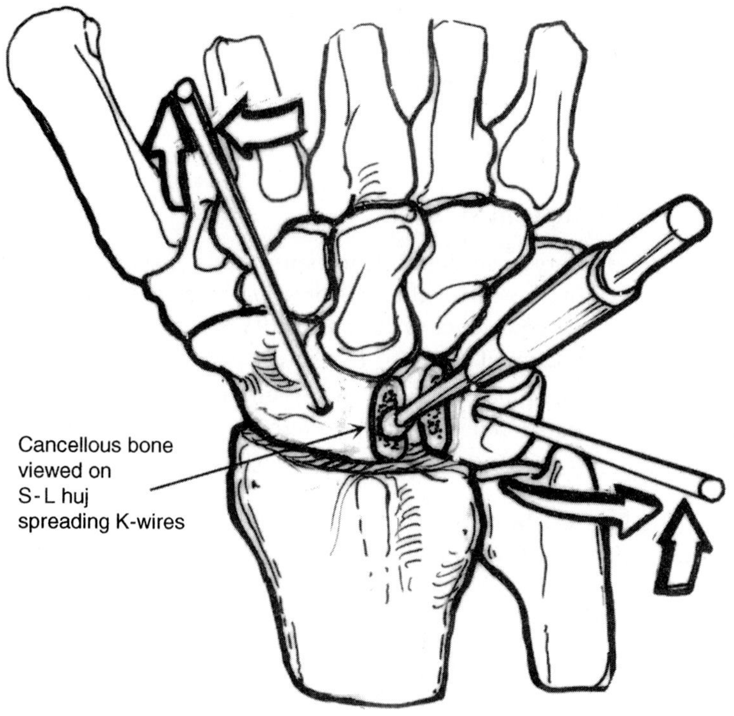

Figure 38–2

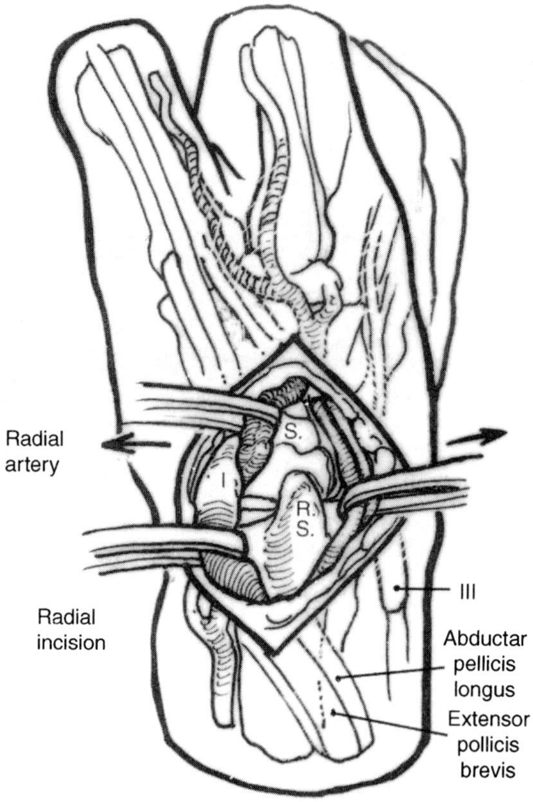

Figure 38–3

- A second 5 cm longitudinal incision is made on the midaxial border of the radius palmar to the first dorsal compartment from 2 cm proximal to the radial styloid to the level of the scaphotrapezial joint (**Fig. 38–3**). Take care to avoid injury to the radial sensory nerve and dorsal branch of the radial artery.
- Open the first dorsal compartment and retract abductor pollicis longus (APL) and extensor pollicis brevis (EPB). Make a longitudinal incision in the radioscaphoid-capsular ligament. Develop this in continuity as a sleeve for repair. Dissect subperiosteally to expose the radial styloid.
- Perform a radial styloidectomy with an osteotome, with care to preserve the radioscaphocapitate ligament. Reduce the scaphoid and lunate with the Kirschner wire joysticks and maintain with a Kocher clamp (**Fig. 38–4**). Extend the scaphoid and flex the lunate to entirely close the SL gap and cover the head of the capitate.
- The Herbert jig is placed through the radial incision and the hook is brought across the dorsoulnar aspect of the lunate under direct vision. Do not violate the lunotriquetral (LT) ligament. The position of the screw should be as central as possible in both the scaphoid and the lunate. The tip of the jig should be at the proximal apex of the lunate when reduced. Alternatively, one can place a guide wire freehand for the Herbert-Whipple cannulated (Zimmer, Warsaw, Indiana) screw system.

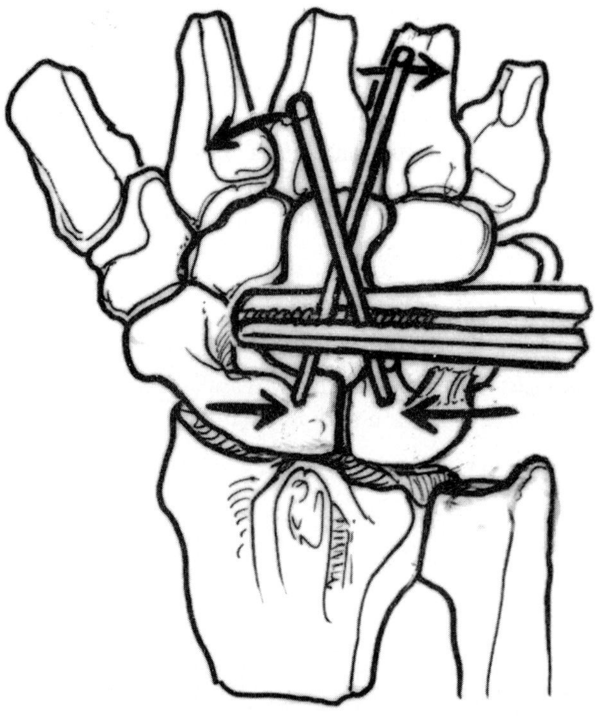

Figure 38–4

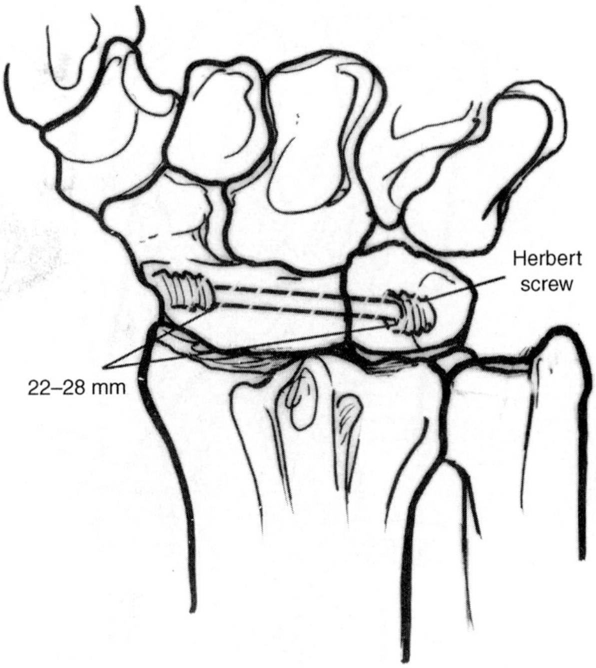

Figure 38–5

- Once the proper position is established and the starting point determined, drill, measure, tap, and insert the correct length Herbert screw. The unthreaded portion of the screw should lie between the two bones. The average length is 22 to 28 mm (**Fig. 38–5**).
- Once the screw is inserted and the jig and Kirschner wires are removed, the wrist may be taken through a full range of motion to confirm that it is unrestricted and that SL reduction is maintained. Confirm with intraoperative imaging. You will note obligatory rotation between the scaphoid and lunate about the instant center of rotation.
- Both dorsal and radial capsular incisions are closed without imbrication to avoid the capsulodesis effect.
- Repair the dorsal retinaculum and close both incisions in standard fashion. Apply a sterile bulky dressing and a palmar gauntlet split.

Postoperative Care

- Short arm thumb spica splint for 4 weeks. The time of immobilization has been progressively shortened as experience with the results of this technique has increased.
- Wrist then placed in removable splint and therapy initiated; range of motion exercises are started, followed by a progressive strengthening program.

■ Pearls

Focal cartilage erosion at distal pole of scaphoid may be seen due to its flexed position; this is not a contraindication to the procedure.

- Several Kirschner wires may be placed in the lunate to "walk up" the reduction.
- Place the Kirschner wires at angles to each other that are equal to the amount of correction desired.
- The radial styloidectomy facilitates placement of the Herbert screw proximal to the site that would be used for fixation of scaphoid fractures. The insertion point of the Herbert screw is proximal to the site that would be used for fixation of scaphoid fractures.
- The Herbert jig tends to slip off the oblique surface of the proximal scaphoid; an awl may be used to create a pilot starting hole.

■ Pitfall

Avoid excessive dissection of dorsal capsule over scaphoid to prevent injury to dorsal blood supply.

Suggested Readings

Rosenwasser MP, Strauch RJ, Miyasaka KC. The RASL procedure: reduction and association of the scaphoid and lunate using the Herbert screw. Techniques in Hand and Upper Extremity Surgery 1997;1:263–272

Section VI.5

The Wrist Joint: Carpal Fracture-Dislocations

39 Open Reduction and Internal Fixation Perilunate Dislocation via Dorsal Approach

Indications

- Any perilunate dislocation

Technique

- Make a longitudinal incision over the third to fourth extensor compartment (**Fig. 39–1**).
- Incise the extensor retinaculum just ulnar to the Lister's tubercle to enter the third extensor compartment.
- Release and retract the extensor pollicis longus (EPL) in a radial direction (**Fig. 39–2**).
- Reflect the extensor digitorum communis (EDC), keeping its tendon sheath intact, and incise the dorsal wrist capsule transversely to protect the dorsal intercarpal ligament, as described by Berger and Weiss.
- Reflect the capsule off the distal radius and carpal bones until the lunate, scaphoid, and proximal two thirds of the capitate are exposed.
- Reduce dorsal perilunate injuries using longitudinal traction and palmar pressure on the distal carpal row. A Freer elevator can be used to shoehorn the lunate to restore the relationship. This is an important step because the dislocation needs to be reduced before fixation can start. A palmar approach may be needed if the lunate is dislocated into the carpal tunnel.
- For palmar lunate dislocations, apply traction and reduce the lunate into place manually or with an elevator.
- After the dislocation is reduced place a 0.045 in. Kirschner wire into the most proximal, dorsal surface of the lunate, avoiding the capitate sulcus. Place a second wire into the distal pole of the scaphoid.
- Rotate the lunate into flexion to cover the head of the capitate. The scaphoid must be extended to complete the reduction.

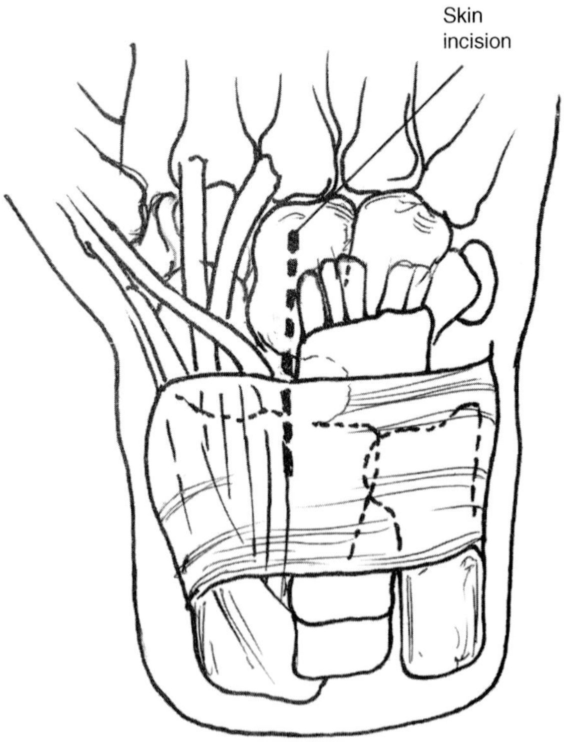

Figure 39–1

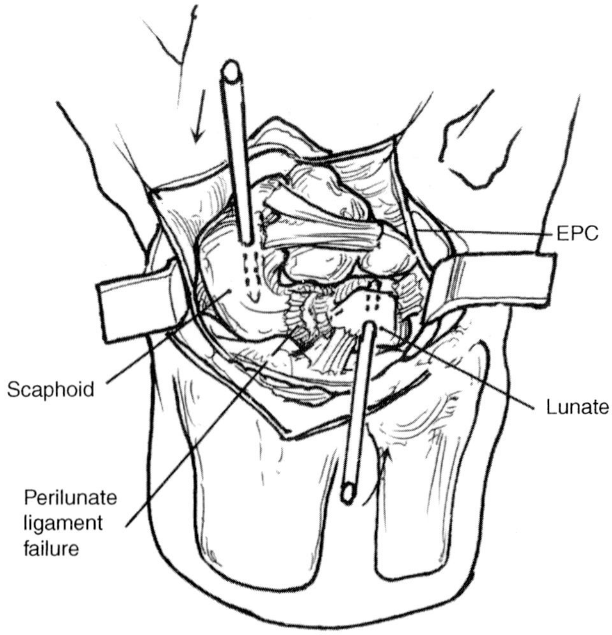

Figure 39–2

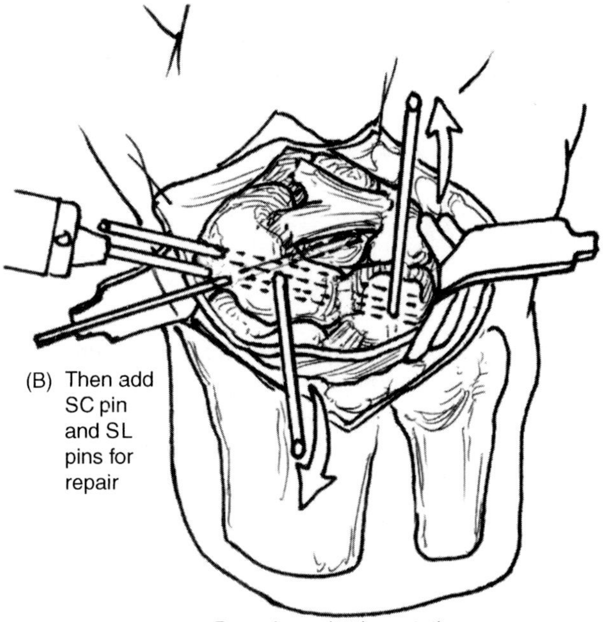

Figure 39–3

- Via a radial approach a 0.062 in. Kirschner wire is placed across the scapholunate (SL) joint paralleling the radial inclination of the radius. A second 0.062 in. wire is placed across the scaphocapitate (SC) articulation (**Fig. 39–3**).
- If there is a residual instability of the capitolunate joint it may signify lono-triquetral (L-T) injury (greater arc) as well and may require an L-T pinning from the ulnar side.
- Remove joystick wires and cut and bend the percutaneous wires.
- Close the dorsal capsule without imbrication.
- Place a short–arm thumb spica splint.

Postoperative Care

- Thumb spica splint for 2 weeks
- Short arm thumb spica cast for 8 weeks
- Active finger motion is encouraged.

■ Pearls

Use joysticks to reduce SLIL. Marked lunate extension can be corrected by placing of 2 sequential dorsal joysticks.

- Rotate the lunate such that the capitate dome is no longer visible, that is, cover the bald head of the capitate.
- Percutaneous Kirschner wires can injure the superficial radial nerve and radial artery and must be carefully placed.
- If reduction of SLIL injury is difficult a combined palmar approach or dorsal capsulodesis must be considered.

■ Pitfall

Percutaneous wires should never cross the radio carpal joint as they loosen and may lead to joint infection.

Suggested Readings

Adkison JW, Chapman MW. Treatment of acute lunate and perilunate dislocations. Clin Orthop 1982;164: 199–207

Berger RA, Weiss AC. Hand Surgery. Vol 1. Philadelphia: Lippincott Williams & Wilkins; 2004

Kozin SH. Perilunate injuries: diagnosis and treatment. J Am Acad Ortho Surg 1998;6:114–120

Melone CP Jr, Murphy MS, Raskin KB. Perilunate injuries: repair by dual dorsal and volar approaches. Hand Clin 2000;16:439–448

40 Open Reduction and Internal Fixation Lunate Dislocation via Combined Dorsal–Palmar Approach

Indications

- Incomplete closed reduction, percutaneous fixation
- Failed closed reduction and percutaneous fixation
- Some authors recommend early open reduction, Kirschner wire fixation, and ligament repair in all lunate dislocations, regardless of the reduction achieved by closed means. Anatomical reduction by closed means is rare because residual carpal instability usually persists.

Technique

- Make a longitudinal incision over the third to fourth extensor compartment (**Fig. 40–1**).
- Incise the extensor retinaculum obliquely.
- Raise a V-shaped flap in the capsule preserving the dorsal intercarpal ligament and dorsal radiolunate-triquetral ligament.
- Expose the palmar capsule using an extended carpal tunnel approach (**Fig. 40–2**).
- Retract the flexor tendons and the median nerve radially. This will reveal the palmarly dislocated lunate and a transverse rent in the capsule (**Fig. 40–3**).
- From the palmar approach the lunate is reduced by manual pressure with gentle longitudinal traction on the wrist (**Fig. 40–4**).
- Place Kirschner wires into the scaphoid (S) and lunate (L) to use as joysticks to reduce the scapholunate (SL) joint. The scaphoid–lunate relationship is restored when the diastasis is reduced and the head of the capitate (C) is contained by the lunate articulation. Kirschner wires are placed across the reduced SL and scaphocapitate articulation.
- Repair the dorsal ligaments. If there is insufficient ligament to suture to, suture anchors are placed in divergent orientations and the ligament is repaired. In rare instances with intersubstance tears a flap of

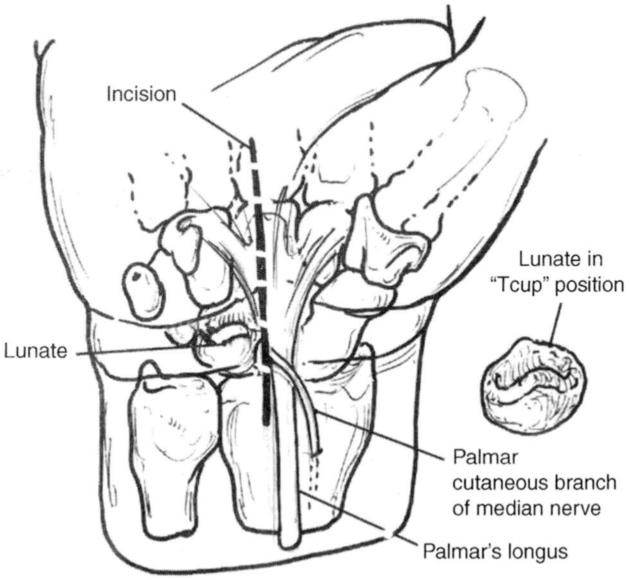

Figure 40–1

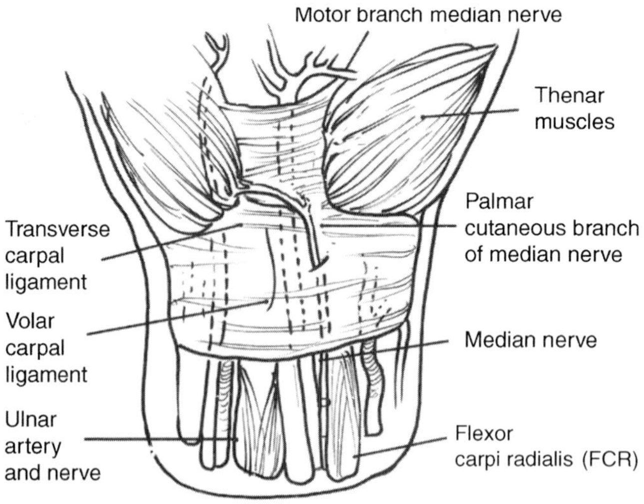

Figure 40–2

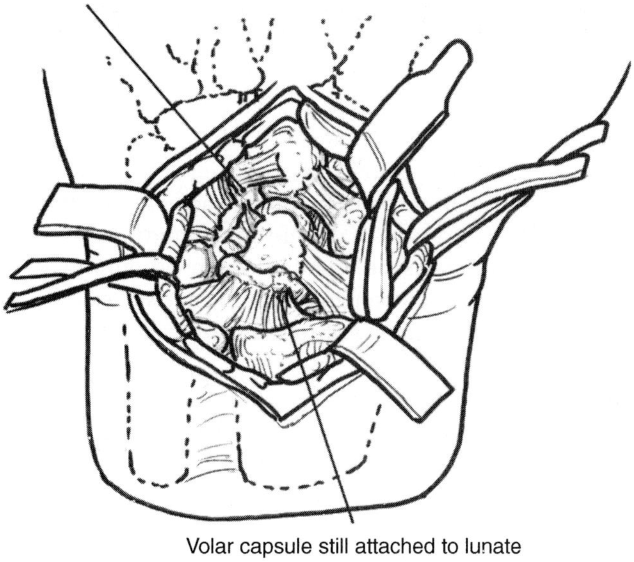

Figure 40–3

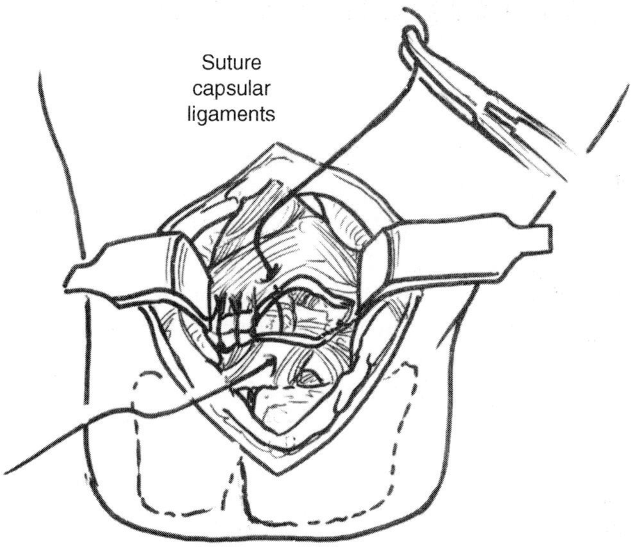

Figure 40–5

dorsal intercarpal ligament can reinforce the dorsal SL ligament (**Fig. 40–5**).

- Use Kirschner wires as joysticks to reduce the lunotriquetral (LT) joint and fix it with divergent percutaneous K-wires. Repair the LT ligament if possible. Repair the dorsal ligaments (**Fig. 40–6**).
- Close the dorsal capsule but do not overly tighten.
- Verify anatomical reduction of the lunate via mini image and repair the palmar rent in the capsule with no. 0 nonabsorbable sutures.
- Close the retinaculum with Z-lengthening.

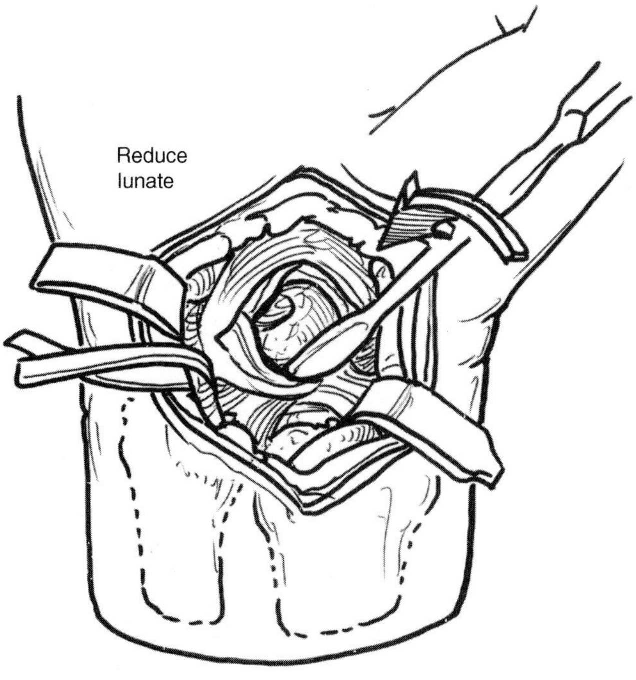

Figure 40–4

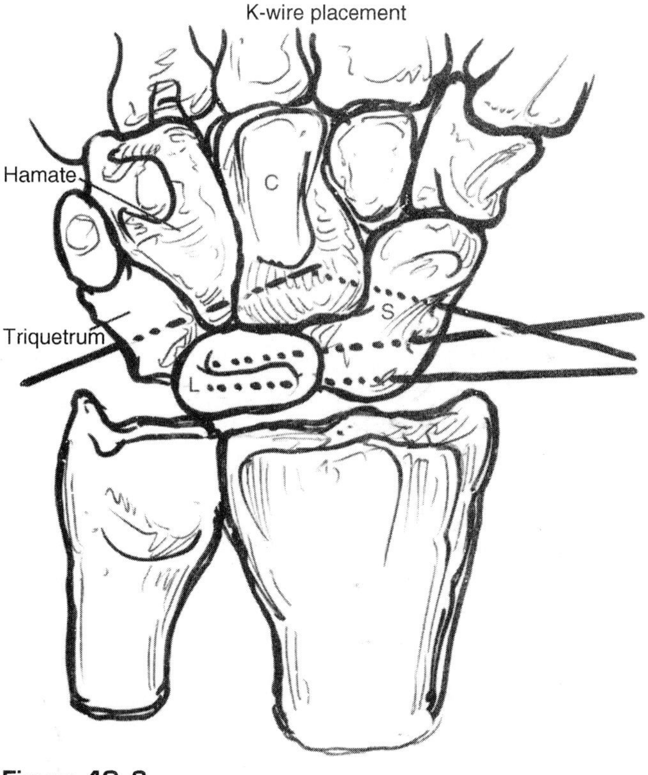

Figure 40–6

Postoperative Care

- Active finger motion is started early and the hand is kept elevated to reduce the swelling that commonly occurs.
- Short arm thumb spica splint for 2 weeks
- Short arm thumb spica cast for 6 weeks
- The wires for lesser arc injuries are removed at 8 weeks and a splint (intermittent use) is continued for another 2 to 4 weeks.
- For greater arc injuries with scaphoid fracture usually a headless screw is used for internal fixation and splints are continued until definite radiographic union, which is often assessed by sagittal CT.

Pearls

Palmarly, the scapholunate interosseous ligament (SLIL) often cannot be repaired because it is covered by the usually intact long radiolunate ligament; attention should be given to the ulnar corner where the LT ligament can be repaired.

Although the LT joint can be pinned first, it is preferable to initially repair the more difficult scapholunate articulation to take advantage of the lunate mobility.

Often, the dorsal ligaments cannot be anatomically reapproximated; Anatomical reduction of carpal bones and removal of loose osteochondral fragments are the primary goals. However, soft tissue augmentation, by either dorsal capsulodesis or tenodesis, can be employed in cases of excessive or irreparable ligament damage.

Suture anchors are easier to use than drill holes.

Pitfalls

If there are any median nerve symptoms do carpal tunnel release.

Avoid transfixation of the radiocarpal joint with Kirschner wires.

Avoid excessive shortening of dorsal capsule.

Suggested Readings

Kozin SH. Perilunate injuries: diagnosis and treatment. J Am Acad Ortho Surg 1998;6:114–120

Melone CP Jr, Murphy MS, Raskin KB. Perilunate injuries: repair by dual dorsal and volar approaches. Hand Clin 2000;16:439–448

41 Open Reduction and Internal Fixation of Trans-scaphoid Perilunate Fracture Dislocation

Indications

Acute carpal fracture dislocations. After 2 to 3 weeks, the surgeon should consider a salvage procedure.

Technique

■ Pearl

Closed reduction of the midcarpal joint just prior to incision will facilitate the dissection.

- Arc of injury noted to enter through the scaphoid (S), extend ulnarly across the midcarpal joint, and exit through the lunotriquetral joint (**Fig. 41–1**).
- Dorsal longitudinal incision
- Release the extensor pollicis longus from the third compartment and retract, with the radial wrist extensors in a radial direction.
- Open the radial wall of the fourth extensor compartment and retract retinaculum and the common extensors in an ulnar direction.
- Inspect the dorsal wrist capsule. The capsule is often avulsed from the distal radius. Identify the radiolunotriquetral ligament so that it can be repaired at the end of the case.
- Split the capsule along the dorsal radiocarpal and intercarpal ligaments raising a radially based flap (**Fig. 41–2**).

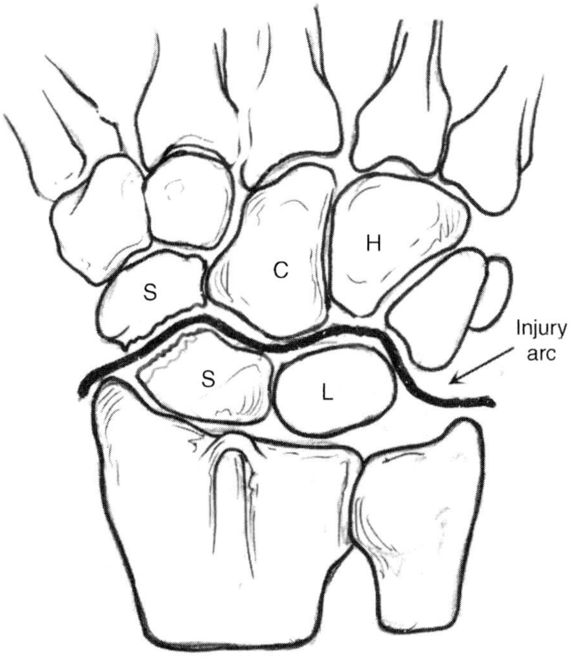

Figure 41–1

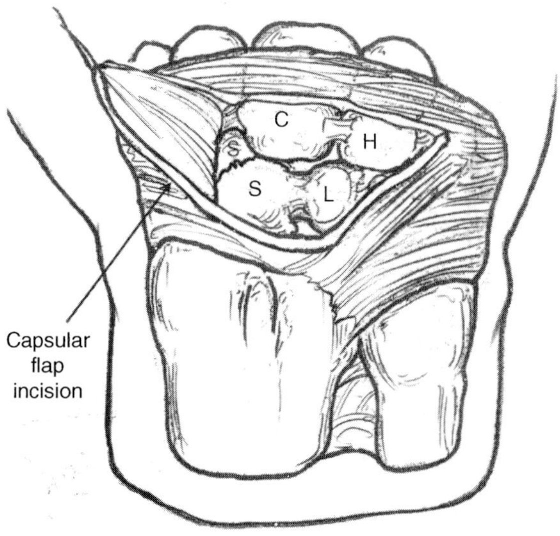

Figure 41–2

- Reduce the radiocarpal and midcarpal joint.
- Flex the wrist to expose and reduce the proximal fragment of the scaphoid.

■ Pearl

Reduction of the scaphoid can be facilitated by placing a 0.045 in. wire in either pole.

- Pin the reduced scaphoid with the pin from a cannulated headless screw (**Fig. 41–3**).

■ Pearl

Provisional stability of comminuted fractures is enhanced by placing a second wire. Align the second wire parallel to the first and place at the margins of the scaphoid so that it does not interfere with screw placement.

- Confirm scaphoid reduction and pin placement with intraoperative fluoroscopy.
- Drill, tap, if necessary, and place the headless screw into the scaphoid.
- Confirm scaphoid reduction and screw placement with intraoperative fluoroscopy.
- Assess and document shearing injuries to the articular surface of the carpus.
- Assess and document ligament injuries.
- Reduce the midcarpal joint and place a 0.045 in. pin across the scaphocapitate joint. The pin should pass through the distal pole of the scaphoid.
- Assess the stability of, and, if necessary, pin the lunotriquetral joint with a 0.045 in. pin.

■ Pitfall

Avoid "backing up" a pin that has been advanced too far. Partial withdrawal leads to premature pin loosening. Advance pins with the assistance of intraoperative fluoroscopy.

- Confirm reduction of the carpus and pin placement with intraoperative fluoroscopy (**Fig. 41–4**).
- Repair the capsulotomy.

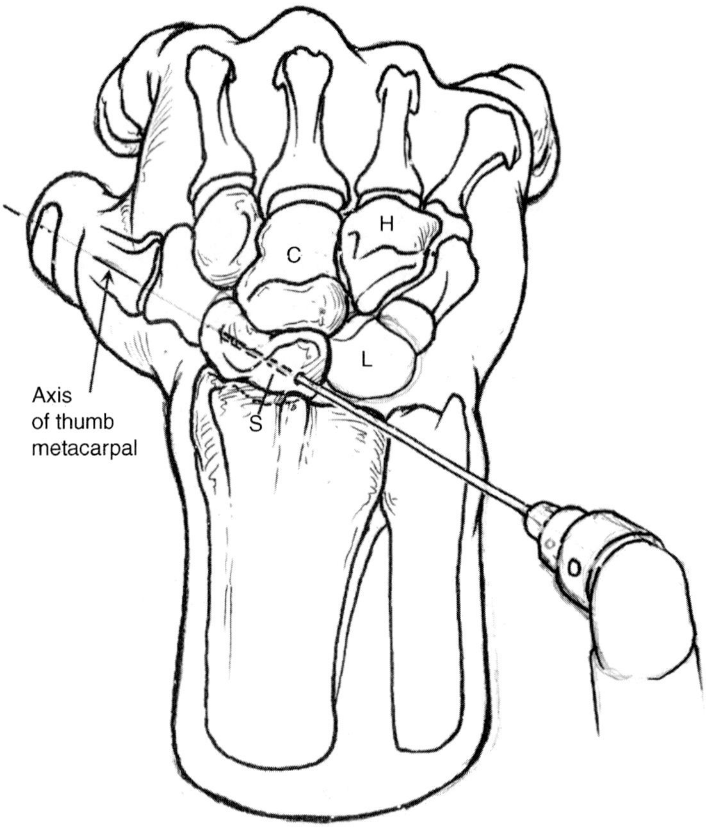

Figure 41–3

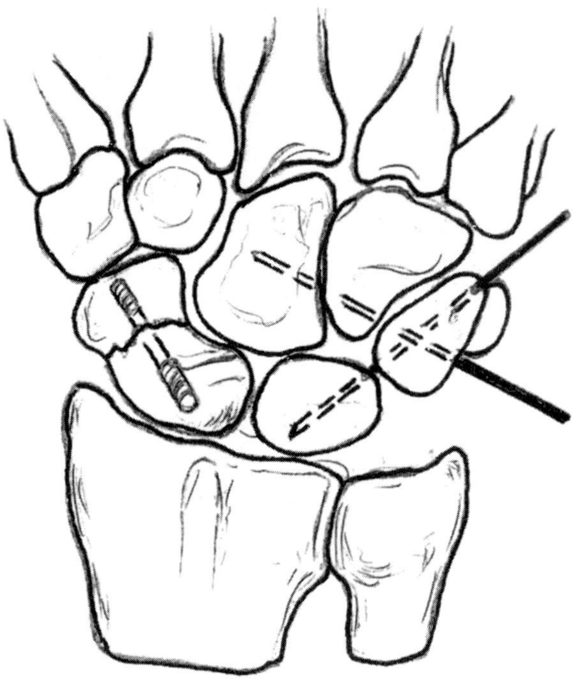

Figure 41–4

- If the radiolunotriquetral ligament was stripped from the radius, use suture anchors to repair it to bone.
- Short arm thumb spica splint

Postoperative Care

- Surgical dressing with short arm thumb spica splint for 10 to 14 days.
- Short arm–thumb spica cast for 6 weeks
- Removable short arm thumb spica splint for 4 weeks. Splint can be removed for gentle wrist range of motion exercises.
- Pins are removed at 3 months.
- Monitor scaphoid healing with plain radiographs and, if necessary, CT scans.
- The time that mobilization is initiated hinges on healing of the scaphoid.

Suggested Readings

Garcia-Elias. Carpal instabilities and dislocations. In: Green DP, Hotchkiss RN, Pederson WC, eds. Green's Operative Hand Surgery 1999:865–881, 914–917

Herzberg G, et al. Perilunate dislocations and fracture-dislocations: a multicenter study. J Hand Surg [Am] 1993;18A:768–779

42 Open Reduction and Internal Fixation of Scaphocapitate Syndrome

Indications

Acute carpal fracture dislocations. After 2 to 3 weeks, the surgeon should consider a salvage procedure.

Technique

- Arc of injury noted to enter through the scaphoid (S), extend across the capitate (C) neck, and exit through the lunotriquetral ligament (**Fig. 42–1A,B**).
- Dorsal longitudinal incision.
- Release the extensor pollicis longus from the third compartment and retract, with the radial wrist extensors in a radial direction.
- Open the radial wall of the fourth extensor compartment and retract retinaculum and the common extensors in an ulnar direction.
- Inspect the dorsal wrist capsule. The capsule is often avulsed from the distal radius. Identify the radiolunotriquetral ligament so that it can be repaired at the end of the case.
- Split the capsule along the dorsal radiocarpal and intercarpal ligaments elevating radially to expose the carpus and the radial styloid (**Fig. 42–2**).
- Assess and document shearing injuries to the articular surface of the carpus.
- Assess and document ligament injuries.
- Small styloid fragments are excised if present.
- Large styloid fragments (>1 cm) should be fixed because most will include part or all of the origin of the radioscaphocapitate ligament.

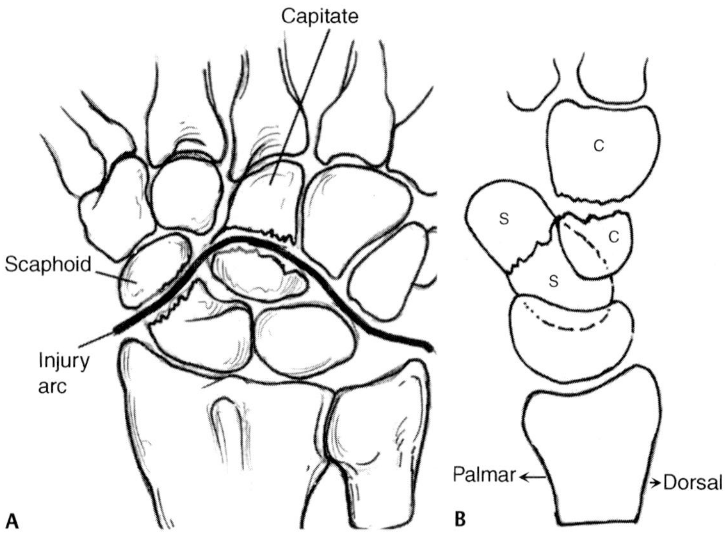

Figure 42–1

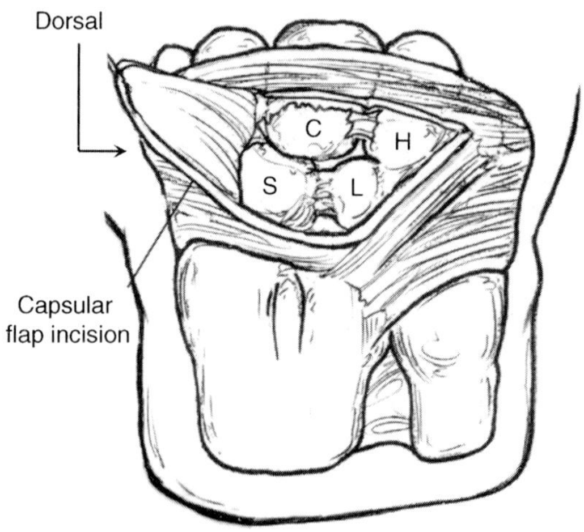

Figure 42–2

Pearl

Large styloid fragments can be fixed with either pins or a cannulated screw. Hardware is placed through a small incision centered over the radial styloid. Protect branches of the radial sensory nerve.

- Flex the wrist to expose and reduce the proximal fragment of the capitate.
- Fix the capitate fracture with two headless screws; if the fragment is small use one screw and a pin or two pins (**Fig. 42–3**).
- Reduce the scaphoid.

Pearl

Reduction of the scaphoid can be facilitated by placing a 0.045 in. wire in either pole.

- Pin the reduced scaphoid with the pin from a cannulated headless screw.

Pearl

Placing a second wire enhances provisional stability of comminuted fractures. Align the second wire parallel to the first and place at the margins of the scaphoid so that it does not interfere with screw placement.

- Confirm scaphoid reduction and pin placement with intraoperative fluoroscopy.
- Drill and place the headless screw into the scaphoid.
- Confirm scaphoid reduction and screw placement with intraoperative fluoroscopy.
- Reduce the midcarpal joint and place a 0.045 in. pin across the scaphocapitate joint. The pin should pass through the distal pole of the scaphoid.
- Assess the stability of, and, if necessary, pin the lunotriquetral joint with a 0.045 in. pin (**Fig. 42–4**).

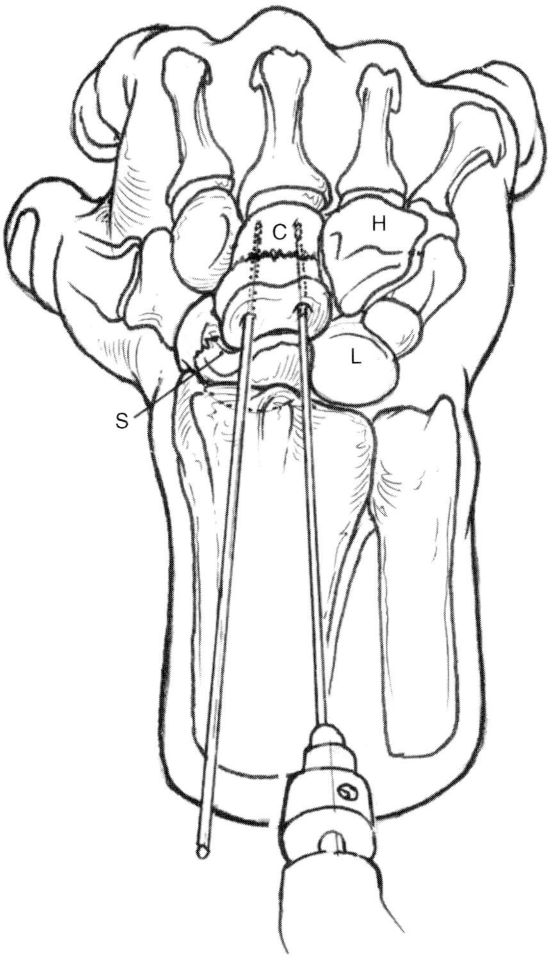

Figure 42–3

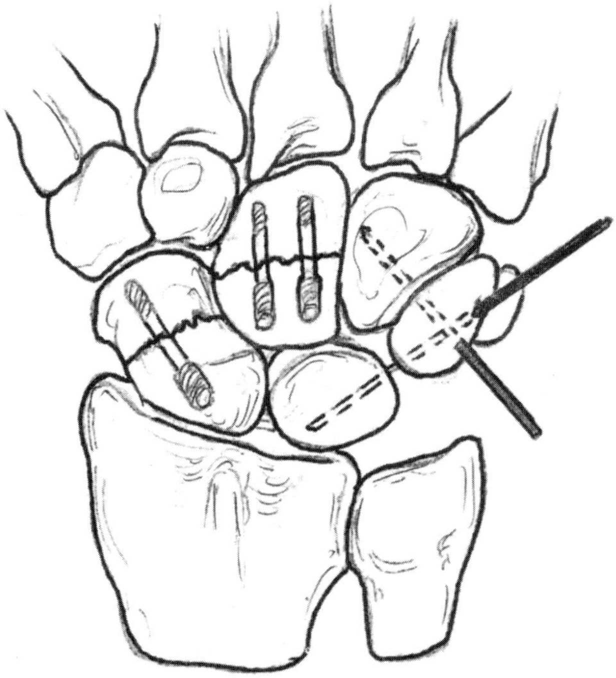

Figure 42–4

■ Pitfall

Avoid "backing up" a pin that has been advanced too far. Partial withdrawal leads to premature pin loosening. Advance pins with the assistance of intraoperative fluoroscopy.

- Confirm reduction of the carpus and pin placement with intraoperative fluoroscopy.
- Repair the capsulotomy.
- If the radiolunotriquetral ligament was stripped from the radius, use suture anchors to repair it to bone.
- Short arm thumb spica splint

Postoperative Care

- Surgical dressing with short arm thumb spica splint for 10 to 14 days
- Short arm thumb spica cast for 6 weeks
- Removable short arm thumb spica splint for 4 weeks. Splint can be removed for gentle wrist range of motion exercises.
- Pins are removed at 3 months.
- Monitor scaphoid healing with plain radiographs and, if necessary, CT scans.
- The time that mobilization is initiated hinges on healing of the scaphoid.

Suggested Readings

Apergis E, Darmanis S, Kastanis G, Papankolaou A. Does the term scaphocapitate syndrome need to be revised? A report of 6 cases. J Hand Surg [Br] 2001;26B:441–445

Vance RM, Gelberman RH, Evans EF. Scaphocapitate fractures. J Bone Joint Surg [Am] 1980;62A:271–276

Section VI.6

The Wrist Joint: Arthritis Due to Scapholunate Advanced Collapse and Scaphoid Nonunion Advanced Collapse

43 Wrist Denervation

Indications

- Symptomatic arthritis in elderly patient with concurrent medical problems that preclude major wrist reconstruction
- Patients of all ages with symptomatic arthritis who want an opportunity to reduce their wrist pain with minimal postoperative morbidity

■ Pitfall

Experience with wrist denervation has been primarily in patients with osteoarthritis. Wrist denervation as an isolated treatment is not recommended in patients with rheumatoid arthritis.

Preoperative Evaluation

- Pain localized to the radiocarpal and midcarpal joints
- Pain diminished with block of the posterior interosseous and anterior interosseous nerves

Technique

- Dorsal midline incision centered two fingerbreadths proximal to radiocarpal joint (**Fig. 43–1**)
- Open the fascia, proximal to the extensor retinaculum between the tendons and muscle bellies of the extensor pollicis longus and tendons of the fourth extensor compartment.
- The posterior interosseous nerve (PIN) lies on the interosseous membrane (**Fig. 43–2**).
- Separate the nerve from the contiguous posterior interosseous artery (PIA).
- Resect a 1 cm segment of the nerve and cauterize the two ends.
- Incise the interosseous membrane over a length of 2 cm.
- The anterior interosseous nerve (AIN) lies directly anterior to the interosseous membrane (**Fig. 43–3**).

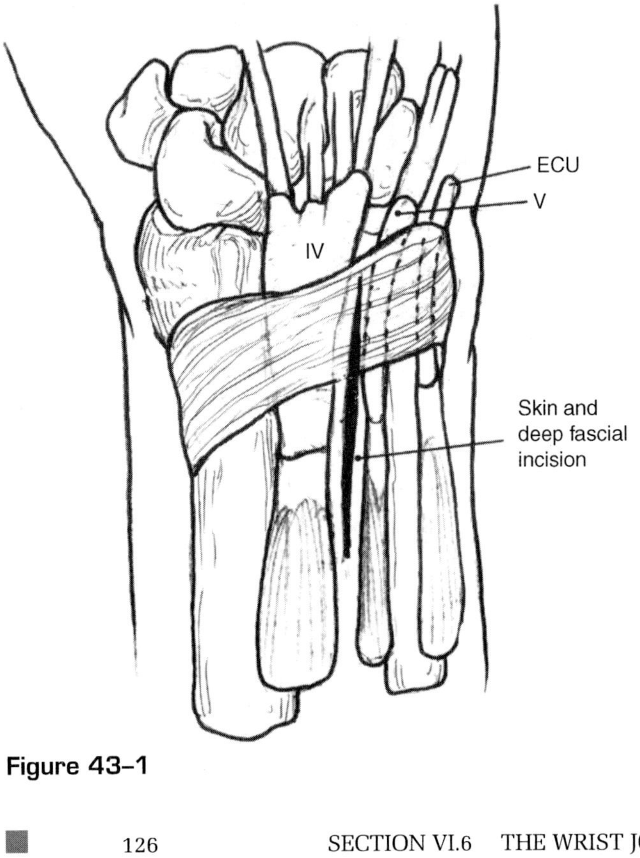

Figure 43–1

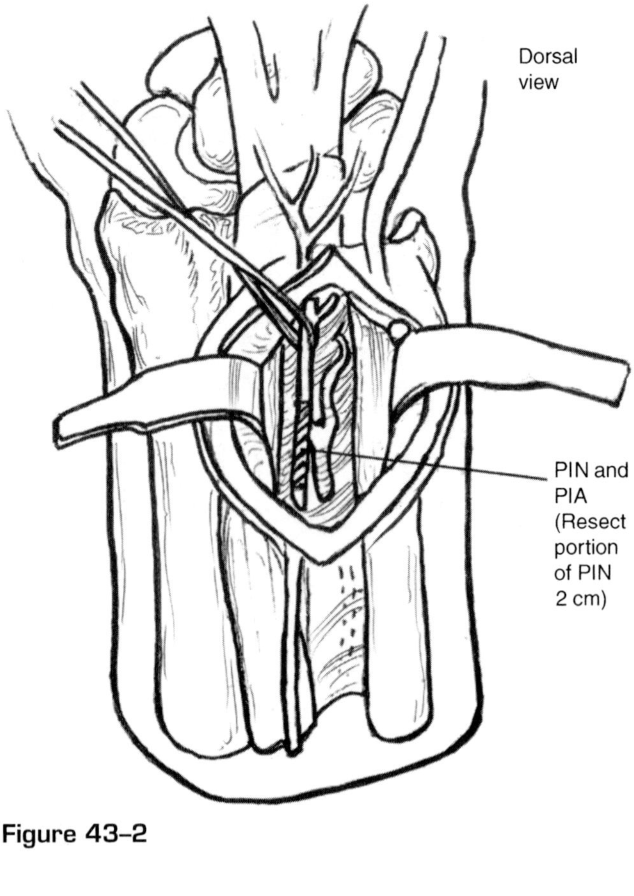

Figure 43–2

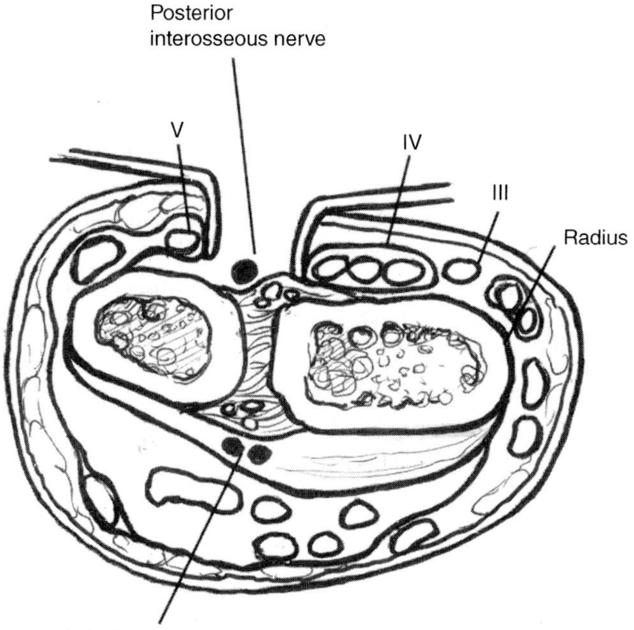

Figure 43–3

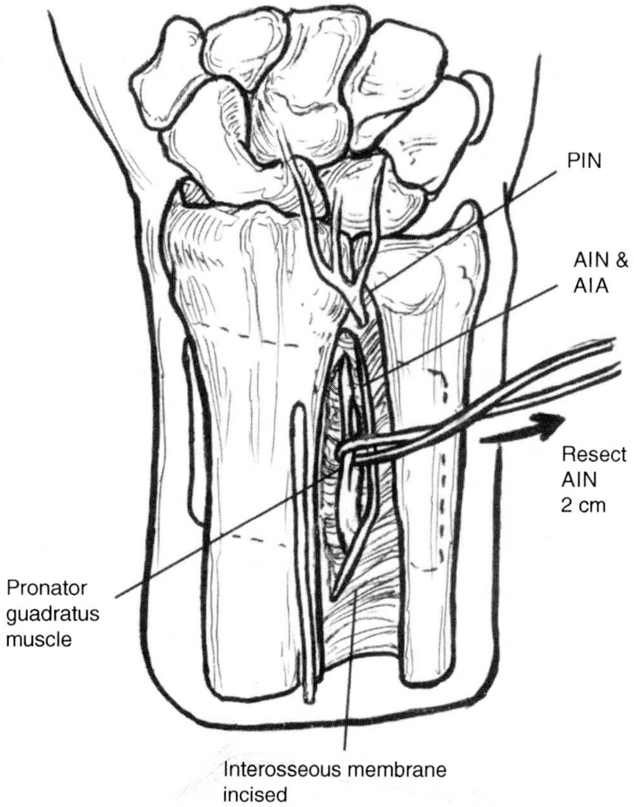

Figure 43–4

- Separate the nerve from the contiguous anterior interosseous artery (AIA).
- Resect a 1 cm segment of the nerve and cauterize the two ends.
- Disrupt small dorsal cutaneous nerves to the wrist by sweeping a finger between the fascia and the subcutaneous tissues, radial, ulnar, and distal to the skin incision (**Fig. 43–4**).
- Close skin and apply a soft dressing.

■ Pearls

An intra-articular injection of cortisone can be given concurrently with the denervation procedure in patients with palpable wrist synovitis.

Postoperative Care

- Immediate wrist motion, gentle use of the wrist and hand until the sutures are removed
- Unrestricted use after suture removal in 10 to 14 days

Suggested Readings

Ishida O, Tsai T-M, Atasoy E. Long-term results of denervation of the wrist joint for chronic wrist pain. J Hand Surg [Br] 1993;18B:76–80

Weinstein LP, Berger RA. Analgesic benefit, functional outcome, and patient satisfaction after partial wrist denervation. J Hand Surg [Am] 2002;27A:833–839

44 Radial Styloidectomy

Indications

- Arthritis between the distal pole of the scaphoid and radial styloid seen in scaphoid nonunion with advanced collapse
- This procedure may relieve pain when performed alone or in conjunction with open reduction and internal fixation (ORIF) of the nonunited scaphoid.
- Impingement between the trapezium and radial styloid recognized intraoperatively following proximal row carpectomy

Technique

- Dorsal approach to the radius (**Fig. 44–1**)
- Incise the capsule between the second and fourth compartments (**Fig. 44–2**).
- Elevate the capsule from the dorsal aspect of the radial styloid working beneath and retracting the tendons of the second dorsal compartment dorsally.
- Dissect around the radial aspect of the styloid elevating the floor of the first extensor compartment and including the insertion of the brachioradialis tendon, retracting these tendons palmarly.

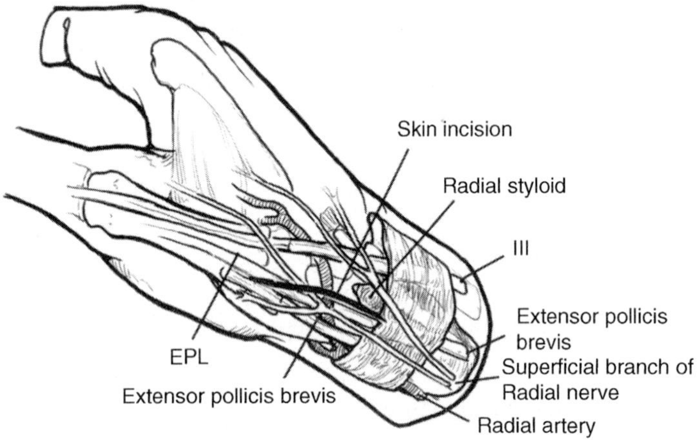

Figure 44–1

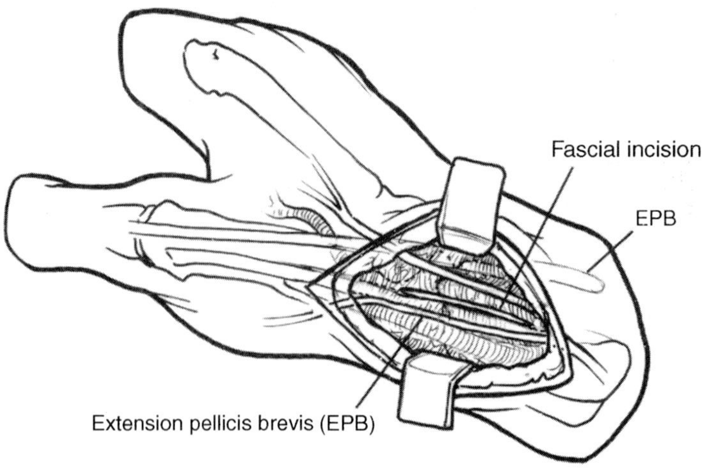

Figure 44–2

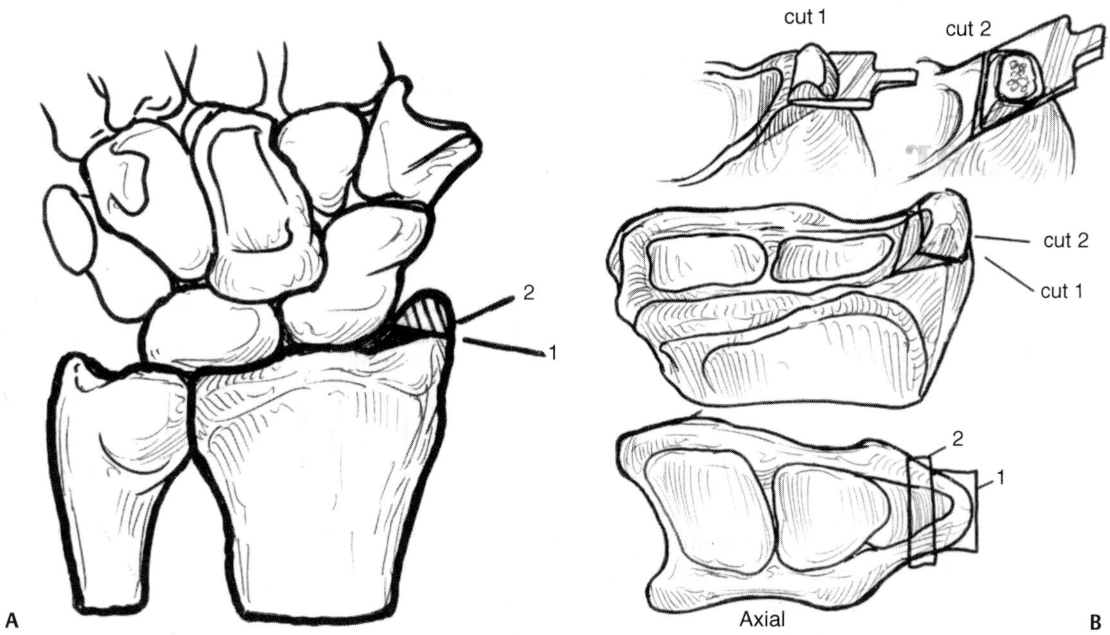

Figure 44–3

■ Pearl

Take care to avoid injury to the tendons of the first dorsal extensor compartment and the radial artery during dissection around the radial aspect of the radial styloid.

- Create two oblique osteotomies at the junction of the worn and intact cartilage in the scaphoid fossa with care to preserve the radioscaphocapitate ligament.
- First osteotomy removes the tip of the radial styloid distal to the radioscaphocapitate ligament origin.
- Second osteotomy removes the worn portion of the scaphostyloid articulation (**Fig. 44–3A,B**).
- Close the capsule.
- Leave the extensor pollicis longus (EPL) in a transposed position between the retinaculum and the subcutaneous tissues.
- Close skin and apply a soft dressing.

Postoperative Care

- Immediate wrist motion, gentle use of the wrist and hand until the sutures are removed
- Unrestricted use after suture removal in 10 to 14 days

Suggested Readings

Barnard L, Stubbins S. Styloidectomy of the radius in the surgical treatment of nonunion of the carpal navicular. J Bone Joint Surg [Am] 1948;30A:98–102

Siegel DB, Gelberman RH. Radial styloidectomy: an anatomical study with special reference to radiocarpal intracapsular ligamentous morphology. J Hand Surg [Am] 1991;16:40–44

45 Proximal Row Carpectomy with Capsular Resurfacing

Indications

- Radioscaphoid arthritis with preservation of the radiolunate and midcarpal joints. This pattern is typically seen in long-standing scapholunate dissociation.

■ Pitfall

Degenerative changes on the capitate may not be apparent on the preoperative radiographs. Patients should be warned about the possibility of an alternative procedure, such as a scaphoid (S) excision and capitate–lunate–triquetral–hamate (CLTH) fusion.

Technique

- A dorsal, longitudinal, 6 to 8 cm skin incision is centered over the capitate (C) (**Fig. 45–1**).
- Release the extensor pollicis longus from the third compartment and retract radially.
- Incise the radial septum of the fourth compartment, elevating the retinaculum as a flap.
- Retract the radial wrist extensors in a radial direction and the extensor digitorum communis in an ulnar direction.
- Create a U-shaped, distally based capsular flap (**Fig. 45–2**).

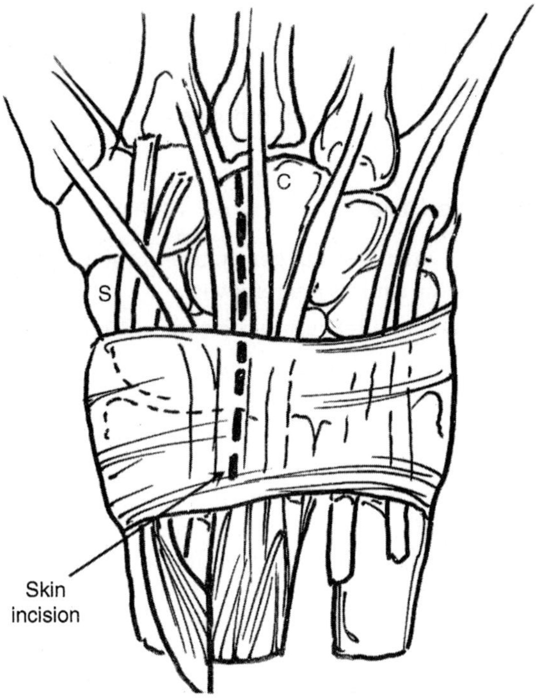

Figure 45–1

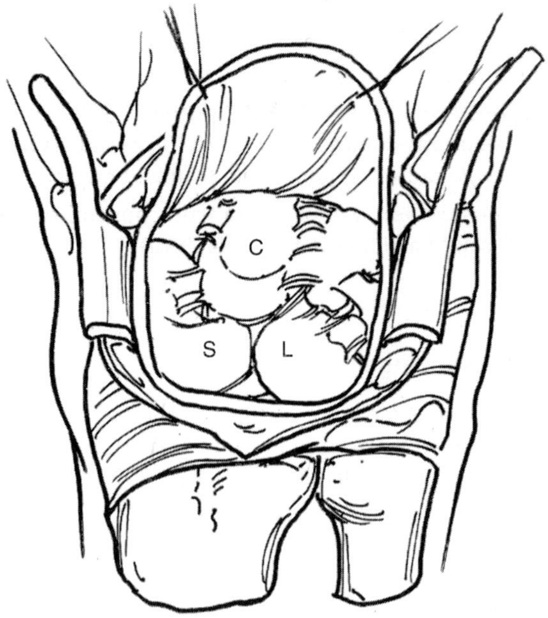

Figure 45–2

Pearl

If unexpected degenerative changes are found on the head of the capitate, the capsular flap can be interposed between the capitate and the lunate (L) fossa.

Pitfall

The flap must be wide enough to completely cover the head of the capitate. The radial margin should be raised beneath the extensor carpi radialis brevis tendon (ECRB); the ulnar margin should be raised just radial to the fifth extensor compartment.

- Inspect the articular surfaces of the capitate and lunate fossa.
- Wear on the capitate is handled in two fashions:

1. Young patient, nonsmoker: scaphoid excision and CLTH fusion.
2. Older patient, smoker: proximal row carpectomy with interposition of the capsular flap.

- Split the scaphoid across its waist with an osteotome and remove the proximal pole of the scaphoid.
- Split remaining distal pole of the scaphoid along its longitudinal axis and remove both pieces with a rongeur.

Pitfall

Avoid injury to the radioscaphocapitate ligament passing palmar to the scaphoid waist.

- Excise osteophytes from the radial styloid.
- Drill a heavy, threaded pin into the lunate and use as a joystick to help remove the lunate with sharp dissection.

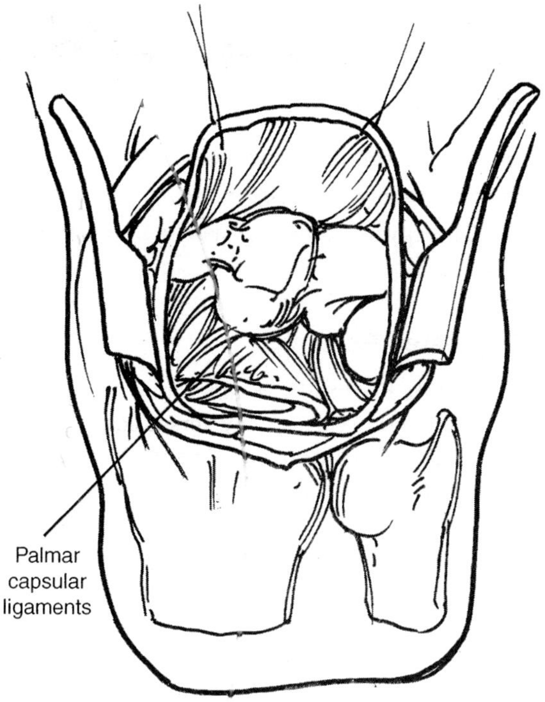

Figure 45–3

- Remove the triquetrum using the same technique as described for removal of the lunate (**Fig. 45–3**).
- If you chose to interpose the capsule, use a 2–0 suture on a short arc needle to suture the dorsal flap to the palmar capsule.
- Use three horizontal mattress sutures with the knot tied dorsally by passing the needle from the dorsal flap through the palmar capsule and back up through the dorsal flap (**Fig. 45–4A,B**).

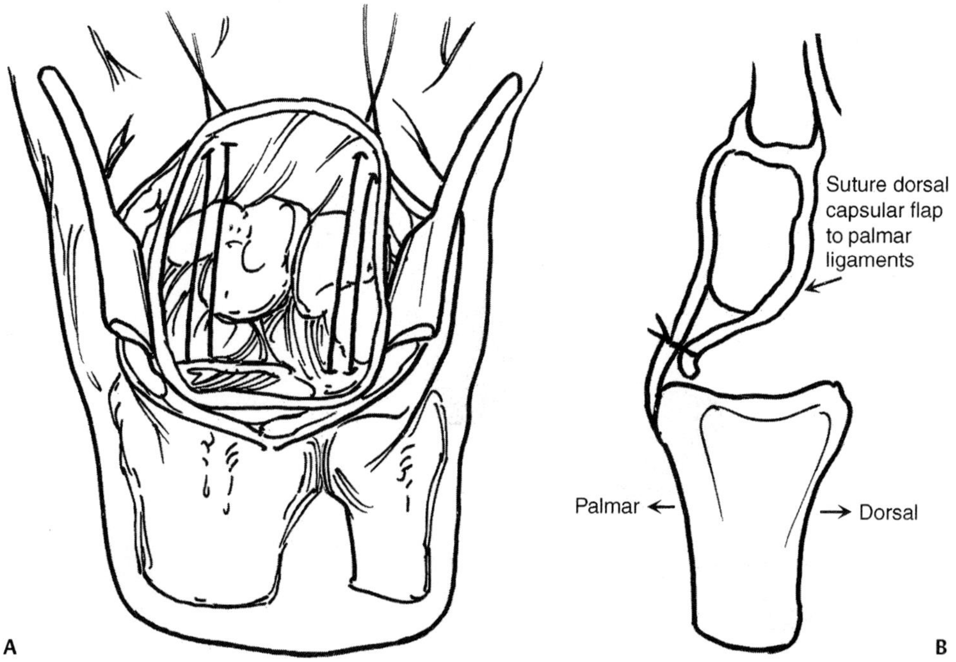

A B

Figure 45–4

- If the cartilage on the head of the capitate is intact close the capsule, retinaculum, and skin.

Postoperative Care

- Palmar splint for 2 weeks
- Short arm cast or thermoplastic splint for 2 weeks
- Therapy as needed for wrist and finger motion

Alternative Techniques

- Scaphoid excision with CLTH fusion
- Complete wrist arthrodesis
- Total wrist prosthetic replacement

Suggested Readings

Cohen MS, Kozin SH. Degenerative arthritis of the wrist: proximal row carpectomy versus scaphoid excision and four-corner arthrodesis. J Hand Surg [Am] 2001;26A:94–104

DiDonna ML, Kiefhaber TR, Stern PJ. Proximal row carpectomy: study with a minimum of ten years of follow-up. J Bone Joint Surg Am 2004;86-A:2359–2365

46 Scaphoid Excision with Capitolunate Triquetrohamate Arthrodesis

Indications

- Radioscaphoid and midcarpal arthritis with preservation of the radiolunate joint. This pattern is typically seen in long-standing scapholunate dissociation or scaphoid nonunion.
- Some surgeons prefer scaphoid excision with capitolunate triquetrohamate (CLTH) arthrodesis to proximal row carpectomy in patients with radioscaphoid arthritis and a midcarpal joint that has no evidence of degenerative changes.

■ Pitfall

Elderly patients and those with severe wrist stiffness have less predictable pain relief and recovery of motion.

Technique

- A dorsal, longitudinal 6 to 8 cm skin incision is made centered over the capitate (C).
- Dissect to the wrist capsule between the second and fourth compartments distal to the extensor pollicis longus tendon.

■ Pearl

Incise the distal edge of the extensor retinaculum between the third and fourth compartments to the level of Lister's tubercle to facilitate exposure.

- Make a transverse capsulotomy across the entire dorsal wrist at the level of the capitolunate joint and reflect the capsule both proximally and distally from the carpus (**Fig. 46–1**).
- Remove the scaphoid (S) piecemeal with a rongeur.
- Excise distally projecting osteophytes from the radial styloid.

■ Pitfall

Avoid injury to the radioscaphocapitate ligament, which passes over the palmar surface of the scaphoid waist.

- Complete the dorsal exposure of the capitate, hamate (H), lunate (L), and triquetrum (T).
- Remove the cartilage and subchondral bone from the intercarpal articulations of the hamate, capitate, triquetrum, and lunate, with the exception of removing only the dorsal half of the capitohamate joint (**Fig. 46–2**).

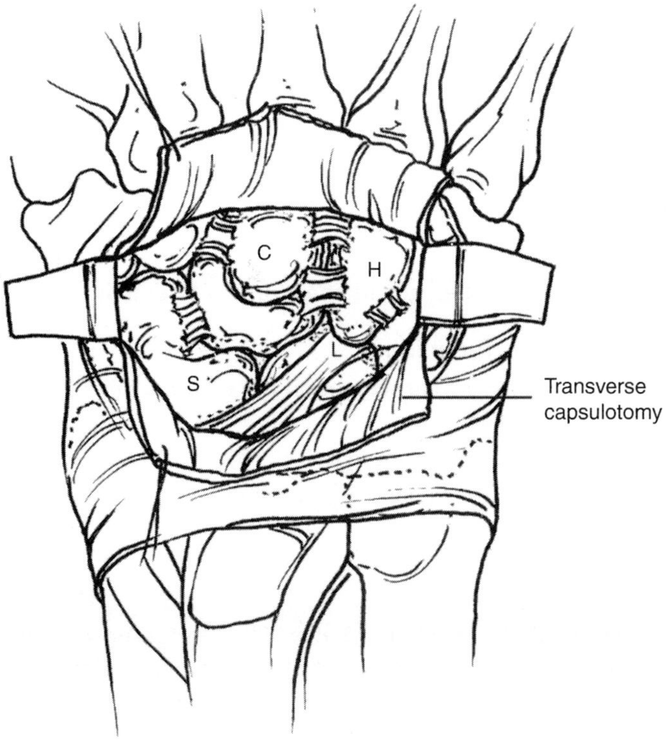

Figure 46–1

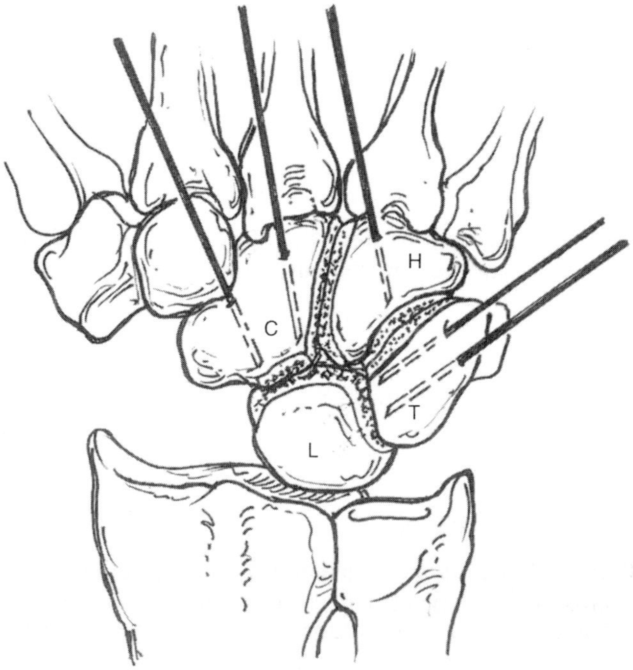

Figure 46–2

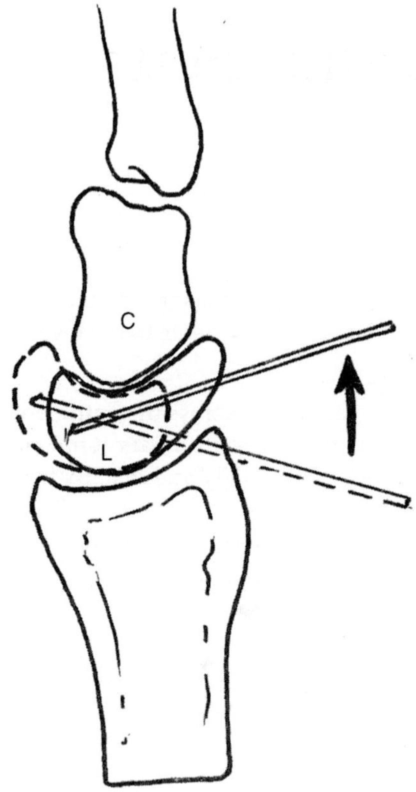

Figure 46–3

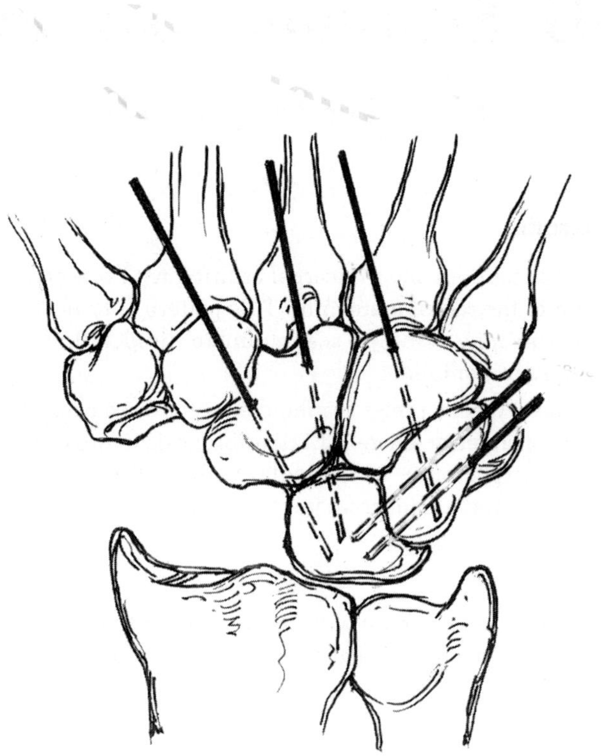

Figure 46–4

- Prepare bone graft from the distal radius or from the iliac crest.
- Insert 0.045 in. K-wires in the carpal bones (two in capitate, two in triquetrum, and one in hamate), checking position via fluoroscopy (**Fig. 46–2**).

■ Pearl

Alternative fixation devices are available such as headless screws and plates.

- Pack bone graft into the intercarpal spaces.
- Reduce the lunate and triquetrum into a neutral position, using joysticks if needed (**Fig. 46–3**).
- Advance the pins into the subchondral bone of the lunate and triquetrum; cut wires beneath skin (**Fig. 46–4**).

■ Pitfall

Failure to correct the lunate's extended position is a common technical error.

- Confirm positions of the carpal bones and fixation devices using fluoroscopy.
- Fill remaining intercarpal gaps with bone graft.
- Close the capsule, retinaculum, and skin.

Postoperative Care

- Wrist is immobilized initially with a plaster splint.
- Convert to a short arm cast for a total of 8 weeks.
- A wrist splint is used with gentle wrist motion until radiographic union.

■ Pearl

Full motion is often not attained for 9 to 12 months.

Alternative Techniques

- Proximal row carpectomy if the capitate head is not degenerated
- Complete wrist arthrodesis
- Total wrist prosthetic replacement

Suggested Readings

Cohen MS, Kozin SH. Degenerative arthritis of the wrist: proximal row carpectomy versus scaphoid excision and four-corner arthrodesis. J Hand Surg [Am] 2001;26A: 94–104

Wyrick JD, Stern PJ, Kiefhaber TR. Motion-preserving procedures in the treatment of scapholunate advanced collapse wrist: proximal row carpectomy versus four-corner arthrodesis. J Hand Surg 1995;20:965–970

47 Excision Distal Pole of the Scaphoid

Indications

- Symptomatic, long-standing scaphoid (S) nonunion with radioscaphoid arthritis
- Margins of scaphoid nonunion sclerotic, with cystic changes in the proximal and distal poles; appearance suggests pseudarthrosis
- Patient who is poor candidate for open reduction and internal fixation (ORIF): heavy smoker, anticipated poor compliance
- No arthritis in the midcarpal joint

■ Pitfall

Patients with a marked dorsal intercalated segmental instability (DISI) deformity and pain emanating from the midcarpal joint are poor candidates for this procedure.

Technique

- A dorsal, longitudinal 6 to 8 cm skin incision centered over the capitate (C) (**Fig. 47–1**)
- Dissect to the wrist capsule using incisions along the dorsal radiocarpal and dorsal intercarpal ligaments creating a radial-based flap between the second and fourth compartments distal to the extensor pollicis longus (EPL) tendon.

■ Pearl

Incise the distal edge of the extensor retinaculum between the third and fourth compartments to the level of Lister's tubercle to facilitate exposure (**Fig. 47–2**).

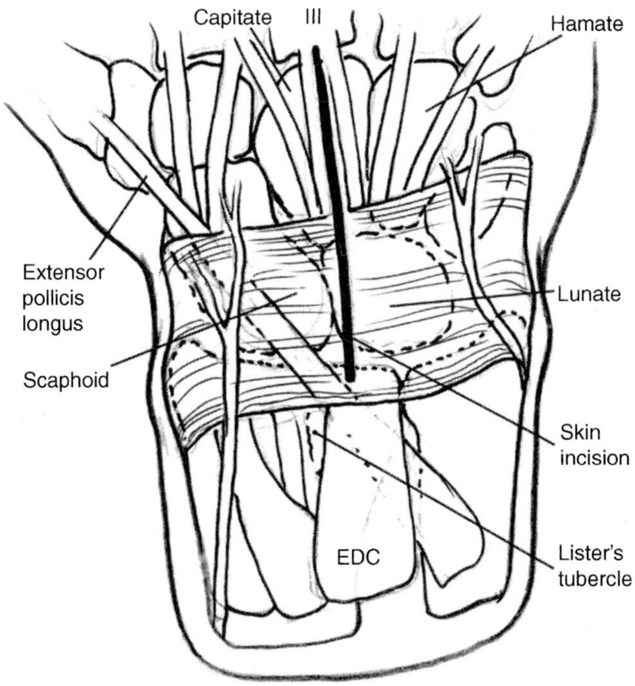

Figure 47–1

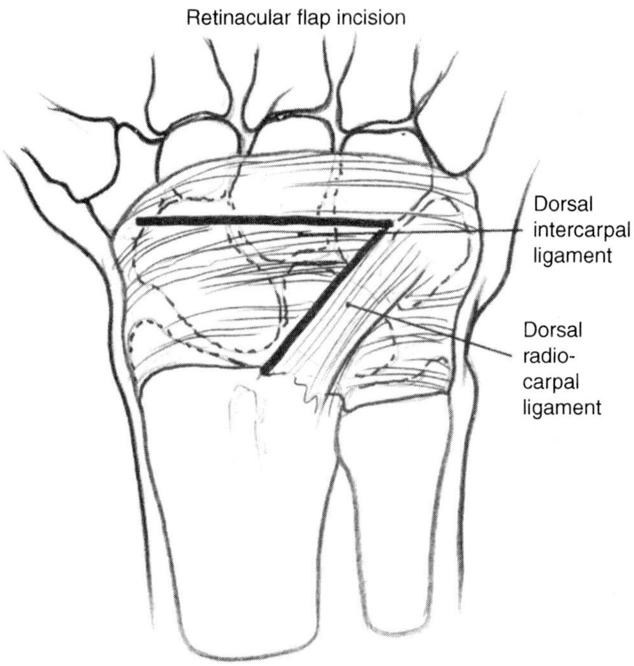

Figure 47–2

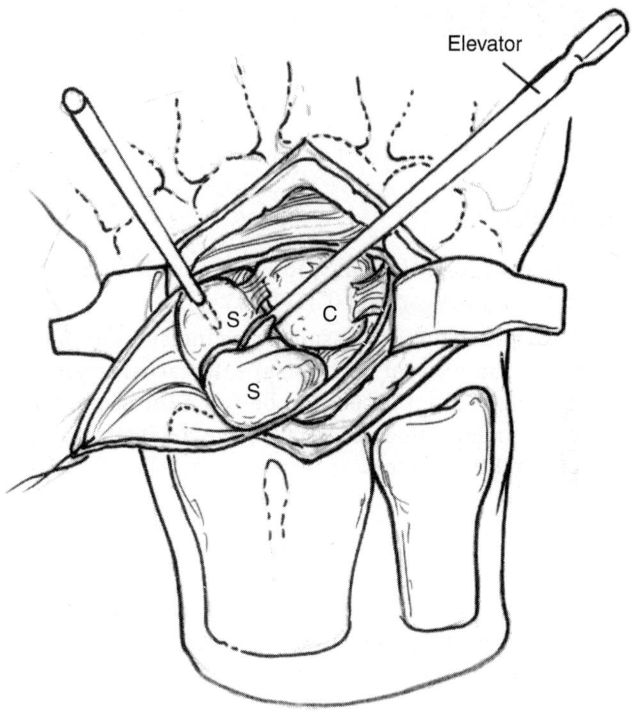

Figure 47–3

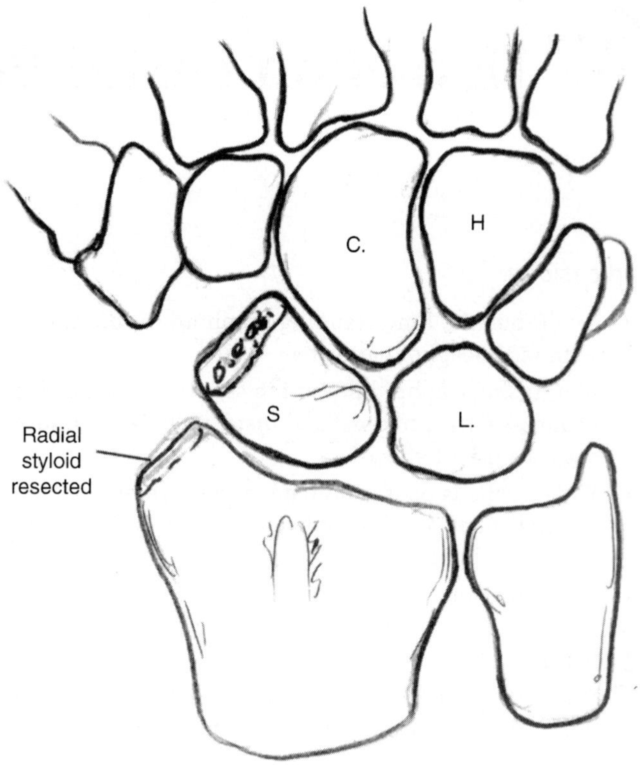

Figure 47–4

- Make a transverse capsulotomy across the entire dorsal wrist at the level of the capitolunate joint and reflect the capsule both proximally and distally from the carpus (**Fig. 47–3**).
- Place a large, threaded Steinmann pin in the distal pole of the scaphoid. Use a scalpel and remove the distal pole of the scaphoid en bloc or piecemeal with a rongeur (**Fig. 47–4**).
- Excise distally projecting osteophytes from the radial styloid.

■ Pitfall

Avoid injury to the radioscaphocapitate ligament passing palmar to the scaphoid waist.

- Confirm adequate resection of the distal pole of the scaphoid using fluoroscopy.
- Close the capsule, retinaculum, and skin.

Postoperative Care

- Wrist is immobilized initially with a plaster splint.
- Convert to a removal splint at 10 to 14 days to be used as needed for support.

Suggested Readings

Malerich MM, Clifford J, Eaton B, et al. Distal scaphoid resection arthroplasty for the treatment of degenerative arthritis secondary to scaphoid nonunion. J Hand Surg [Am] 1999;24:1196–1205

Malerich MM, Littler JW, Eaton R. Distal scaphoid resection arthroplasty for the treatment of patients with degenerative arthritis secondary to scaphoid nonunion. Techniques in Hand and Upper Extremity 2002;6: 98–102

Section VI.7

The Wrist Joint: Scaphotrapeziotrape-zoid Arthritis

48 Scaphotrapeziotrapezoid Joint Fusion

Indications

Long-standing scaphotrapeziotrapezoid (STT) arthritis recalcitrant to nonoperative treatment

Technique

- Dorsoradial incision that begins at Lister's tubercle, traverses the anatomical snuffbox, and ends at the STT joint. Incision can be curved or designed with a zigzag configuration. Exposure can also be accomplished via a dorsal transverse incision (**Fig. 48–1**).
- Protect the radial sensory nerves and lateral antebrachial cutaneous branches using loupe magnification. The dorsal approach exposes the STT joint between the extensor carpi radialis longus and brevis tendons through a transverse capsular incision. The radial approach is more extensive and performed between the extensor pollicis brevis (EPB) (first compartment) and extensor pollicis longus (EPL) (third compartment) tendons (**Fig. 48–2**).
- The deep branch of the radial artery resides just proximal to the STT joint and must be protected in both approaches.
- Using the radial approach, a longitudinal arthrotomy is performed from the radial styloid to the distal scaphoid (S). The distal scaphoid, trapezium (Tm), and trapezoid (Td) are identified. The articular and subchondral surfaces of the scaphoid, trapezium, and

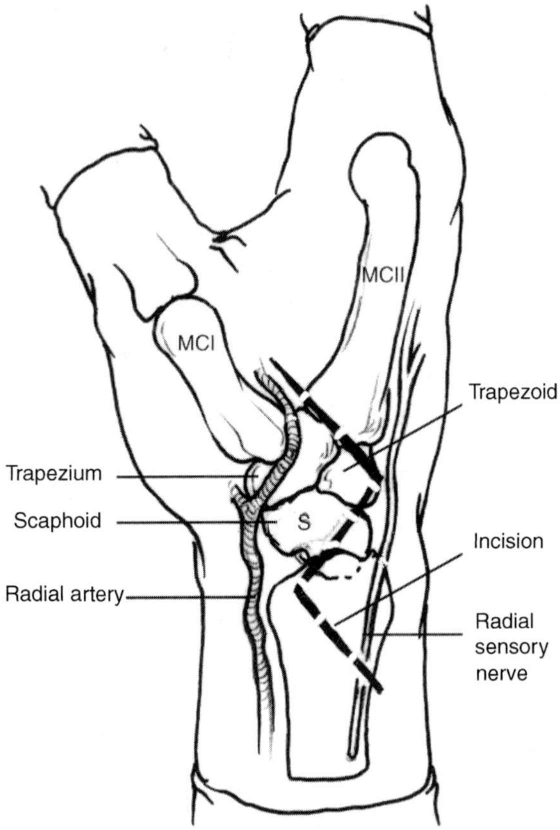

Figure 48–1

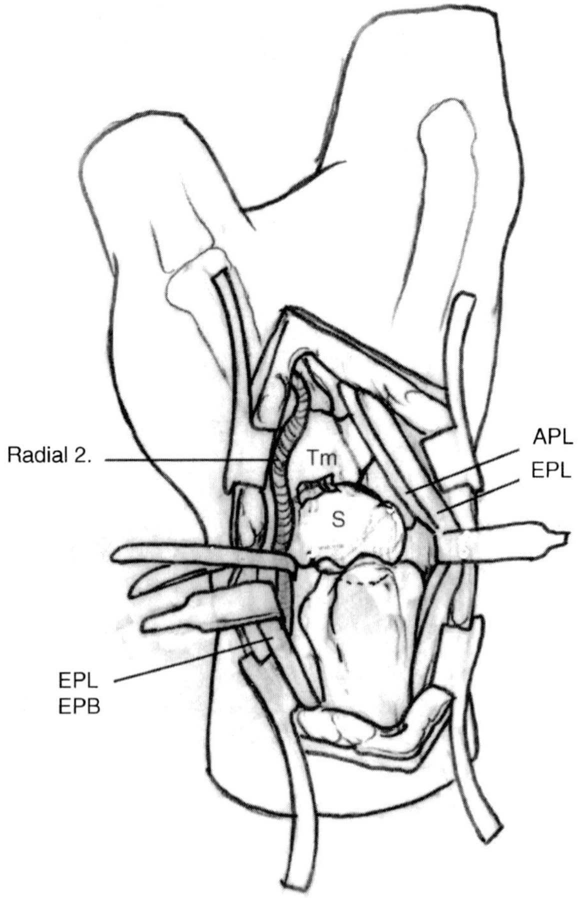

Figure 48–2

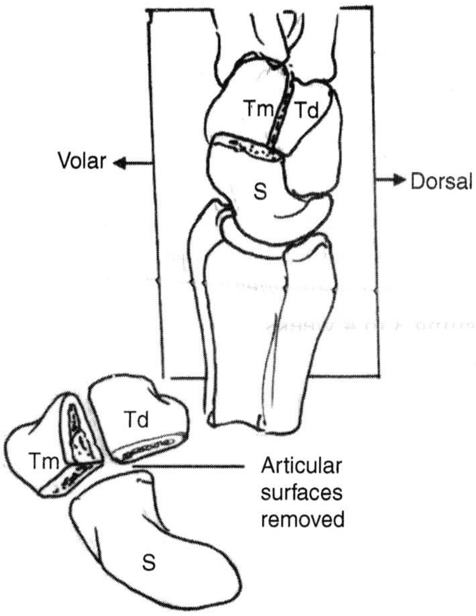

Figure 48–3

trapezoid are removed until cancellous bone is exposed (**Fig. 48–3**).

- A rongeur and small curved osteotomes are employed to prevent thermal necrosis and maximized bone carpentry. Certain patients will have extremely hard bone, and a high-speed bur will be required.
- Two to three double-ended trocar-tipped 0.45 in. (1.1 mm) wires are preset into position after the bony surface has been prepared and prior to bone grafting. This can be accomplished using one of two techniques; the wires can be driven through the trapezium or trapezoid from within the STT joint into a percutaneous position or the wires can be placed from a percutaneous position through the trapezium or trapezoid (**Fig. 48–4**).

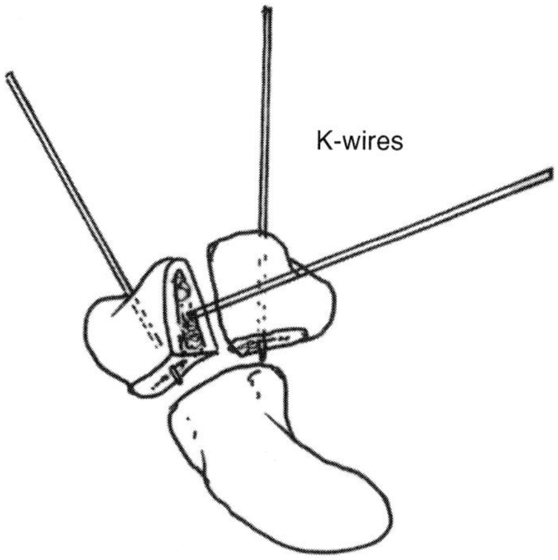

Figure 48–4

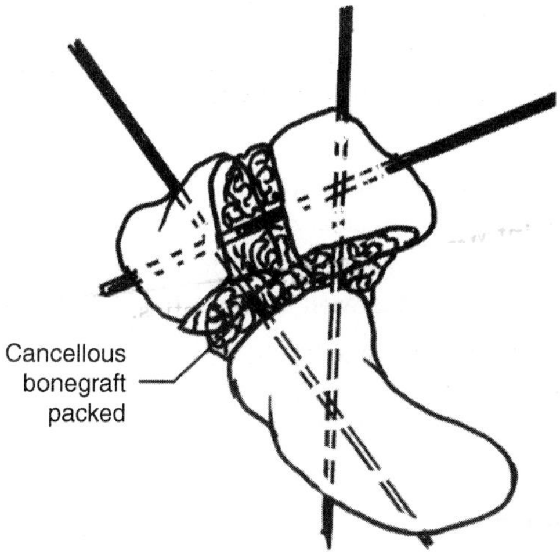

Figure 48–5

- The wire positions are adjusted to ensure passage across the arthrodesis site and engagement of the scaphoid. The wire lengths are adjusted to reside just within the trapezium or trapezoid bone. Accurate placement of the wires is essential because subsequent bone grafting will obscure visualization of wire alignment.
- Bone graft is harvested from the distal radius from either a second transverse incision over the distal radius or a proximal extension of the radial zigzag incision.
- The bone graft is packed into the depths of the fusion site to maintain the external dimensions of the STT joint. The preset wires are advanced into the scaphoid to secure the arthrodesis site (**Fig. 48–5**).
- Additional bone graft is densely packed into the spaces between the scaphoid, trapezium, and trapezoid. The position of the wires is verified using fluoroscopy from AP, lateral, and oblique projections.
- The pins are cut beneath the skin.
- A radial styloidectomy is performed to prevent radial styloid impingement. The styloid is exposed by subperiosteal elevation of the first compartment. Removal of 5 to 8 mm is performed to relieve scaphoid impingement without detachment of the radioscaphocapitate or radiolunate ligament.

■ Pearls

Use a high-speed burr in patients with extremely hard bone.

- Accurate placement of the preset Kirschner wires is essential because subsequent bone grafting obscures visualization of wire position and x-rays are hard to interpret.
- Scaphoid reduction is usually not required when performing STT arthrodesis for STT osteoarthritis. The scaphoid is already positioned in the recommended 45 to 50 degree angle to the long axis of the radius.

Pitfalls

Injury to either or both the radial sensory nerves and the lateral antebrachial cutaneous branches can lead to painful neuromas.

- Avoid narrowing of the STT joint because the surrounding joint will be adversely affected.
- Screw fixation is not recommended for fear of midcarpal compression and altered kinematics.
- Excessive radial styloidectomy will detach the radioscaphocapitate or radiolunate ligament or both.
- Nonunion rates are high (4–20%). Proper bone resection and accurate internal fixation are mandatory.

Postoperative Care

- The extremity is initially immobilized in a compressive dressing and short arm thumb spica splint with the thumb interphalangeal joint free.
- Elevation and finger motion are encouraged immediately following the procedure.
- Ten to 14 days after surgery, the sutures are removed and the splint changed to a short arm thumb spica cast. This cast must provide proper padding over the pins, which are frequently palpable beneath the skin.
- The pins are removed 8 weeks after the procedure if radiographs show adequate healing. A thermoplastic splint is then fabricated and active wrist motion initiated. The patient is gradually weaned from the splint over the ensuing 3 to 4 weeks.
- Strengthening and passive motion are commenced 12 weeks after surgery.

Alternative Techniques

- Scaphotrapezial fusion can be performed via a volar trans–flexor carpi radialis approach.
- Distal scaphoid excision
- Carpo-metacarpal joint arthroplasty for pantrapezial disease

Suggested Readings

Kozin SH. The surgical treatment of scaphotrapeziotrapezoid osteoarthritis. Hand Clin 2001;17:303–314

Watson HK, Weinzweig J, Guidera PM, et al. One thousand intercarpal arthrodeses. J Hand Surg [Br] 1999; 24(3): 307–315

49 Scaphotrapeziotrapezoid Joint Arthroplasty

Indications

Long-standing scaphotrapeziotrapezoid (STT) arthritis recalcitrant to nonoperative treatment

Technique

- Dorsoradial incision that begins at Lister's tubercle, traverses the anatomical snuffbox, and ends at the scaphotrapeziotrapezoid (STT) joint. Incision can be curved or zigzag configuration **(Fig. 49–1).**
- Protect the radial sensory nerves and lateral antebrachial cutaneous branches using loupe magnification.
- Expose the STT joint between the extensor pollicis brevis (EPB) (first compartment) and extensor pollicis longus (EPL) tendons. The deep branch of the radial artery resides just proximal to the STT joint and must be protected **(Fig. 49–2)**.
- A longitudinal arthrotomy is performed from the radial styloid to the distal scaphoid (S). The distal scaphoid fragment is identified.

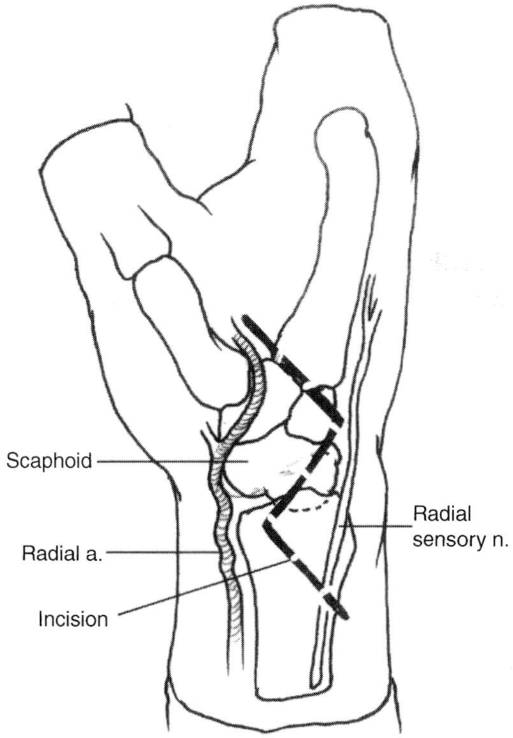

Figure 49–1

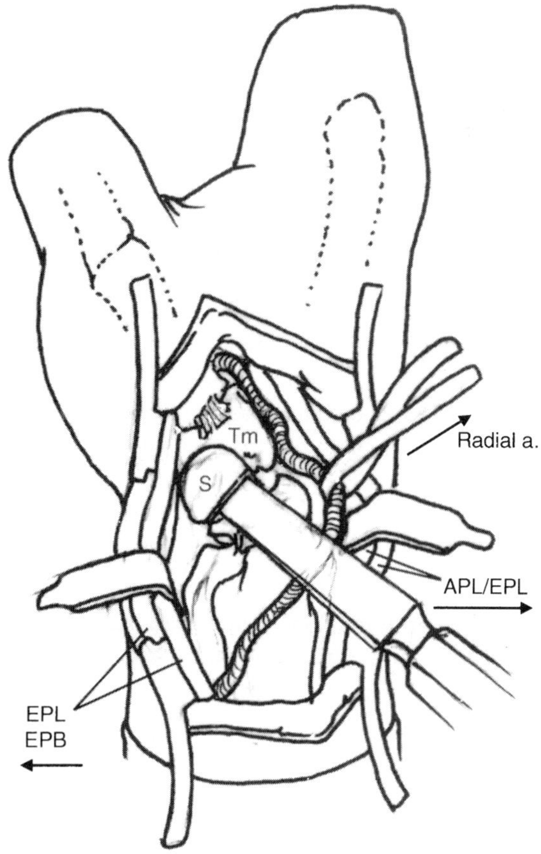

Figure 49–2

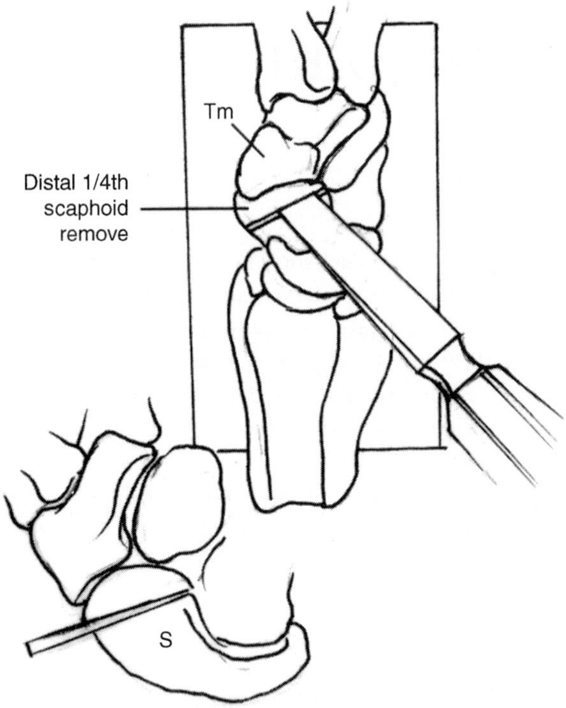

Figure 49–3

- The distal one fourth to one third of the scaphoid is removed with an oscillating saw or osteotome. Sharp dissection of the volar carpal ligaments around the distal scaphoid is required (**Fig. 49–3**).
- An elongated radial styloid may prevent adequate exposure of the scaphoid. This enlarged styloid can be removed by subperiosteal exposure of the first compartment followed by radial styloidectomy.
- Adequate excision has been performed when there is no impingement between the remaining scaphoid and the trapeziotrapezoid joint during on wrist motion.
- The arthrotomy is closed by reapproximation of the capsular flap. The EPL is left transposed from its third compartment if transposition is needed for exposure.

■ Pearls

A needle can be inserted into the STT joint to verify its location by fluoroscopy and facilitate exposure.

- A threaded pin can be inserted into the distal fragment to facilitate excision.

■ Pitfall

Injury to either or both the radial sensory nerves and the lateral antebrachial cutaneous branches can lead to painful neuromas.

Postoperative Care

- Splint wrist in neutral position for two weeks.
- Subsequent active and active-assisted range of motion
- Strengthening is instituted as motion improves over time.

Alternative Techniques

- Distal scaphoid excision can also be performed via a volar trans–flexor carpi radialis approach (similar to a volar exposure for a scaphoid nonunion). The distal scaphoid is excised in a similar fashion and the adequacy of resection evaluated by any residual impingement during wrist during motion. The volar approach is reserved for cases with concomitant flexor carpi radialis tendonitis requiring decompression.
- STT joint arthrodesis
- Carpo-metacarpal joint arthroplasty for pantrapezial disease

Suggested Readings

Garcia-Elias M, Lluch AL, Farreres A, et al. Resection of the distal scaphoid for scaphotrapeziotrapezoid osteoarthritis. J Hand Surg [Br] 1999;24: 448–452

Section VI.8

The Wrist Joint: Rheumatoid and Post-traumatic Arthritis

50 Arthroscopic Synovectomy

Indications

- Chronic synovitis from inflammatory arthritis that is unresponsive to medical management

Pitfall

Results are less predictable if radiographs demonstrate joint erosions.

Technique

- Standard wrist arthroscopy setup is used.
- Use the 3–4, 4–5 or 6R, and radial and ulnar (RMC-UMC) midcarpal portals to inspect the joint and for synovectomy (**Fig. 50–1**).
- Shaver, punch, and radiofrequency devices can all be used.

Pitfall

Establish high fluid outflow to avoid excessive heat if radiofrequency devices are used.

- Use a systematic approach beginning from the center of the radiocarpal joint and progressing radial and ulnar.

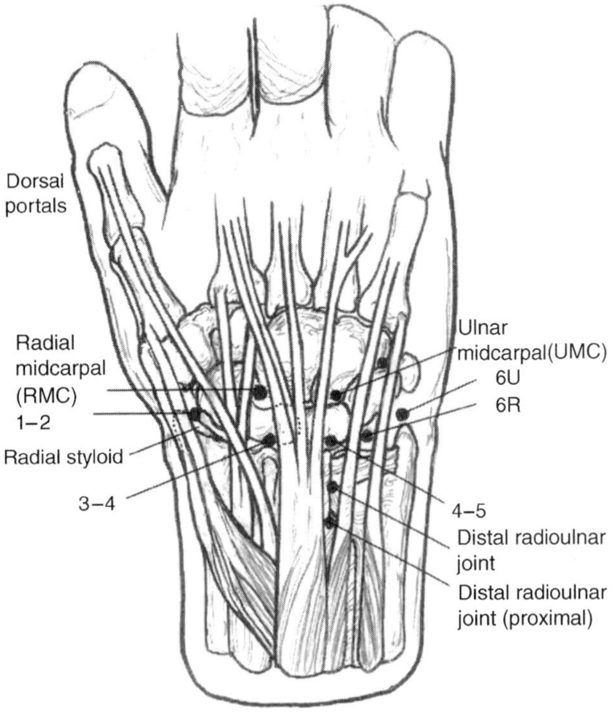

Figure 50–1

- Synovitis is typically greatest in the prestyloid recess, along the dorsal capsule, and near the radial styloid (**Fig. 50–2A–C**).

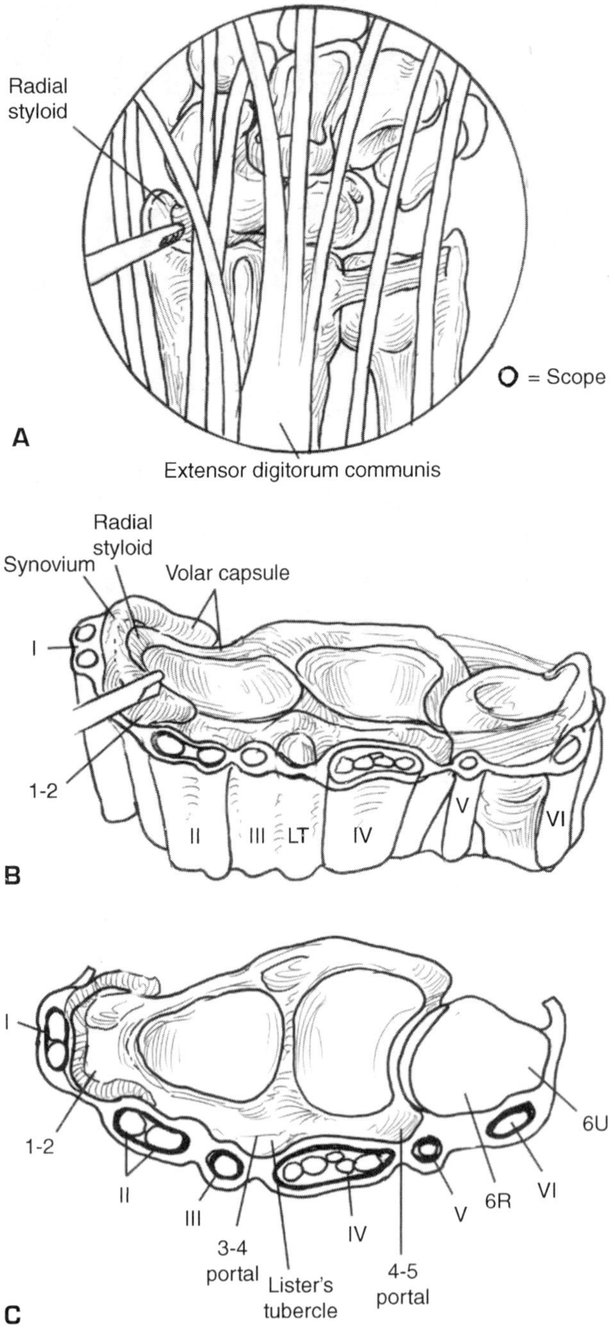

Figure 50–2

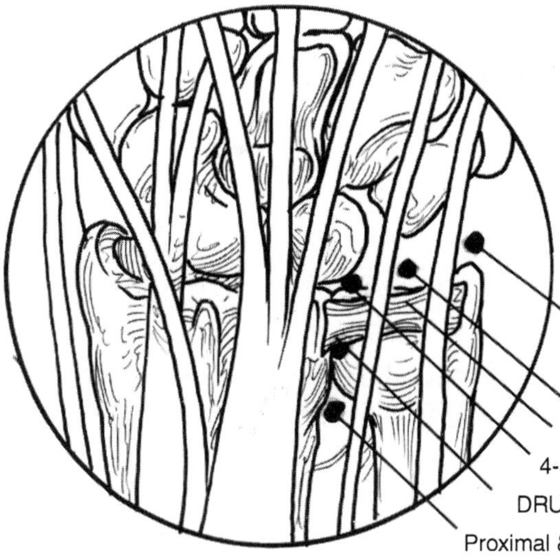

Figure 50–3

■ Pearl

To complete the synovectomy in the radial aspect of the wrist, a 1–2 portal may be needed.

- If the distal radioulnar joint (DRUJ) is involved, combined proximal and distal DRUJ portals are established.
- The arthroscope and shaver are interchanged to complete the synovectomy of the proximal DRUJ pouch and beneath the triangular fibrocartilage complex (TFCC) (**Fig. 50–3**).

■ Pearl

Arthroscopic DRUJ synovectomy is difficult; as an alternative, a dorsal open approach to the DRUJ can be done safely following radiocarpal and midcarpal arthroscopy.

Postoperative Care

- Apply a soft dressing and begin gentle motion immediately.
- Strengthening exercises are begun at the first postoperative visit.

Alternative Technique

- Open synovectomy

Suggested Readings

Adolfsson L, Frisen M. Arthroscopic synovectomy of the rheumatoid wrist: a 3.8-year follow-up. J Hand Surg [Br] 1997;22B:711–713

Adolfsson L, Nylander G. Arthroscopic synovectomy of the rheumatoid wrist. J Hand Surg [Br] 1993;18B:92–96

51 Extensor Carpi Radialis Longus to Extensor Carpi Ulnaris Tendon Transfer

Indications

- Radial deviation of the wrist with reduced capacity for active ulnar deviation due to an inflammatory arthropathy.
- Post-traumatic extensor carpi ulnaris (ECU) disruption with radial deviation of the wrist.

■ Pitfall

Inability to passively correct the wrist deformity and diminished extensor carpi radialis longus (ECRL) or extensor carpi radialis brevis (ECRB) function are contraindications.

Technique

- A dorsal, midline, longitudinal 6–8 cm incision is made, centered over the rim of the radius.
- Full-thickness skin flaps are raised, including the veins, nerves, and subcutaneous fat.
- The sixth extensor compartment is opened, the ECU is extracted, and a tenosynovectomy is performed.

■ Pearl

The entire retinaculum is raised as a radially based flap to the septum between the first and second compartments if a more complete dorsal tenosynovectomy is necessary.

- The ECRL is sharply released from its insertion on the base of the second metacarpal.
- If the second compartment has been opened for a tenosynovectomy, the ECRL is dissected free from surrounding tissue.
- When the second compartment is intact, the tendon is identified proximal to the retinaculum and carefully dissected from within the compartment while applying traction until it is free.
- Repair the retinaculum leaving the ECU and ECRL tendons superficial to it (**Fig. 51–1**).

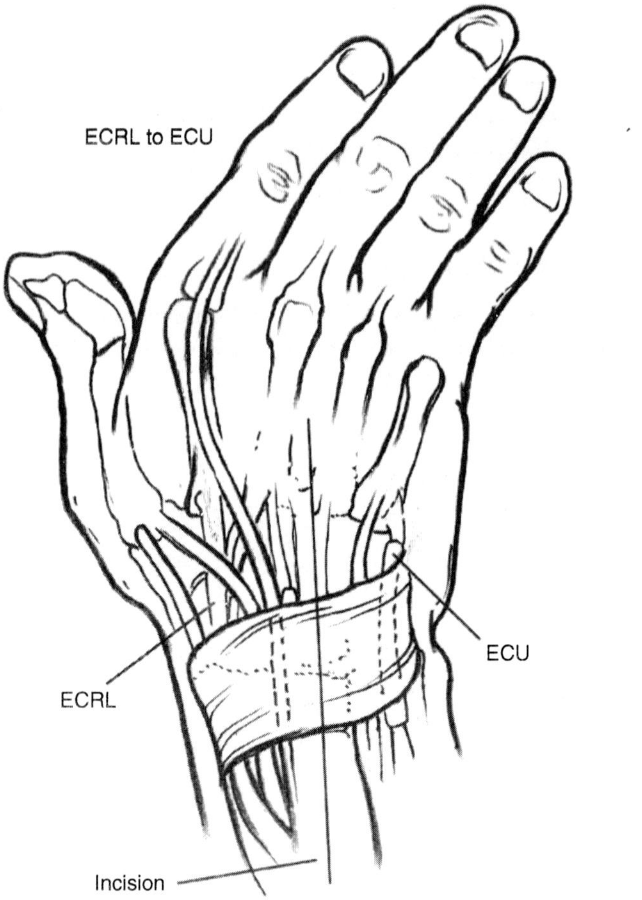

Figure 51–1

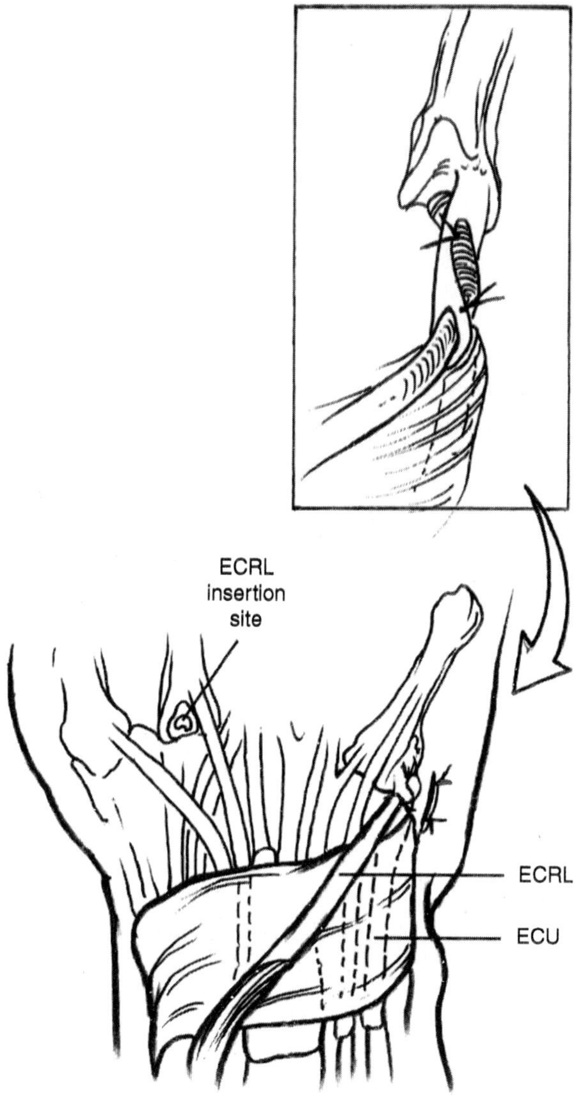

Figure 51–2

■ Pearl

One half of the extensor retinaculum can be placed deep to all tendons to reinforce an attenuated wrist capsule.

- The free distal end of the ECRL tendon is woven into the ECU tendon ~1 cm proximal to its insertion and secured with sutures.
- The transfer is tensioned to hold the wrist in neutral position (**Fig. 51–2**).

■ Pitfall

Make sure the ECRL tendon is not kinked by fascia, especially near its musculotendinous junction.

- A suction drain is inserted if needed and the skin closed.

Postoperative Care

- A standard dressing with a wrist plaster splint is applied with the wrist in 30 degrees of extension.
- Convert to a short arm cast with the wrist maintained in 30 degrees of extension until 4 weeks postoperative.
- Begin gentle range of motion exercises while using a splint for an additional 2 weeks.

Alternative Techniques

1. Radiocarpal fusion, total wrist arthrodesis, or wrist implant arthroplasty may be required in more advance disease.

Suggested Readings

Boyce T, Youm Y, Sprague BL, Flatt AE. Clinical and experimental studies on the effect of extensor carpi radialis longus transfer in the rheumatoid hand. J Hand Surg [Am] 1978;3A:390–394

Clayton ML, Ferlic DC. Tendon transfer for radial rotation of the wrist in rheumatoid arthritis. Clin Orthop 1974;100:176–185

52 Radiocarpal Fusion

Indications

- Radioscapholunate (RSL) fusion for post-traumatic radiocarpal arthritis
- Radiolunate (RL) fusion to prevent ulnocarpal subluxation in rheumatoid arthritis (RA).

Technique

- Remove articular cartilage and subchondral plate down to bleeding cancellous bone from reciprocal surfaces of scaphoid (S), lunate (L), and radius (**Fig. 52–1**).
- Retrograde 0.062 in. pins through scaphoid and lunate.

■ Pearl

Pins in lunate pass through triquetrum without fusing lunotriquetral joint.

- Reduce lunate and scaphoid so that the radiolunate
- Radiolunate (RL) angle is 0 degrees on a lateral radiograph.
- Advance pins. Check reduction with intraoperative imaging (**Fig. 52–2**).
- For RL fusion, remove articular cartilage and subchondral bone from reciprocal surfaces of lunate and radius.

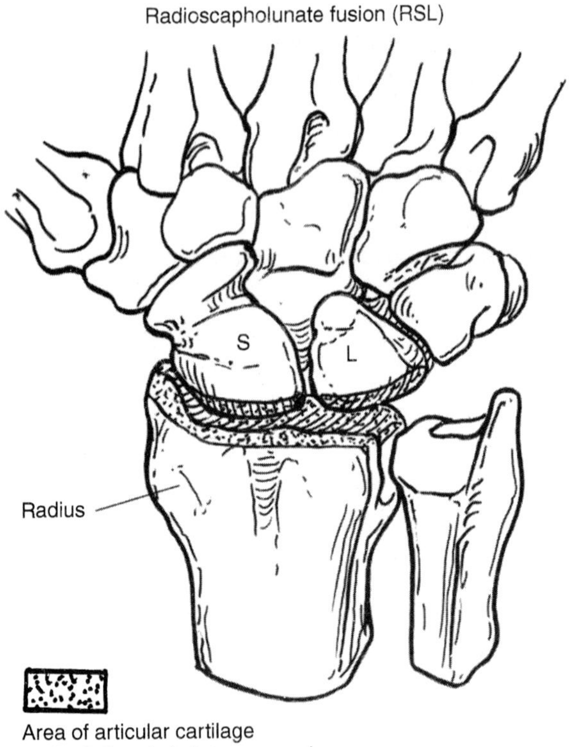

Figure 52–1

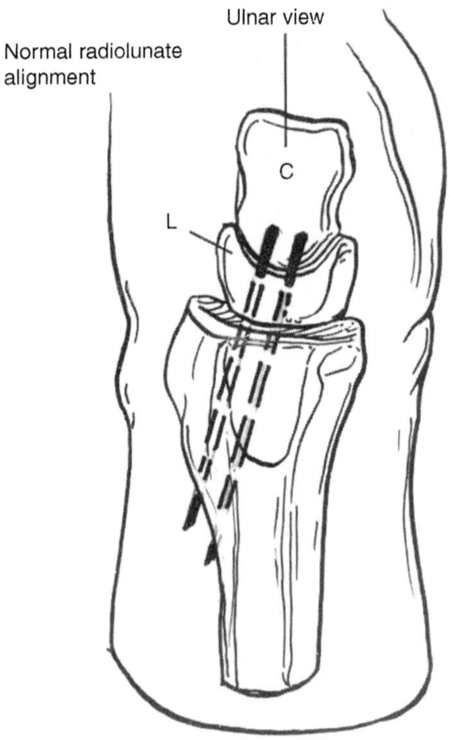

Figure 52–2

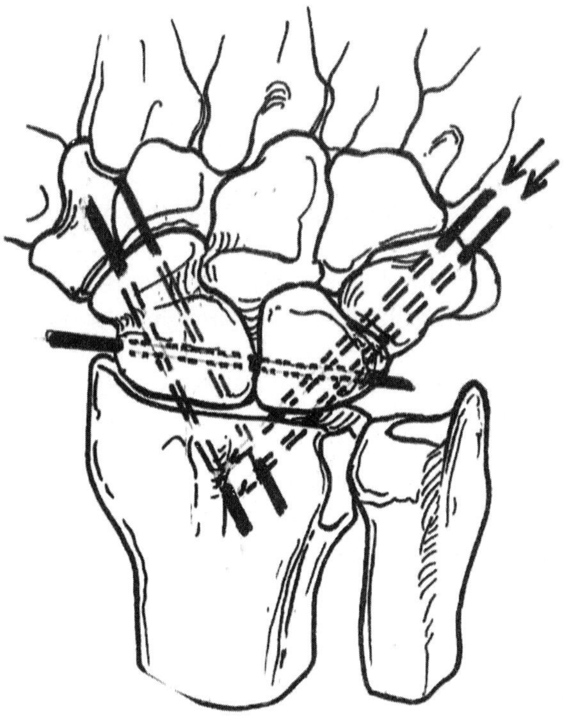

Figure 52–3

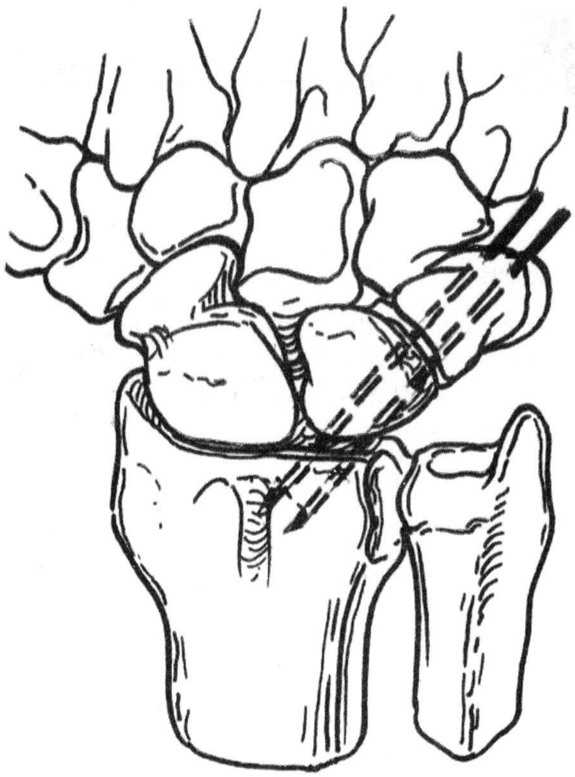

Figure 52–4

- Retrograde two 0.062 in. pins into lunate (**Fig. 52–3**).
- Reduce lunate on radius.
- Advance pins across RL joint (**Fig. 52–4**).
- Check image.
- Assess distal radioulnar joint (DRUJ). Decide if hemi- or complete resection of distal ulna is necessary.
- For both fusions cut pins beneath skin.

■ Pearl

Ensure that cut ends of pins don't interfere with extensor tendon excursion.

Alternative Technique

- Can consider screw or plate fixation
- Resection of the distal pole of the scaphoid may improve wrist motion post-operatively by unlocking the midcarpal joint.

Postoperative Care

- Encourage finger motion.
- Short arm splint for 2 weeks
- Short arm cast until fusion healed, usually 6 to 8 weeks

Suggested Readings

Halikis MN, Colello-Abraham K, Taleisnik J. Radiolunate fusion: the forgotten partial arthrodesis. Clin Orthop 1997;341:30–35

Linscheid RL, Dobyns JH. Radiolunate arthrodesis. J Hand Surgery [Am] 1985;10A:821–829

Nagy L, Buchler U. Long-term results of radioscapholunate fusion following fractures of the distal radius. J Hand Surg [Br] 1997;22(6):705–710

53 Total Wrist Arthrodesis

Indications

- Post-traumatic, rheumatoid, or osteoarthritis with radiocarpal and midcarpal degeneration
- Bone loss or deformity due to infection or tumor
- Fixed wrist deformity from neurological deficit

Technique

- A dorsal, longitudinal 10 to 12 cm skin incision is centered over Lister's tubercle (**Fig. 53–1**).
- The extensor retinaculum is incised through the third dorsal compartment.
- Extensor pollicis longus (EPL) is transposed radially.
- Make a longitudinal incision through the periosteum and capsule from the midshaft of the third metacarpal, across the wrist joint, and in the floor of the third extensor compartment.
- Capsular flaps are raised off the carpus in both the radial and ulnar directions.
- Resect a segment of the posterior interosseous nerve as it enters the dorsal wrist capsule.
- The dorsal surface of the distal radius is exposed by subperiosteal elevation of the second and fourth extensor compartments (**Fig. 53–2**)

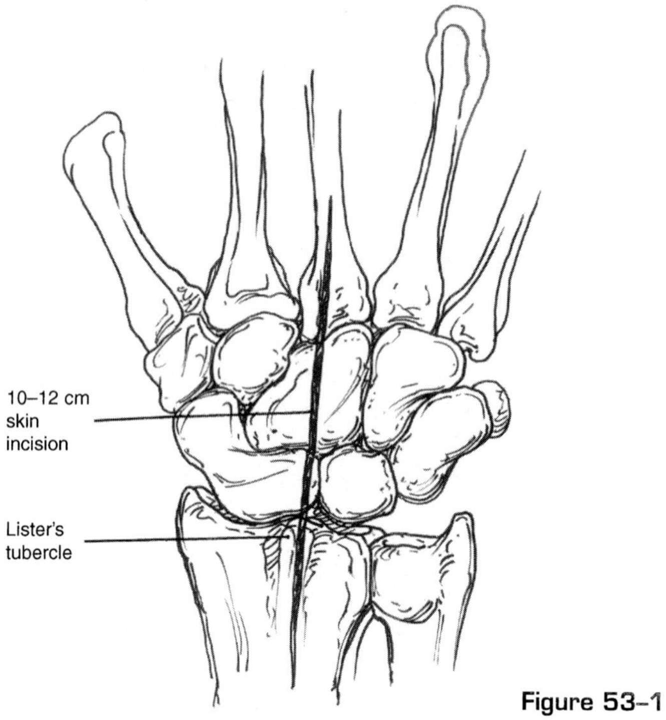

Figure 53–1

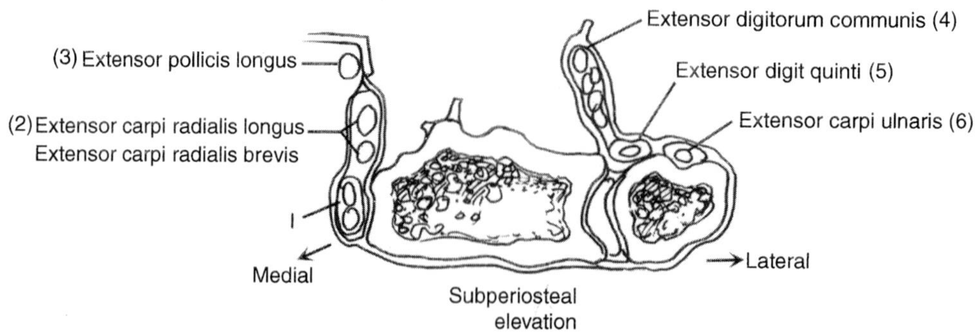

Figure 53–2

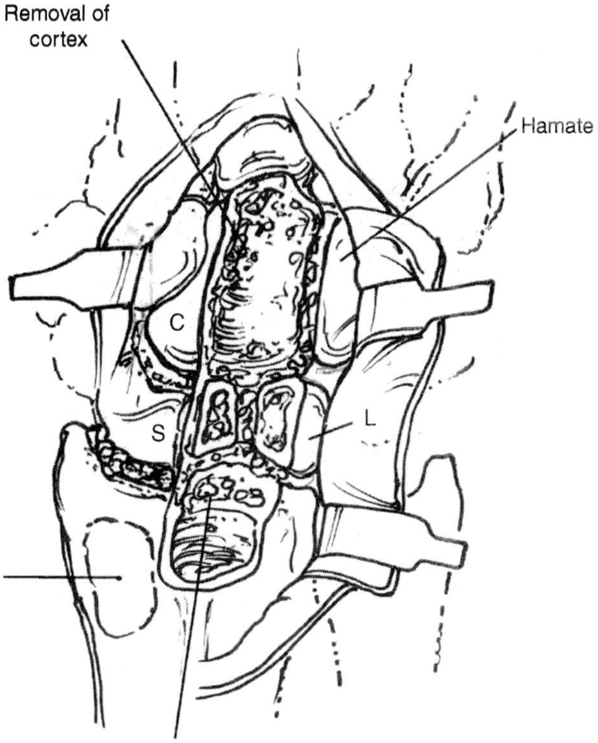

Figure 53–3

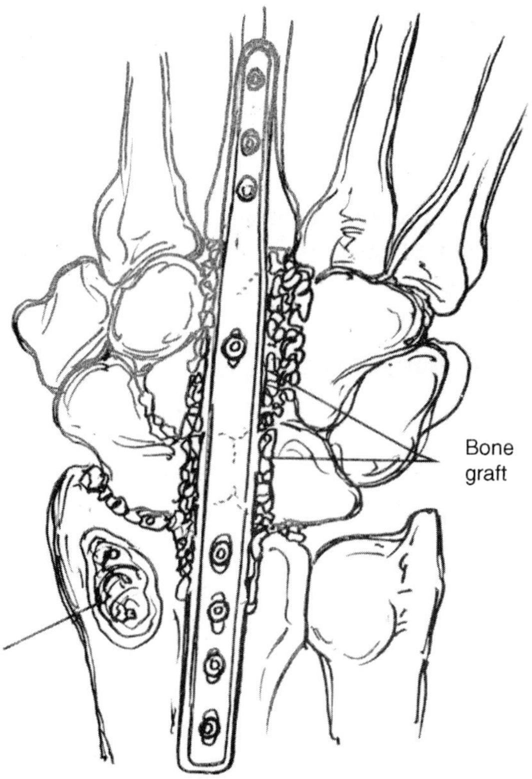

Figure 53–4

Pitfall

With the exception of the third compartment, do not open the extensor compartments. This reduces the risk of tendon adhesions.

- Remove Lister's tubercle to provide a flat surface over the dorsal aspect of the distal radius.
- The dorsal surfaces of the scaphoid (S), lunate (L), capitate (C), and third carpometacarpal joint are removed.
- Excise the remaining cartilage and subchondral bone from the articular surfaces of the intercarpal, third carpometacarpal, and radiocarpal joints (**Fig. 53–3**).
- In some cases, the volar-most portions of the intercarpal and carpometacarpal joint surfaces can be retained to maintain anatomical intercarpal spacing and wrist height.

Pitfall

Include the third carpometacarpal joint in the fusion to reduce the risk of fatigue fracture of the plate.

- Bone graft is obtained from the distal radius or from the iliac crest if there are large bone defects.
- A wrist arthrodesis plate is chosen to span from the third metacarpal shaft to the distal radius. Attempt to engage six cortices with screws through the plate into both the metacarpal and distal radius.

Pearl

A precontoured, dedicated wrist arthrodesis plate will reduce the risk of tendon irritation.

- Pack bone graft into the previously prepared spaces intended for fusion.
- Insert screws in the metacarpal first to ensure proper length and fit of the plate.
- The proximal screws are then inserted, which should put the wrist in ~15 degrees of extension (**Fig. 53–4**).

Pitfall

Ensure the joint is not distracted following insertion of the proximal screws.

- The distal ulna is retained unless there is arthritis of the distal radioulnar joint.
- Confirm proper plate position and screw lengths with fluoroscopy.
- Fill remaining gaps in the fusion site with bone graft.

- Close the capsule over the plate.
- Partially close the retinaculum, leaving the EPL superficial to it.
- Close the skin over a suction drain.

Postoperative Care

- A bulky dressing is applied with a plaster splint to support the wrist.
- A removable wrist splint is used for 6 weeks.
- Full activity is allowed at 12 weeks if radiographs show fusion.

Alternative Techniques

- Intramedullary rods, staples, or large corticocancellous grafts with screws can be used for fixation.
- Total wrist prosthetic replacement

Suggested Readings

Millender LH, Nalebuff EA. Arthrodesis of the rheumatoid wrist: an evaluation of sixty patients and a description of a different surgical technique. J Bone Joint Surg Am 1973;55:1026–1034

Weiss AP, Hastings H II. Wrist arthrodesis for traumatic conditions: a study of plate and local bone graft application. J Hand Surg [Am] 1995;20A:50–56

54 Total Wrist Arthroplasty

Indications

- Rheumatoid arthritis and low-demand patients with post-traumatic or osteoarthritis involving both the radiocarpal and midcarpal joints

Technique

- A dorsal, longitudinal 10 to 12 cm skin incision is made centered over Lister's tubercle.
- The extensor retinaculum is raised as a radially based flap from the sixth to the second compartments.
- The entire dorsal wrist capsule is raised as a distally based rectangular flap, including the periosteum over the distal radius, and, if the ulna is to be resected, the dorsal distal radioulnar joint (DRUJ) capsule (**Fig. 54–1**).
- For the Universal 2 total wrist system (KMI; Kinetos Medical Inc., Carlsbad, California), the intramedullary guide rod is inserted and the radial cutting guide is applied to resect the radius distal articular surface (**Fig. 54–2A,B**).

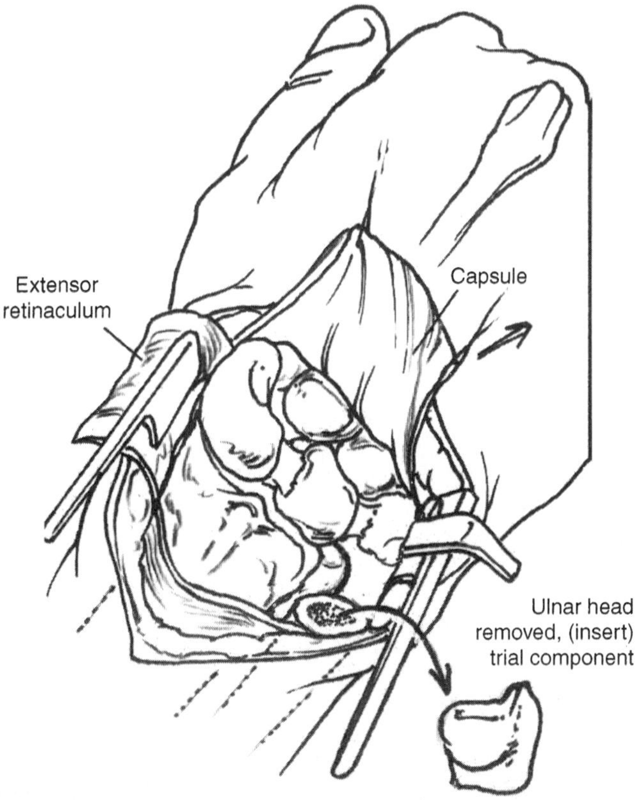

Figure 54–1

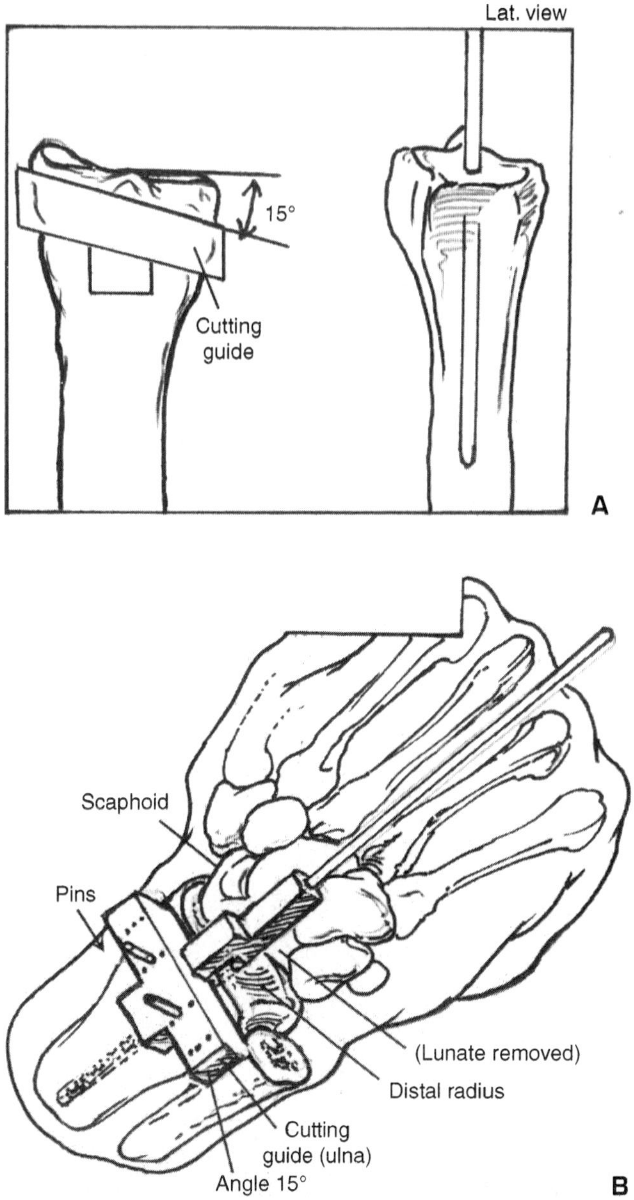

Figure 54–2

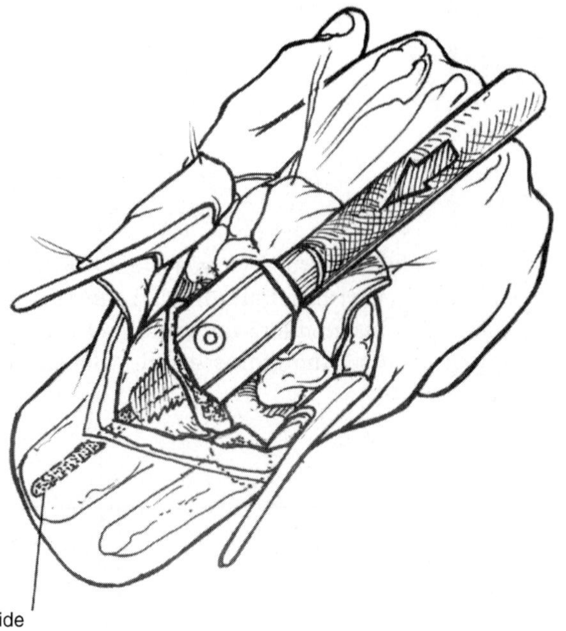

Figure 54–3

- Reinsert the guide rod and broach the radius to the proper size (**Fig. 54–3**).
- Insert the radial component trial; remove after confirming proper fit.

Pearl

The articular surface of the distal ulna is removed if there is distal radioulnar joint (DRUJ) arthrosis or severe erosion of the radius.

- The lunate (L) is removed by sharp dissection.
- Using the drill guide, a hole is created in the capitate (C) in line with the third metacarpal (**Fig. 54–4**).
- The carpal cutting guide is applied and the carpal osteotomy is made at the level of proximal pole of the hamate (H) (**Fig. 54–5A,B**).

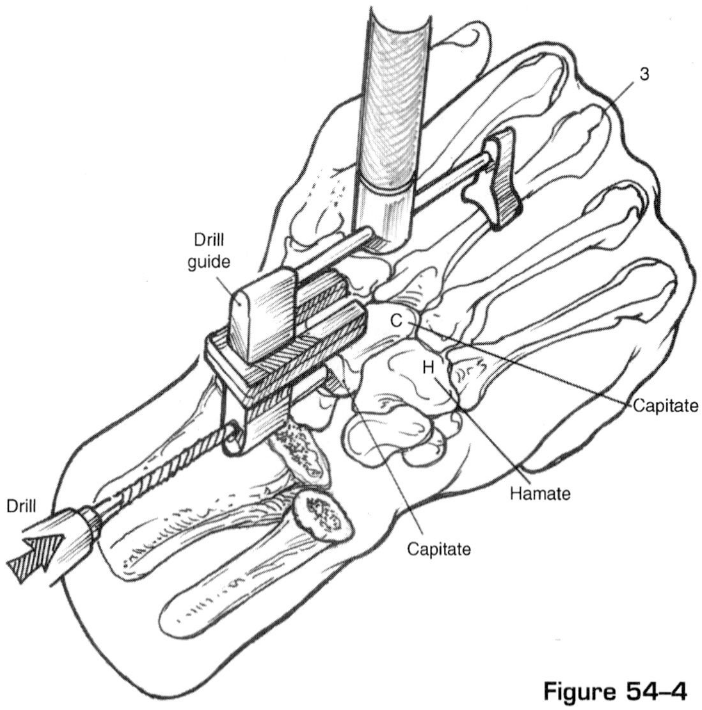

Figure 54–4

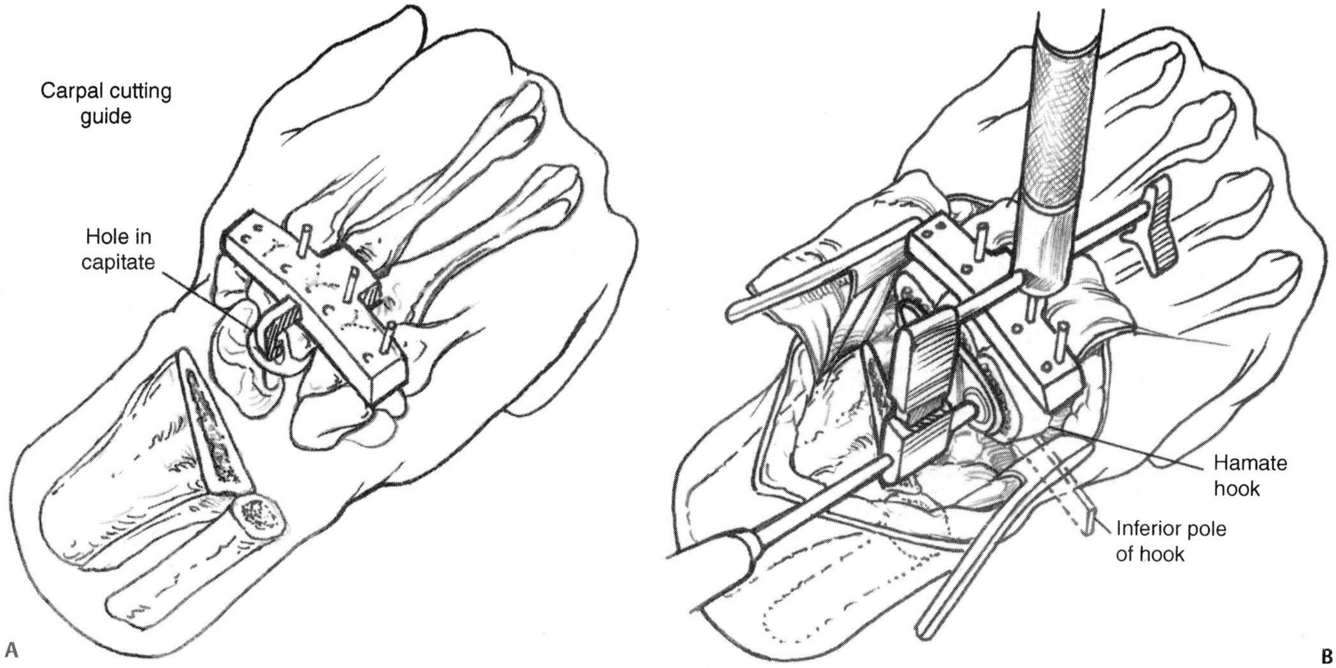

Figure 54–5

Pearl

Pinning the triquetrum to the hamate and the scaphoid(S) to the capitate will help maintain carpal alignment while making the saw cut.

- Insert the carpal component trial.
- Apply the drill guide to the carpal component and second metacarpal shaft; drill the hole for the radial screw and insert a trial screw (30–35 mm).
- Similarly, apply the drill guide to the carpal component and fourth metacarpal shaft; drill the hole for the ulnar screw, and insert a trial screw (15–20 mm) (**Fig. 54–6**).

Pitfall

Extend and hold the mobile fourth metacarpal in extension while drilling for the ulnar screw to avoid inserting it in a volar direction.

- Reinsert the radial trial component and apply the carpal polyethylene trial.
- Reduce the joint and test prosthetic stability and motion, which should be ~35 degrees each of flexion and extension.

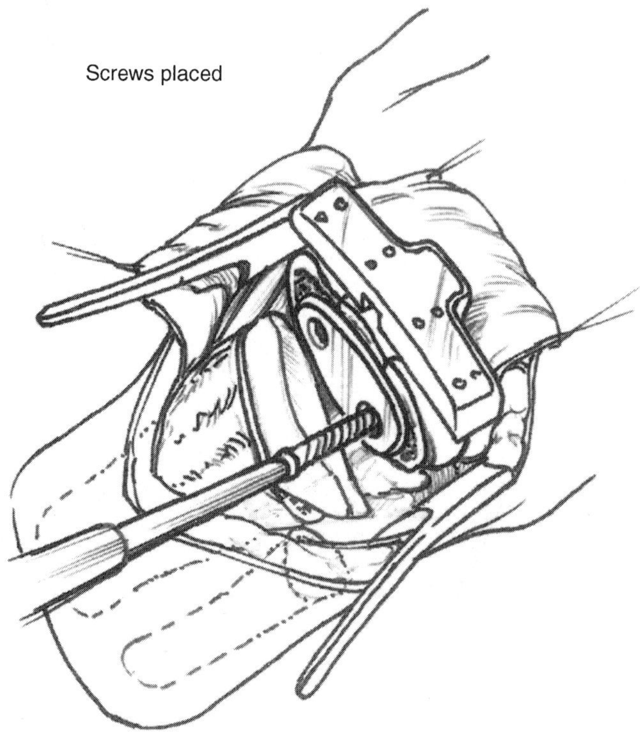

Figure 54–6

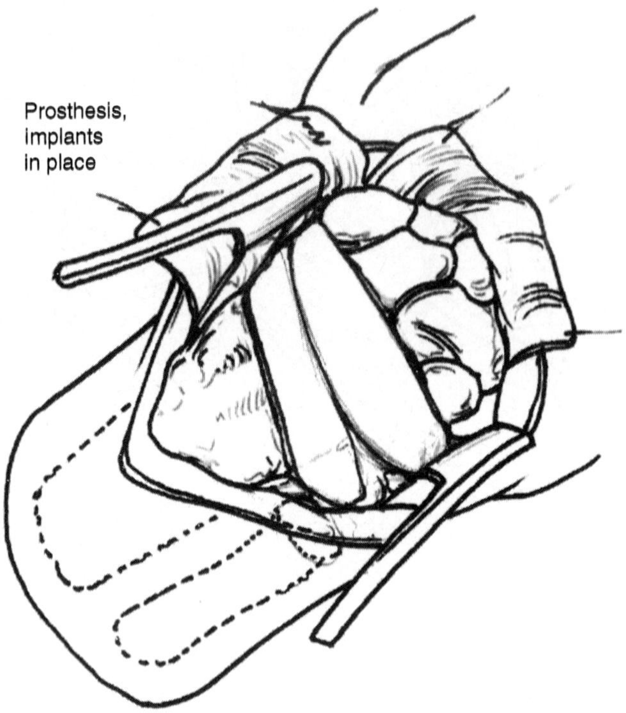

Figure 54–7

■ Pitfall

If the joint is too tight, remove more radius but do not release the palmar capsule or remove more carpus.

- Remove the trial components.
- Using a bur or curette, remove remaining cartilage and subchondral bone from the intercarpal surfaces between the scaphoid, capitate, hamate, and triquetrum and pack with cancellous bone chips.
- Insert the final metal components using the impactors and insert the final carpal screws.
- Apply the final polyethylene component; reduce the joint, and test motion and stability (**Fig. 54–7**).
- Close the capsule completely, augmenting with half of the extensor retinaculum or tensor fascia lata allograft if necessary.
- Close the skin over a suction drain.

Postoperative Care

- A bulky dressing is applied with a plaster splint to support the wrist.
- A removable wrist splint is used for 4 weeks.
- Gentle motion is started during the first week.
- Avoid strenuous activities for 8 weeks.

Alternative Techniques

- Total wrist arthrodesis

Suggested Readings

Cobb TK, Beckenbaugh RD. Biaxial total-wrist arthroplasty. J Hand Surg [Am] 1996;21(6):1011–1021

Divelbiss BJ, Sollerman C, Adams BD. Early results of the Universal total wrist arthroplasty in rheumatoid arthritis. J Hand Surg [Am] 2002;27(2):195–204

Section VI.9

The Wrist Joint: Kienböck Disease

55 Radial Shortening

Indications

Symptomatic Kienböck disease without lunate collapse (stages 0, I, or II) in a wrist with a positive ulnar variance

Technique

- Palmar incision over the flexor carpi radialis (FCR) tendon beginning at wrist crease and extending 8 to 10 cm up the forearm
- Open FCR tendon sheath and retract tendon in ulnar direction. Incise the floor of the tendon sheath.
- Identify and incise the pronator quadratus (PQ) along its radial margin and elevate from the distal radius (**Fig. 55–1A,B**).
- Place retractors on both sides of the radius. Expose enough of the radius to accommodate a six-hole dynamic compression plate (DCP) (**Fig. 55–2**). This exposure may require partial elevation of flexor pollicis longus (FPL) origin.
- Apply the six-hole DCP along distal radius. The distal aspect of the plate may have to be bent to match the palmar slope of the distal radius.

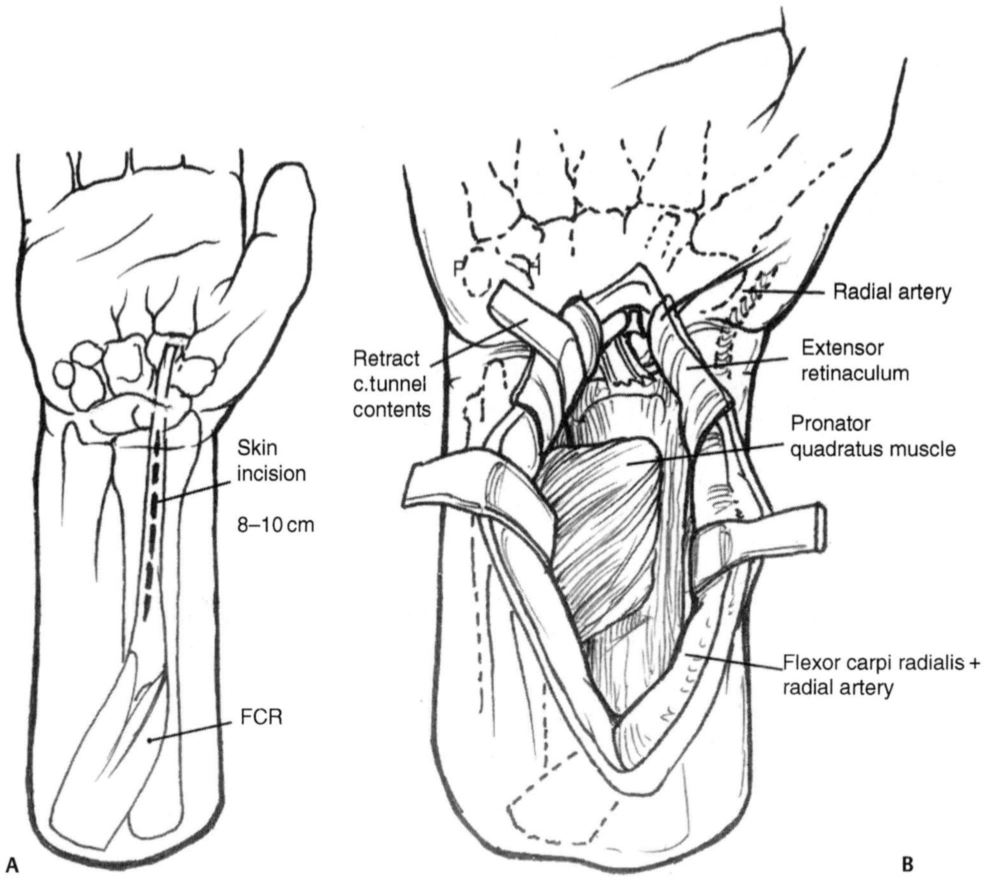

Figure 55–1

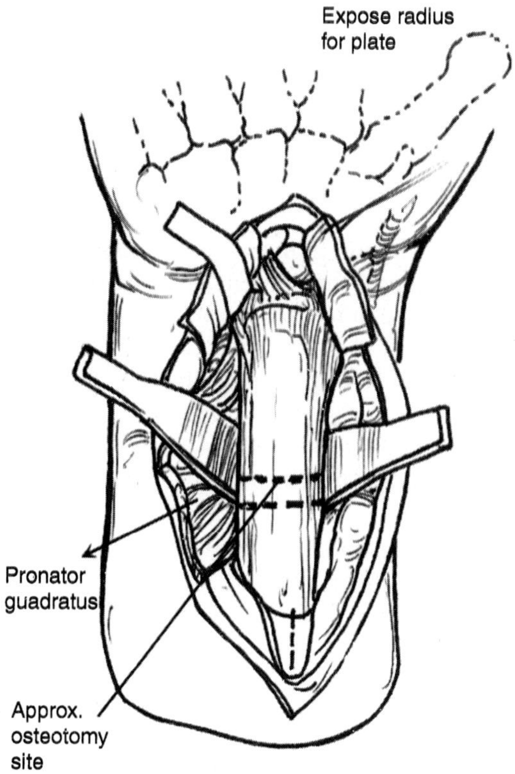

Figure 55–2

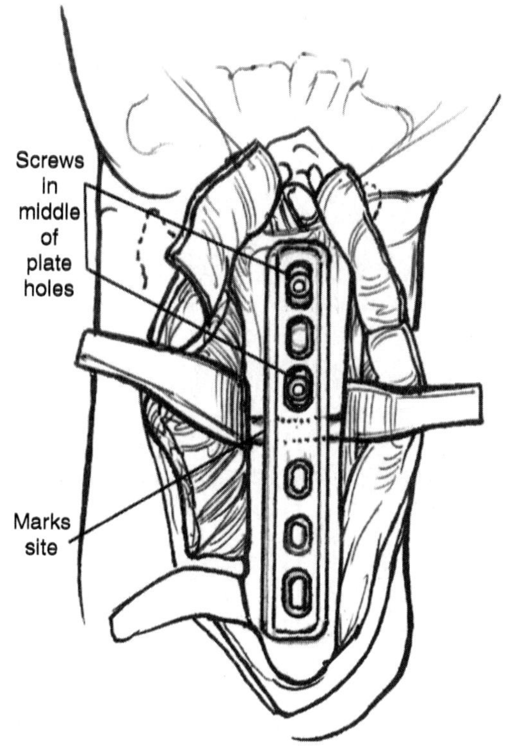

Figure 55–3

- Mark the osteotomy site between third and fourth holes in the plate. Place bicortical screws distal to the planned site of the osteotomy.

■ Pearl

The osteotomy should be performed in the metaphysis to increase the chance and rate of healing.

- Remove the screws and plate. Elevate the periosteum at osteotomy site.
- Make the first cut two thirds of the way through the radius. This cut can be either transverse or oblique to the long axis of the radius. A second cut is made parallel to the first, 2 to 4 mm proximal to the initial osteotomy. Complete the first cut and remove wafer of radius.
- Reapply the plate and distal screws. Compress the osteotomy by manual pressure until bone ends approximate. Hold with reduction clamp applied between the proximal plate and radius (**Fig. 55–3**).
- Secure the proximal portion of the plate using one or two compression screws to compress the osteotomy site. Place the remaining screws in neutral compression (**Fig. 55–4**).

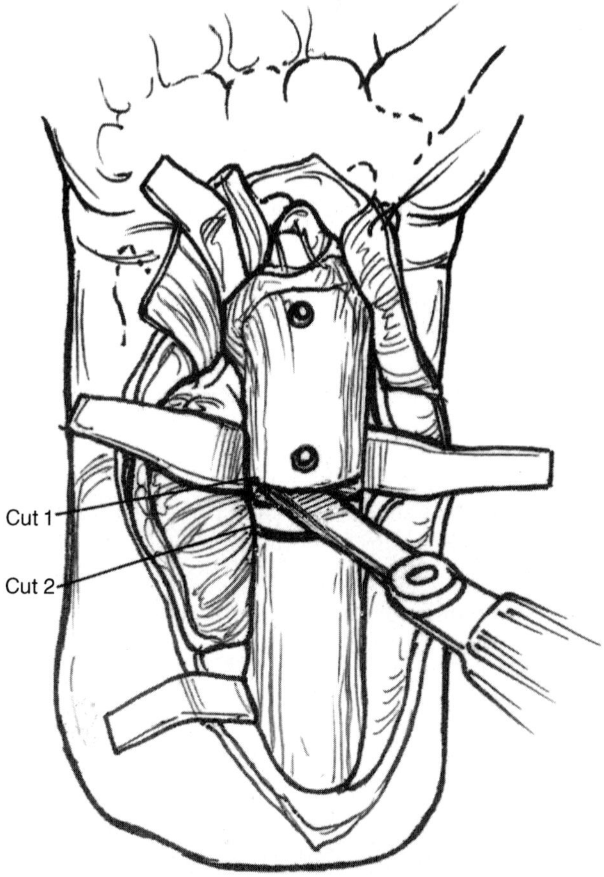

Figure 55–4

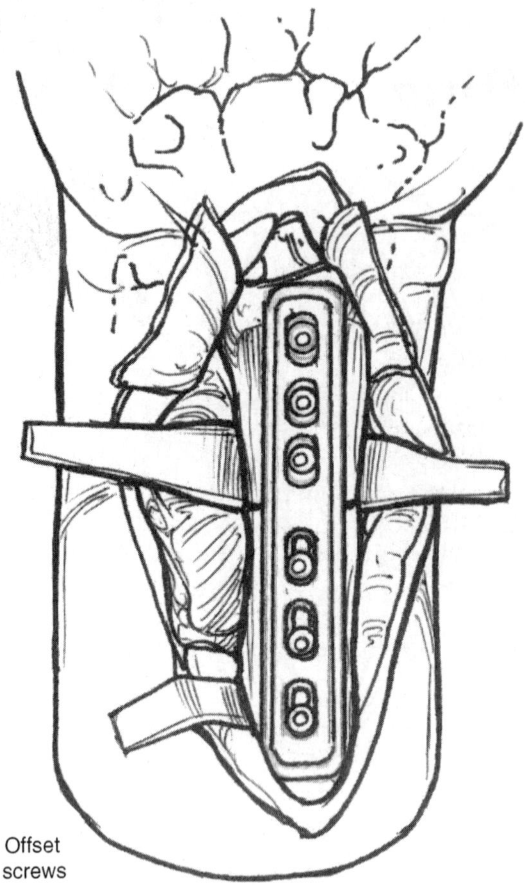

Figure 55–5

- Check the alignment of the osteotomized radius and the plate and screw position with fluoroscopy (**Fig. 55–5**).

■ Pearl

An oblique osteotomy made at a 45 degree angle to the long axis of the radius increases the surface available for healing and allows the surgeon to enhance compression across the osteotomy using a lag screw.

■ Pitfall

Avoid marginal fixation with a small plate.

Postoperative Care

- The extremity is initially immobilized in a compressive dressing and sugar-tong thumb spica splint. The forearm is positioned in neutral and the wrist slightly extended. Elevation and finger motion are encouraged immediately following the procedure.
- Ten to 14 days after surgery, the sutures are removed and the splint changed to a short arm cast. A reliable patient can be placed directly into a thermoplastic splint.
- The extremity is immobilized for 4 weeks. A thermoplastic splint is then fabricated and active and active-assisted motion instituted.
- Strengthening and passive motion are commenced 12 weeks after surgery.

Alternative Techniques

- Use compression device via unicortical screw placed proximal to plate to enhance compression across osteotomy site.
- Oblique osteotomy with interfragmentary fixation
- Jig designed for shortening osteotomies
- Osteotomy can be designed to change the radial inclination. Various authors recommend a decrease or increase in radial inclination. Most favor an increase in slope via a medial closing wedge.
- Ulna lengthening

Suggested Readings

Nakamura T, Imaeda T, Miura T. Radial shortening for Kienböck's disease: factors affecting the operative result. J Hand Surg [Br] 1990;15(1):40–45

Nakamura R, Satoshi T, Watanabe K, Tsunoda K. Radial wedge osteotomy for Kienböck's disease. J Bone Joint Surg Am 1991;73A:1391–1396

Weiss APC, Weiland AJ, Moore R, Wilgis EFS. Radial shortening for Kienböck's disease. J Bone Joint Surg Am 1991;73A:384–391

56 Vascularized Bone Grafting for Kienböck Disease

Indications

Vascularized bone grafts (VBGs) can be used for revascularization in early or advanced Kienböck disease with an ulnar neutral or plus variance as long as the cartilage shell is intact and no arthrosis is found. VBGs can also be used as an adjunctive procedure to radial shortening in patients with an ulnar minus variance. This technique is not indicated when there is fragmentation of the lunate or arthritis.

Technique

- Longitudinal dorsal incision that begins just ulnar to Lister's tubercle and extends to the base of the third metacarpal (**Fig. 56–1**)
- Protect the radial sensory nerves and lateral antebrachial cutaneous branches using loupe magnification. Elevate flaps at the level of the extensor retinaculum.
- The extensor digitorum communis compartment is identified and opened. The fourth extensor compartment artery (ECA) is identified deep to the tendons along the radial aspect. The fourth ECA is adjacent to the posterior interosseous nerve (PIN) (**Fig. 56–1**).
- The fourth ECA is dissected in a proximal direction to its origin from the posterior division of the anterior interosseous artery (AIA). At this site, the fifth ECA is located as it connects to the same division. The fifth ECA is dissected in a distal direction toward the dorsal intercarpal arch.
- The anterior interosseous artery is ligated proximal to the origins of the fourth and fifth ECAs to create a single pedicle (**Fig. 56–2**).
- A VBG is configured 1 cm proximal to the radiocarpal joint and centered over the fourth ECA. The

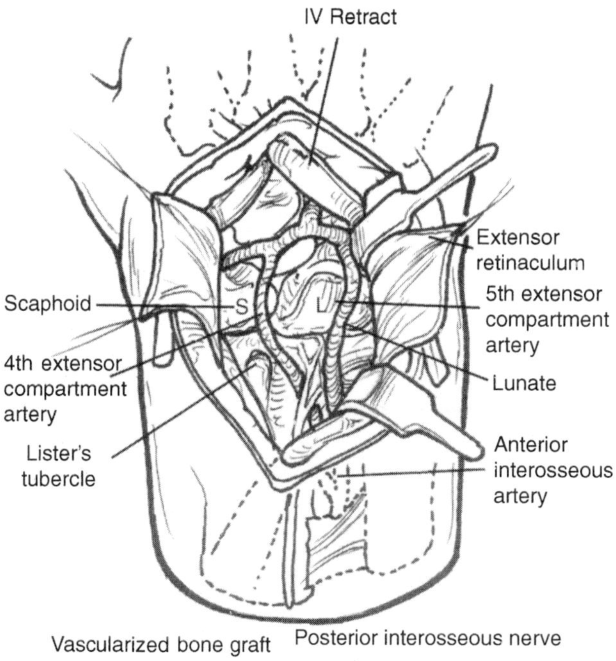

Figure 56–1

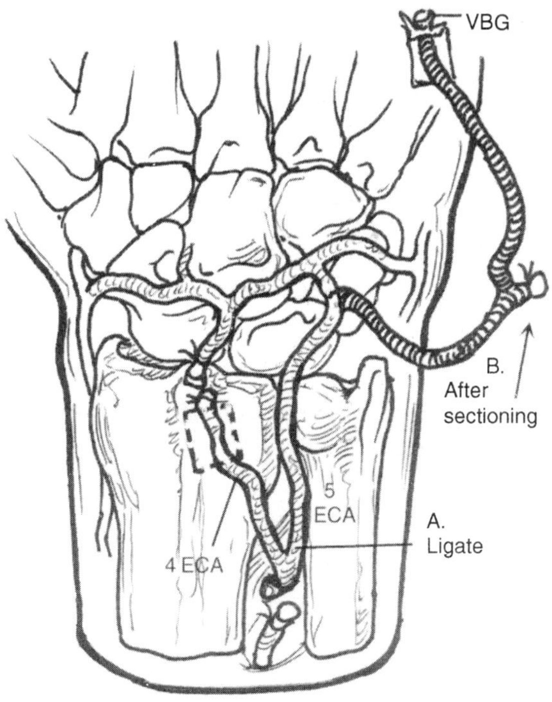

Figure 56–2

VBG is carefully harvested using small curved and straight osteotomes. The vascular pedicle is protected. The VBG is elevated on its common pedicle and retracted in an ulnar direction (**Fig. 56–2**).

- A longitudinal arthrotomy is performed over the lunate, which is inspected for shape and configuration. The cartilage shell of the lunate should be intact to accept a VBG. The shell must be preserved during manipulation of the lunate. The necrotic bone is removed using curettes via a dorsal window (**Fig. 56–3**). Any collapse is gently expanded in a sequential fashion.
- Additional cancellous bone graft is harvested from the distal radius using the cortical defect created by the harvest of the VBG. The bone graft is packed within the lunate.
- The tourniquet is deflated to verify blood flow with the VBG. The VBG is fashioned to wedge within the lunate and dorsal window. The cortical surface serves as a strut across the reconstituted lunate. The pedicle is protected during the insertion of the VBG (**Fig. 56–4**). Internal fixation is not used.
- An external fixator is applied to bridge the radiocarpal joint and unload the lunate during revascularization. Pins are inserted into the second metacarpal and radius using small incisions. A small amount of distraction is applied.

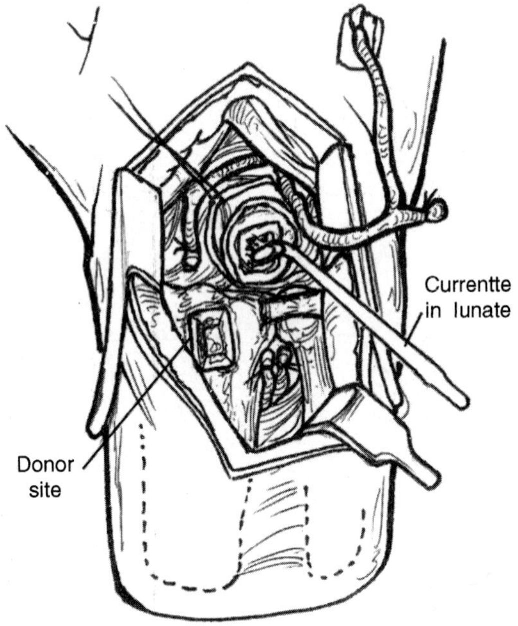

Figure 56–3

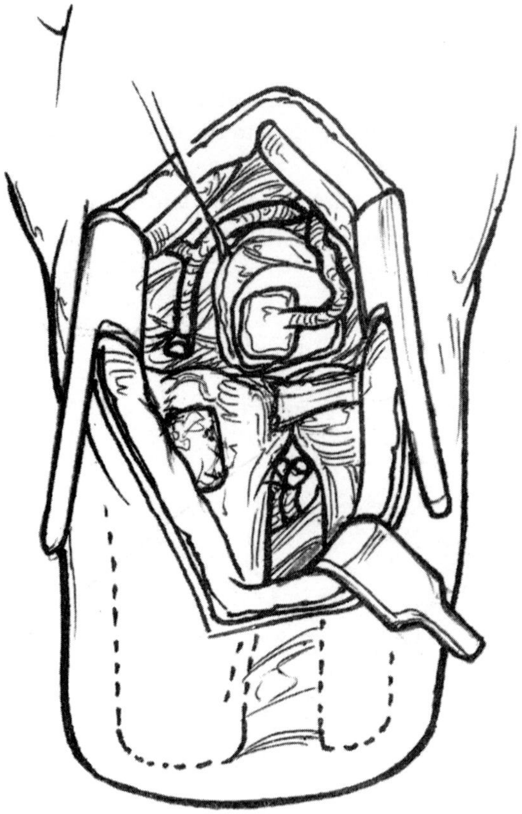

Figure 56–4

Pearls

Gentle exsanguination of the limb with an Ace bandage is used to facilitate identification of the vascular pedicles.

- The fourth and fifth ECAs are the preferred pedicle for Kienböck disease. The fourth can be used as a single pedicle or combined with the fifth ECA. This combination allows retrograde flow from the fifth ECA to flow orthograde into the fourth ECA via their common anterior interosseous artery.

Pitfalls

Failure to identify the VBG before capsulotomy may result in injury to its pedicle.

- Internal fixation of the VBG can disrupt limited blood supply and result in failure.
- Failure to unload the lunate during the revascularization process

Postoperative Care

- The extremity is initially immobilized in a compressive dressing and sugar-tong splint.
- Elevation and finger motion are encouraged immediately following the procedure.
- Ten to 14 days after surgery, the splint and sutures are removed. A splint is fabricated to protect the external fixator, and pin care is initiated.
- External fixator is removed 10 to 12 weeks after surgery. Active and active-assisted motion and therapy are started.
- Magnetic resonance imaging can be used to follow the revascularization process.

Alternative Techniques

- Alternative sources of VBGs are available, including alternative dorsal grafts and volar sources (e.g., the pronator quadratus and pisiform).
- The lunate must be unloaded during the revascularization process. This can be accomplished by a variety of techniques, including external fixation, intercarpal arthrodesis, or temporary scaphocapitate pinning.

Suggested Readings

Leung PC, Hung LK. Use of the pronator quadratus bone graft in bony reconstruction around the wrist. J Hand Surg [Am] 1990;15(4):637–640

Sheetz KK, Bishop AT, Berger RA. The arterial blood supply of the distal radius and ulna and its potential use in vascularized pedicled bone grafts. J Hand Surg [Am] 1995;20(6):902–914

Shin AY, Bishop AT. Pedicled vascularized bone grafts for disorders of the carpus: scaphoid nonunion and Kienböck's disease. J Am Acad Orthop Surg 2002;10:210–216

57 Capitate Shortening with Capitohamate Fusion

Indications

Symptomatic Kienböck disease without lunate (L) collapse (stages 0, I, or II) in a wrist with neutral or positive ulnar variance.

Technique

- Longitudinal dorsal incision that begins just ulnar to Lister's tubercle and extends to the base of the third metacarpal
- Protect the radial sensory nerves and lateral antebrachial cutaneous branches using loupe magnification. Elevate flaps at the level of the extensor retinaculum.
- The extensor pollicis longus (EPL) tendon is identified and the third compartment opened. The EPL tendon is transposed in a radial direction from the third compartment.
- The second compartment is elevated in a radial direction and the fourth compartment in an ulnar direction. The posterior interosseous nerve is located under the fourth compartment and resected.
- A longitudinal capsulotomy is performed to expose the underlying radiocarpal and midcarpal joints. The capsule may have to be elevated from the radius (inverted T capsulotomy) for adequate carpal exposure (**Fig. 57–1**).
- The capitate (C) and hamate (H) are exposed by capsular elevation. A capitate shortening (2–4 mm) is desegned at the level of the distal articular surface of the scaphoid (S).
- A thin osteotome is used to remove a wafer of bone from the capitate via two parallel cuts. The osteotome is driven partially through the capitate during the first cut and completely for the second. The osteotome is then replace into the first cut and the osteotomy completed followed by removal of the intervening bone fragment (**Fig. 57–2**). The volar capsule is not disrupted.

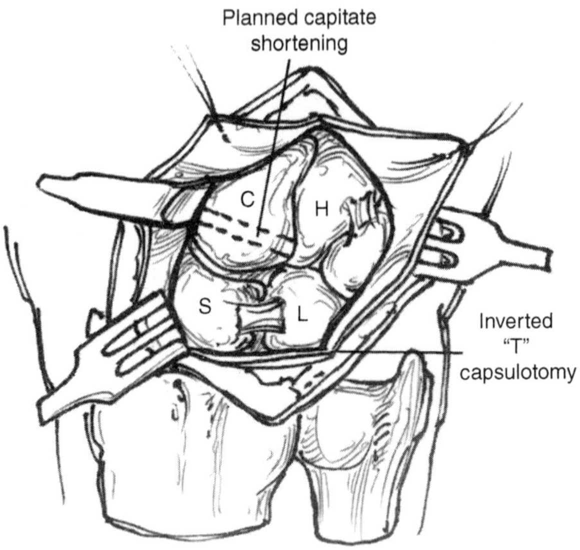

Figure 57–1

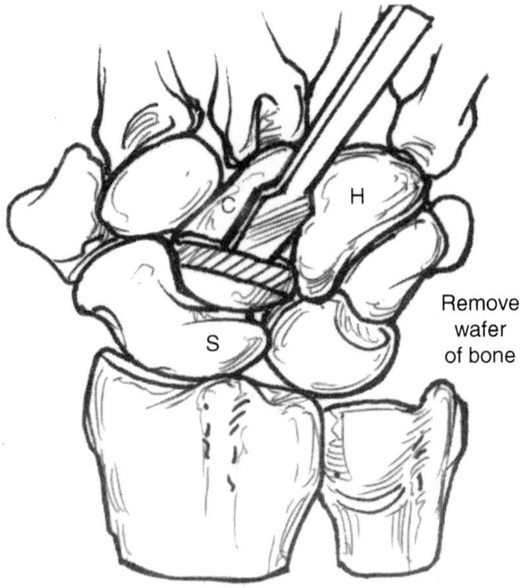

Figure 57–2

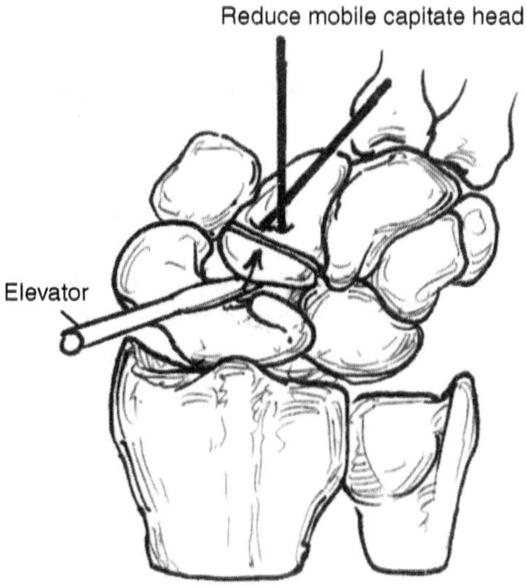

Figure 57–3

- The mobile capitate head is reduced onto the distal fragment using an elevator placed into the midcarpal joint. Two 0.045 in. or 0.062 in. wires are placed across the osteotomy site in a crossed configuration (**Fig. 57–3**).
- The articular and subchondral surfaces between the capitate and hamate are removed using curettes, rongeurs, and osteotomes (**Fig. 57–4**).

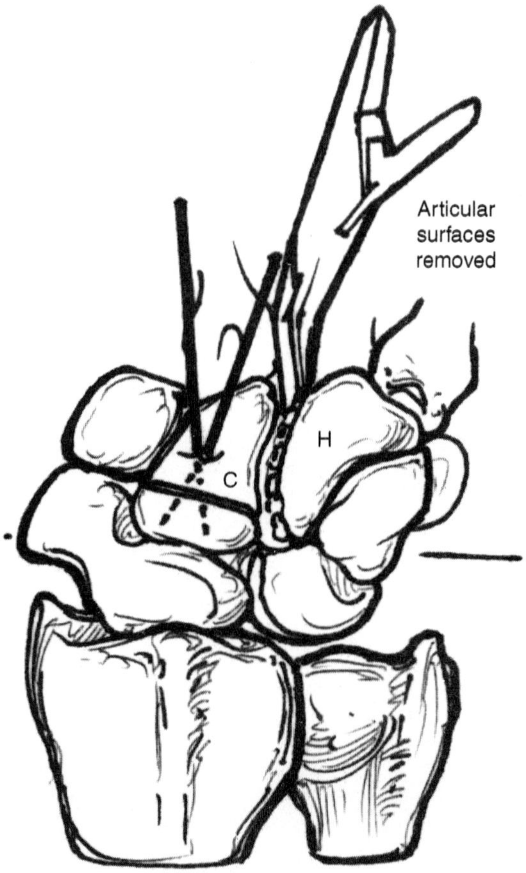

Figure 57–4

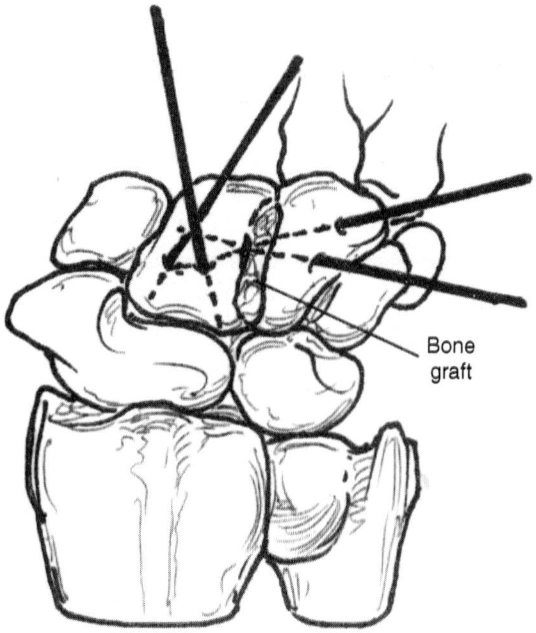

Figure 57–5

- Two percutaneous 0.045 in. or 0.062 in. Kirschner wires are placed across the capitohamate joint. Bone graft is harvested from the distal radius. Cancellous bone graft is packed into the depths of the fusion site within the denuded capitohamate surfaces (**Fig. 57–5**).
- Verify pin placement using minifluoroscopy and make necessary adjustments. Pins are usually cut beneath the skin.
- The capsule is reapproximated and standard closure is performed and the EPL tendon is transposed dorsal to its compartment.

■ Pearls

Elevation of full-thickness flaps at the level of the extensor retinaculum prevents inadvertent injury to the cutaneous nerves.

- Denude capitohamate articulation down to cancellous bone to enhance fusion rate.
- Use thin osteotomes to avoid fracturing of the bone surrounding the osteotomy site.

■ Pitfalls

Avascular necrosis of the capitate is a concern, although this complication is unlikely.

- Nonunion rates are fairly high (up to 20%). Proper bone resection and accurate internal fixation are mandatory.
- Avoid ulnar sensory nerve during percutaneous Kirschner wire placement.

Postoperative Care

- The extremity is initially immobilized in a compressive dressing and sugar-tong thumb spica splint with the thumb interphalangeal joint not included. The forearm is positioned in neutral and the wrist slightly extended. Elevation and finger motion are encouraged immediately following the procedure.
- Ten to 14 days after surgery, the sutures are removed and the splint changed to a short arm thumb spica cast.
- The extremity is immobilized for 8 weeks. A thermoplastic splint is then fabricated and active and active-assisted motion instituted.
- Pin removal after healing appears evident, usually ~10 weeks after surgery
- Strengthening and gentle passive motion are commenced 12 weeks after surgery.

Alternative Techniques

- Other means of internal fixation, including Kirschner wires, bone plug, miniplate, and staple
- Vascularized bone grafting
- Scaphocapitate arthrodesis
- Joint leveling procedures in ulnar negative variance

Suggested Readings

Almquist EE. Capitate shortening in the treatment of Kienböck's disease. Hand Clin 1993 Aug; 9(3):505–512

Almquist EE. Kienböck's disease. Hand Clin 1987;3(1): 141–148. J Hand Surg [Am] 1993;18A: 26–33

Horii E, et al. Effect of force transmission across the carpus in procedures used to treat Kienböck's disease. J Hand Surg 1990;15:393–400

Inoue G. Capito-hamate fusion for Kienböck's disease: good results in 8 cases followed for 3 years. Acta Orthop Scand 1992;63:560–562

58 Scaphocapitate Fusion with Lunate Excision

Indications

Kienböck disease with the following:

1. Stage IIIB disease. (See **Table 58–1**.)
2. Stage IIIA disease with neutral or positive ulnar variance
3. After unsuccessful joint leveling procedure

Technique

- Longitudinal dorsal incision that begins just ulnar to Lister's tubercle and extends to the base of the third metacarpal (**Fig. 58–1**).
- Protect the radial sensory nerves and lateral antebrachial cutaneous branches using loupe magnification. Elevate flaps at the level of the extensor retinaculum.
- The extensor pollicis longus (EPL) tendon is identified and the third compartment opened. The EPL tendon is transposed in a radial direction from the third compartment.
- The second compartment is elevated in a radial direction and the fourth compartment in an ulnar direction. The posterior interosseous nerve is located under the fourth compartment and resected.
- A capsulotomy is performed to expose the underlying radiocarpal and midcarpal joints. The capsular incision is created along the dorsal radiocarpal and

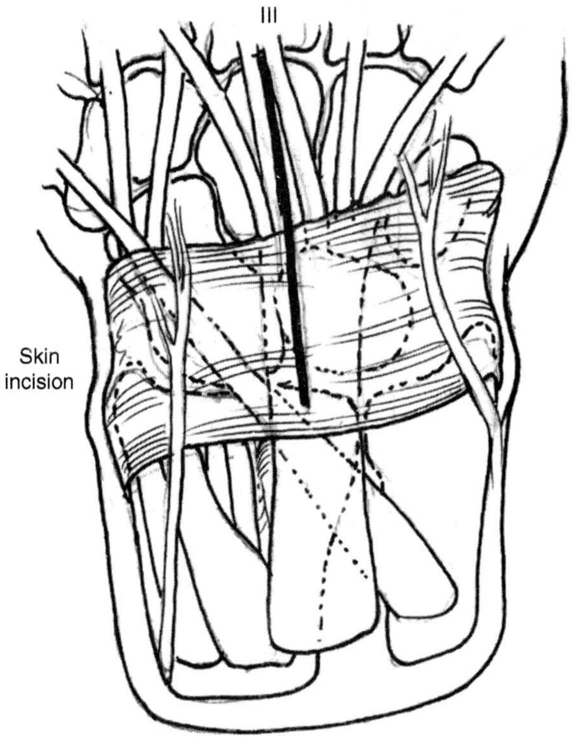

Figure 58–1

Table 58–1 Lichtman's Radiographic Classification of Klinbock's Disease

Stage	Description	Additional Significance
I	Normal except for possible linear or compression fracture	
II	Density changes apparent in lunate	
IIIA	Collapse of lunate without fixed scaphoid rotation	
IIIB	Collapse of lunate plus fixed scaphoid roattion	The load is shifted over to the lunate which will speed up collapse
IV	Stage III plus generalized degenerative changes throughout the carpus	

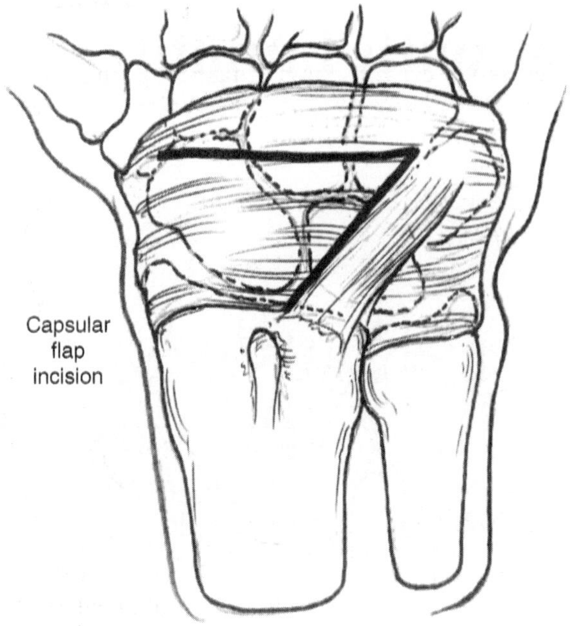

Figure 58–2

intercarpal ligaments. This capsulotomy incision provides adequate carpal exposure (**Fig. 58–2**).

- Synovectomy is performed to facilitate visualization. The lunate (L) is examined for fragmentation and collapse. A grossly deformed lunate is removed using a rongeur; otherwise, the lunate can be retained.
- The articular and subchondral surfaces between the scaphoid (S) and capitate (C) are removed using curettes, rongeurs, and thin osteotomes. The volar rim of articular surface is not violated to maintain midcarpal dimensions (**Fig. 58–3**).

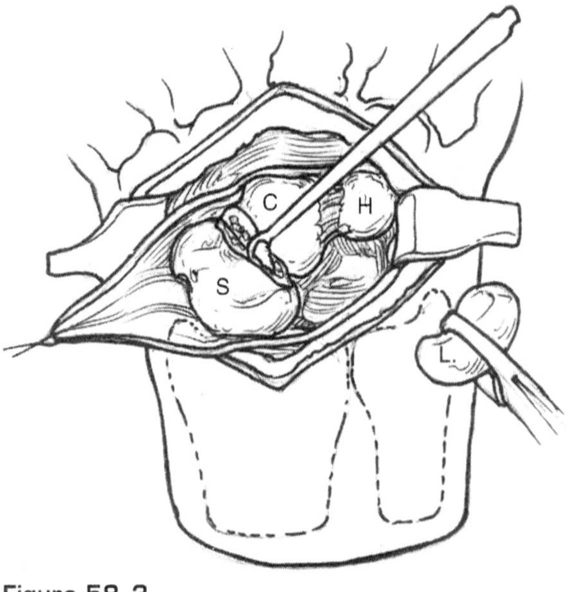

Figure 58–3

- Bone graft is harvested from the distal radius. Iliac crest bone graft is an alternative option.
- Prior to fixation, any intercarpal malalignment should be corrected. The scaphoid should align ~45 degrees relative to the radius in the sagittal plane. This reduction can be accomplished by manual pressure or by using 0.45 to 0.62 in. (1.1–1.5 mm) wires as joysticks.
- Two guide wires for cannulated compression screw fixation are used for provisional fixation. These wires are directed from a radial to ulnar direction and may require a separate radial small incision. The wires are visualized across the scaphocapitate joint and driven into the capitate. An elongated radial styloid will require removal to facilitate guide wire placement.
- The carpal reduction and wire position are verified by fluoroscopy.
- Cancellous bone graft is packed into the depths of the fusion site within the denuded scaphocapitate surfaces.
- The cannulated drill is placed over the guide wire with careful protection of the soft tissues. The cannulated headless screw is also placed over the guide wire and scaphocapitate joint (**Fig. 58–4**).
- Additional bone graft is densely packed into the spaces between the scaphoid and capitate. The position of the screws is verified using fluoroscopy and anteroposterior, lateral, and oblique projections.
- The capsule is reapproximated and closure is performed with the EPL tendon transposed into the subcutaneous tissues.

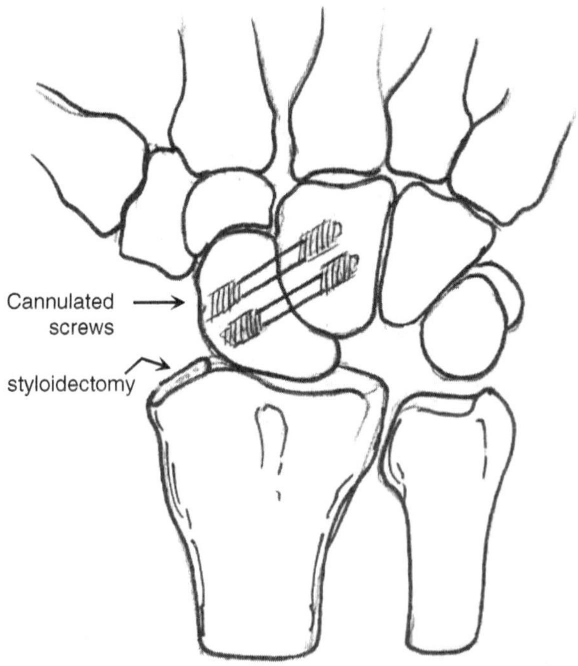

Figure 58–4

Pearls

Elevation of full-thickness flaps at the level of the extensor retinaculum prevents inadvertent injury to the cutaneous nerves.

- Reduce any intercarpal malalignment, such that the scaphoid aligns 45 degrees relative to the radius.
- Denude scaphocapitate articulation down to cancellous bone to enhance fusion rate.
- Accurate positioning of the guide wires is critical. Removal of an elongated radial styloid facilitates placement.

Pitfalls

Guide wires to cannulated screw systems can be fragile. Drill and screw must be carefully inserted with coaxial alignment to prevent breakage of guide wire.

- Radial incision for guide wire and screw placement should be large enough to avoid inadvertent injury to the sensory nerves.
- Nonunion rates are fairly high (up to 20%). Proper bone resection and accurate internal fixation are mandatory.

Postoperative Care

- The extremity is initially immobilized in a compressive dressing and sugar-tong thumb spica splint with the thumb interphalangeal joint not included. The forearm is positioned in neutral and the wrist slightly extended. Elevation and finger motion are encouraged immediately following the procedure.
- Ten to 14 days after surgery, the sutures are removed and the splint changed to a short arm–thumb spica cast.
- The extremity is immobilized for 6 weeks. A thermoplastic splint is then fabricated and active and active-assisted motion instituted.
- Strengthening and passive motion are commenced 12 weeks after surgery.

Alternative Techniques

- Scaphocapitate fusion can be performed with other means of internal fixation, including wires, bone plug, mini plate, and staples.
- Scaphotrapeziotrapezoid joint fusion
- Proximal row carpectomy

Suggested Readings

Moy OJ, Peimer CA. Scaphocapitate fusion in the treatment of Kienböck's disease. Hand Clin 1993;9:501–504

Pisano SM, Peimer CA, Wheeler DR, Sherwin F. Scaphocapitate intercarpal arthrodesis. J Hand Surg [Br] 1991;16(2):328–333

Rotman MB, Manske PR, Pruitt DL, Szerzinski J. Scaphocapitolunate arthrodesis. J Hand Surg [Am] 1993;18(1):26–33

Section VI.10

The Wrist Joint: The Pediatric Wrist

59 Fractional Lengthening

Indications

Spastic, flexed fingers with inadequate finger extension and the inability to release objects. This spasticity is usually associated with cerebral palsy or traumatic brain injury.

Technique

- Longitudinal incision (6–8 cm) over distal third of forearm just ulnar to palmaris longus tendon (**Fig. 59–1**). Bluntly dissect through subcutaneous incision to identify flexor tendons and neurovascular bundles. Identify flexor digitorum superficialis (FDS) tendons palmar to median nerve.
- Isolate each FDS tendon proximal at its muscle–tendon junction. Incise tendinous portion within the muscle–tendon junction, such that intact muscle remains on both sides of the cut tendon (**Fig. 59–2A,B**). Gently extend finger to separate cut ends of FDS tendons ~1 to 1.5 cm.

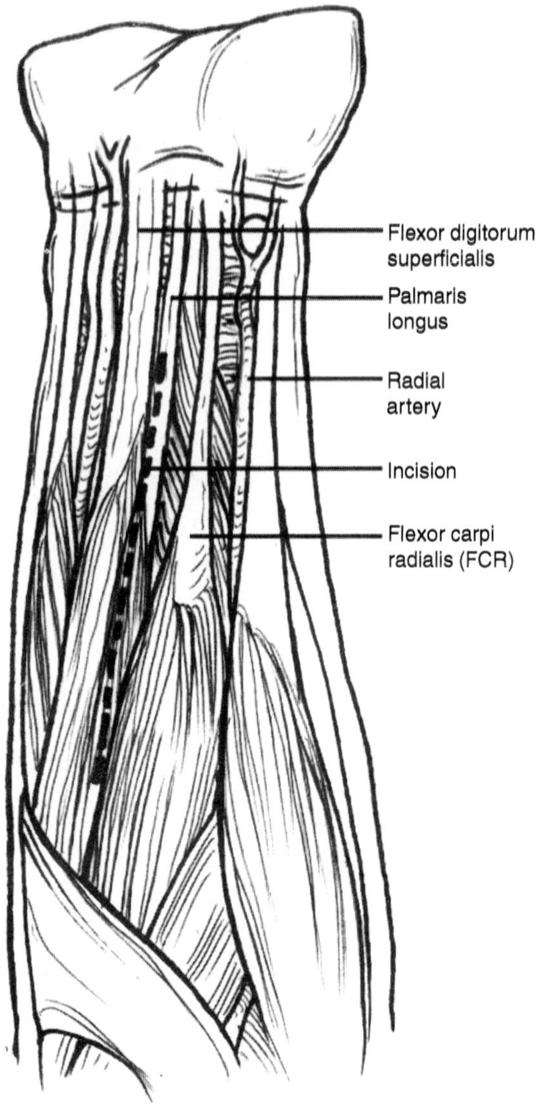

Figure 59–1

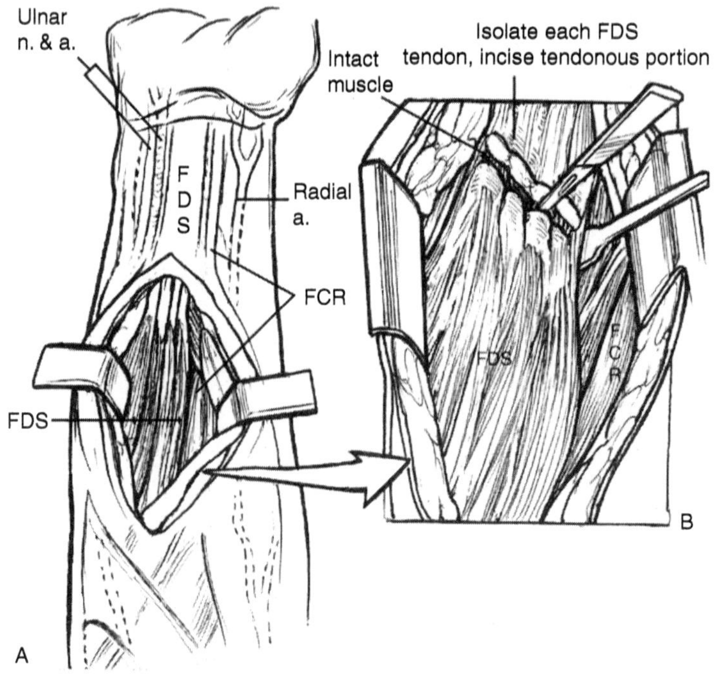

Figure 59–2

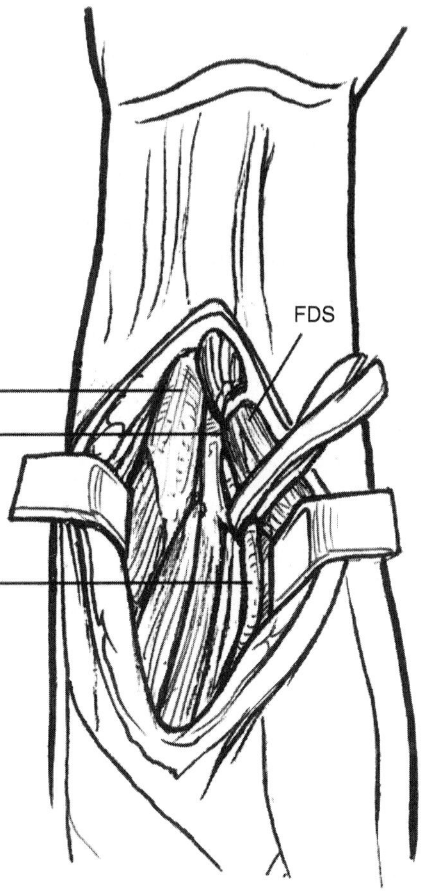

Figure 59–3

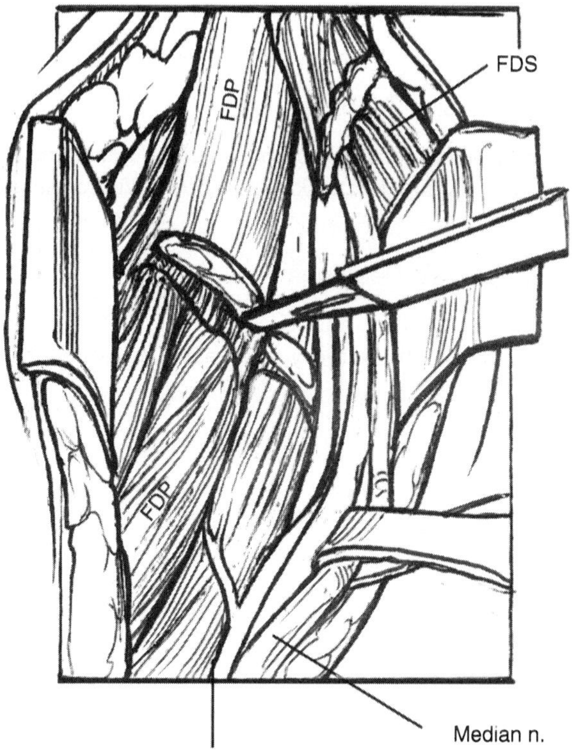

Figure 59–4

- Isolate flexor digitorum profundus (FDP) tendons deep to median nerve. Long, ring, and small fingers always have common muscle belly and can be fractionally lengthened together at muscle–tendon junction (**Fig. 59–3**). Index FDP tendon often has a separate muscle–tendon belly and requires individual lengthening.
- Incise tendinous portion of FDP tendons within the muscle–tendon junction, such that intact muscle remains on both sides of the cut tendon (**Fig. 59–4**). Gently extend finger to separate cut ends of FDP tendons ~1 to 1.5 cm.
- Perform concomitant wrist flexor tendon lengthening, tendon transfer, or fusion as indicated.
- Close subcutaneous tissue and skin with absorbable suture.

■ Pearls

FDS tendons reside superficial to median nerve, and FDP tendons are deep.

- FDS tendons require individual fractional lengthening. FDP tendons to ulnar three digits can be lengthened together.

■ Pitfalls

Overextension of wrist and fingers in severely contracted FDS or FDP muscle–tendon units can result in discontinuity between tendon and muscle.

- Injury to either or both the median nerve or ulnar neurovascular bundle during isolation of tendons

Postoperative Care

- The extremity is initially immobilized in a compressive dressing and short arm splint with the wrist in extension and hand in position of function.
- Remove splint 5 to 7 days after surgery and fabricate splint that replicates position of immobilization.

- Begin active finger motion out of splint three to four times a day.
- Wean daytime wearing of splint over 3 to 6 weeks depending on progress.
- Wear splint at night for 12 weeks.

Alternative Technique

- Superficialis to profundus tendon transfer in nonfunctional hand with skin breakdown within the palm
- Flexor–pronator slide to improve both wrist flexion and forearm pronation
- Wrist fusion for uncontrollable spasticity and skin breakdown within the palm; may be combined with flexor digitorum superficialis to flexor digitorum profundus tendon transfer
- Tendon transfer to augment finger extension. Finger flexion deformity must be easily correctable by passive positioning.

Suggested Readings

Keenan MAE, Kozin SH, Berlet AC. Manual of Orthopaedic Surgery for Spasticity. New York: Raven; 1993

Van Heest AE, House JH, Cariello C. Upper extremity surgical treatment of cerebral palsy. J Hand Surg [Am] 1999;24A:323–330

60 Closing Wedge Osteotomy of Carpus

Indications

Arthrogryposis with a fixed flexion and ulnar deviation deformity of the wrist

Technique

- Dorsal transverse or semicircular incision across the midcarpal joint (**Fig. 60–1**)
- Protect the cutaneous branches using loupe magnification. Elevate flaps at the level of the extensor retinaculum.
- Isolate the wrist and finger extensor tendons. Identify the extensor pollicis longus (EPL) tendon and open the third compartment. Mobilize the EPL in a radial direction. The radial wrist extensors are usually hypoplastic and adherent to the dorsal capsule. Attempt to mobilize these tendons in a radial direction.
- Isolate extensor carpi ulnaris (ECU) tendon. Palpate muscle–tendon junction ~6 to 8 cm above wrist. Make transverse incision at this level and identify proximal tendon. Incise distal aspect of tendon. Pull cut end of tendon into proximal incision (**Fig. 60–2.** S, scaphoid; H, hamate; Tg, triquetum).
- Retract the extensor digitorum communis tendons in an ulnar direction. Identify the extensor carpi ulnaris tendon and divide at its insertion into the fifth metacarpal.
- Make a transverse arthrotomy at the midcarpal joint. Elevate the capsule in a proximal and distal direction to expose the radiocarpal and midcarpal joint.
- Place a 0.045–in. wire into the lunate (L) perpendicular to the long axis of the forearm. Place a second 0.045–in. wire into the capitate (C) perpendicular to the long metacarpal. The wires should converge at the base of the midcarpal joint. Verify wire position by fluoroscopy. The angle created by these wires outlines the wedge resection.

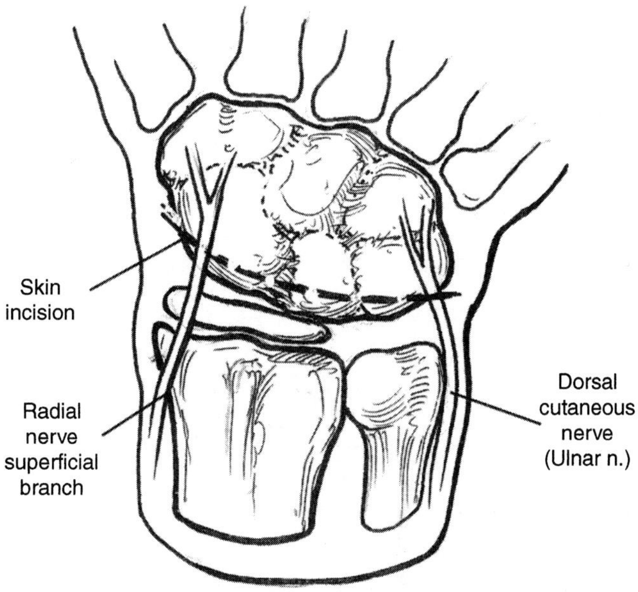

Figure 60–1

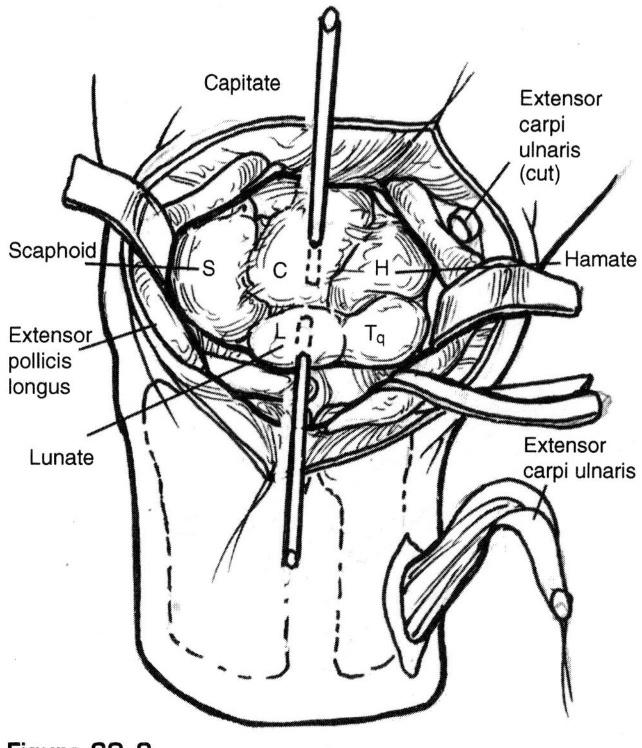

Figure 60–2

- Cut the proximal carpal row parallel to the first wire and the distal carpal row parallel to the second wire. A scalpel is used in the young child and an osteotome or saw is used in older patient. The wedge can be slightly greater at the radial carpus to correct any ulnar deviation deformity (i.e., biplanar correction) **(Fig. 60–3A–D)**.
- Remove the intervening bone and close the osteotomy site by placing the wrist into extension. Place nonabsorbable sutures across the osteotomy site.

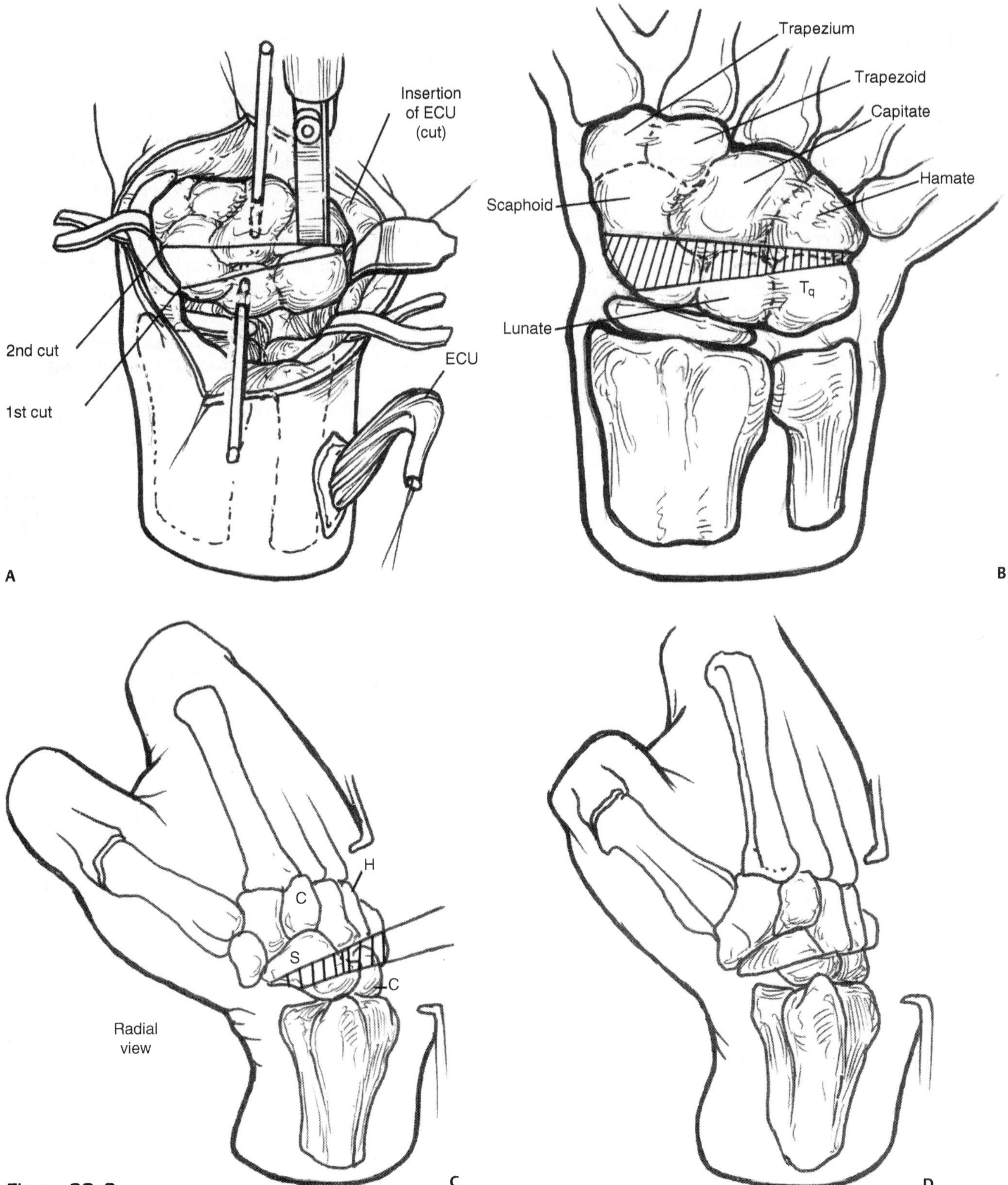

Figure 60–3

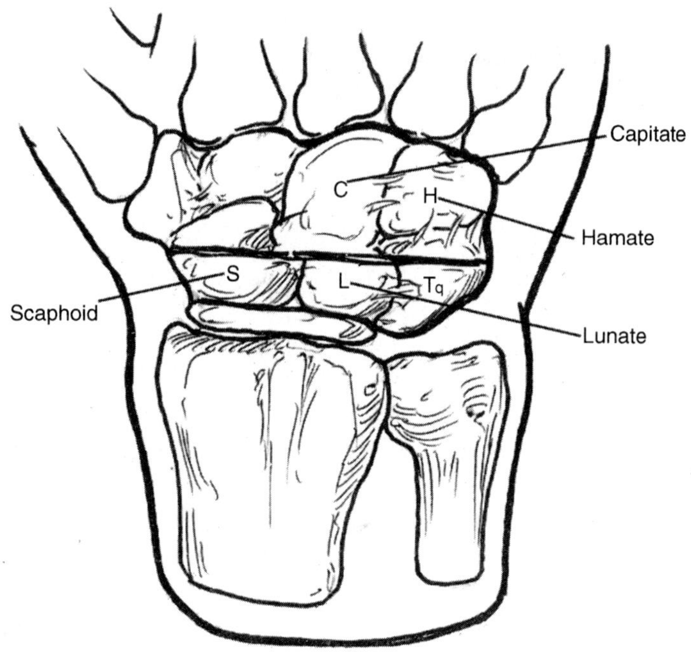

Figure 60–4

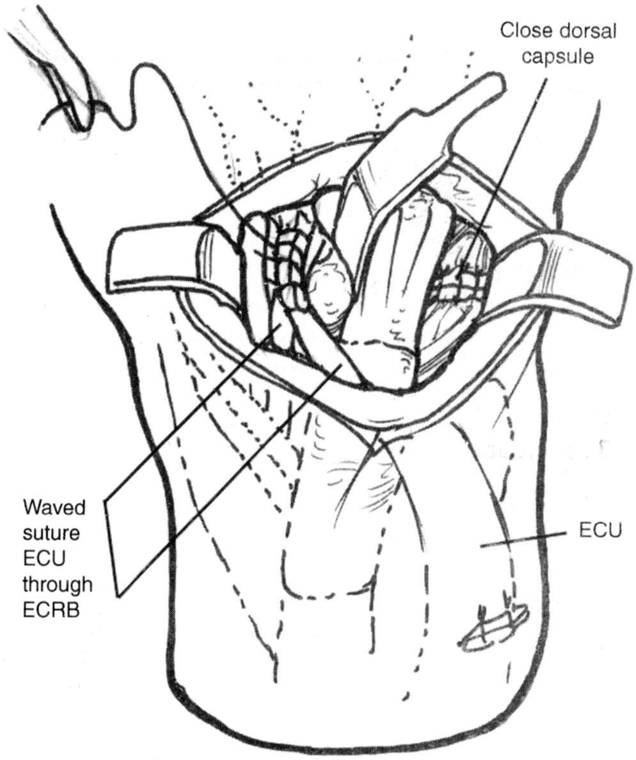

Figure 60–5

Supplemental wire fixation can be added (**Fig. 60–4**).

- Close the dorsal capsule. Transfer the extensor carpi ulnaris to the radial wrist extensors (**Fig. 60–5**). Close subcutaneous tissue and skin. Redundant skin can be excised through the ECRB.

■ Pearls

Identify all extensor tendons prior to arthrotomy.

- Careful wire placement prior to osteotomy. Use fluoroscopy to verify wire position.

■ Pitfalls

Protect extensor tendons during wedge resection.

- Identify midcarpal joint and protect radiocarpal joint to eliminate any chance of radiocarpal resection.

Postoperative Care

- The extremity is initially immobilized in a compressive dressing and sugar-tong splint with the wrist in extension.
- The forearm is positioned in neutral.
- Elevation and finger motion are encouraged immediately following the procedure.
- Ten to 14 days after surgery, the sutures are removed and the splint changed to a short arm cast.
- The extremity is immobilized for 6 to 8 weeks. Any supplemental wires are removed at this time.
- A thermoplastic splint is fabricated, and active and active-assisted motion is instituted. Passive wrist flexion is avoided. The splint is worn full-time for 3 months.
- Part-time splinting is continued for 6 months and at night for up to 1 year.

Alternative Techniques

- Proximal row carpectomy
- Dorsal wedge osteotomy of the distal radius
- Arthrodesis at maturity

Suggested Readings

Ezaki M. Treatment of the upper limb in the child with arthrogryposis. Hand Clin 2000;16:703–711

Mennon U. Early corrective surgery of the wrist and elbow in arthrogryposis multiplex congenita. J Hand Surg [Br] 1993;18B:304–307

61 Tendon Transfer for Wrist Extension

Indications

Wrist in a flexed posture with inadequate wrist extension due to spasticity, paresis, or paralysis. Flexor carpi ulnaris (FCU) or extensor carpi ulnaris (ECU) or both are usually used as donors.

Technique

- Harvest ECU tendon via multiple transverse incisions. Begin with 1.5 cm transverse incision over distal ulna. Bluntly dissect through subcutaneous incision to identify sixth extensor compartment. Incise retinaculum and isolate ECU tendon. Palpate muscle–tendon junction ~6 to 8 cm above wrist. Make transverse incision at this level and identify proximal tendon (**Fig. 61–1**).
- Place Allis tissue forceps (Jarit Surgical Instruments, Hawthorne, New York) around tendon and position wrist into extension. Turn forceps to pull tendon in a proximal direction. Incise distal aspect of tendon (**Fig. 61–2**). Pull cut end of tendon into proximal incision (**Fig. 61–3**).
- Harvest FCU tendon via 1.5 cm transverse incision over volar wrist crease and proximal to pisiform

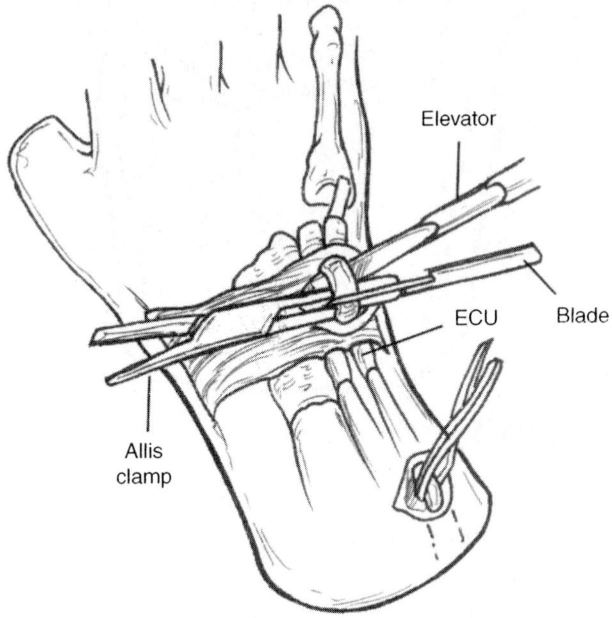

Figure 61–2

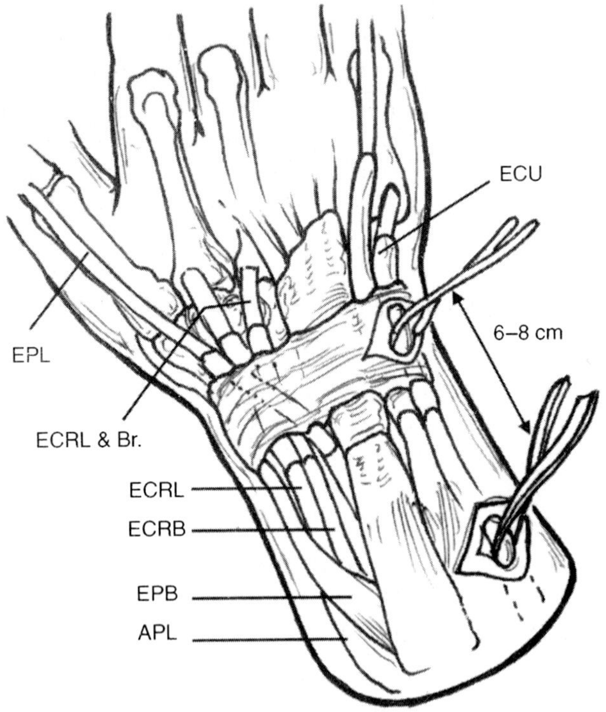

Figure 61–1

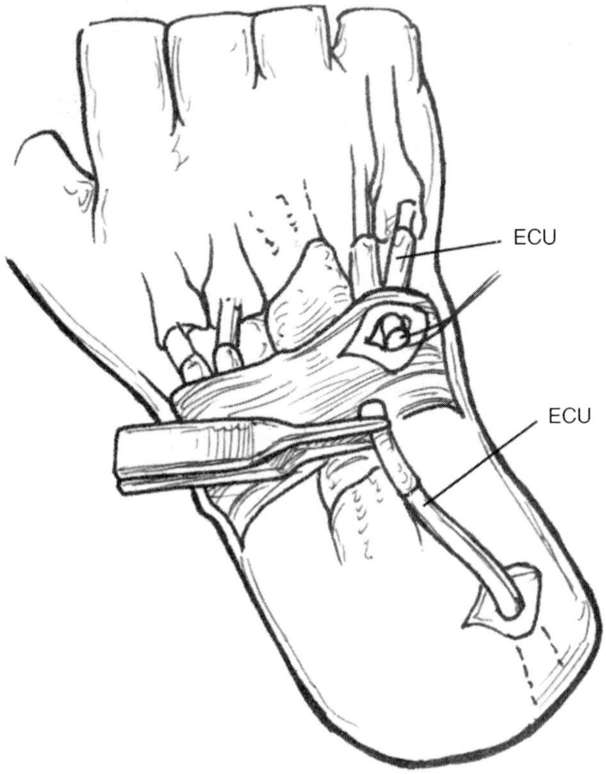

Figure 61–3

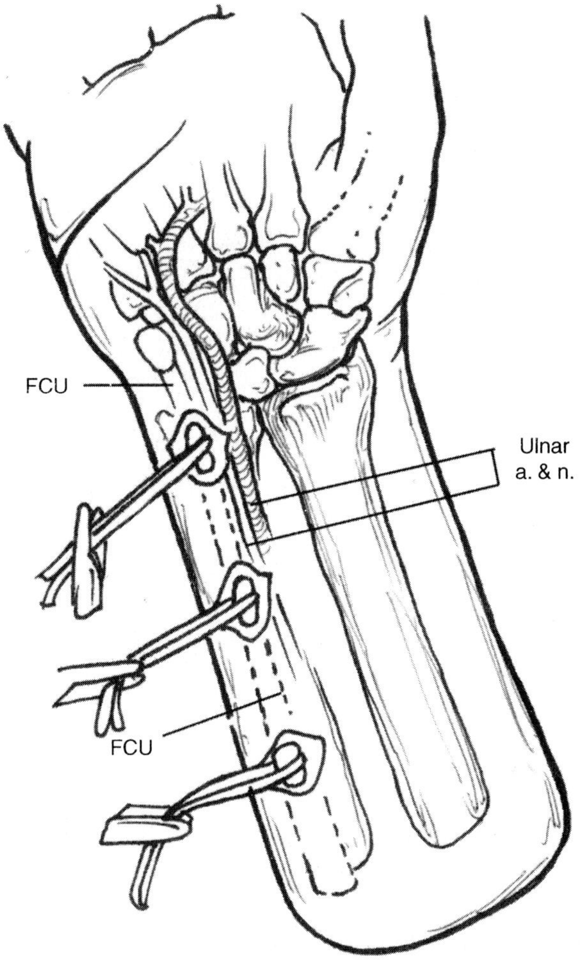

Figure 61–4

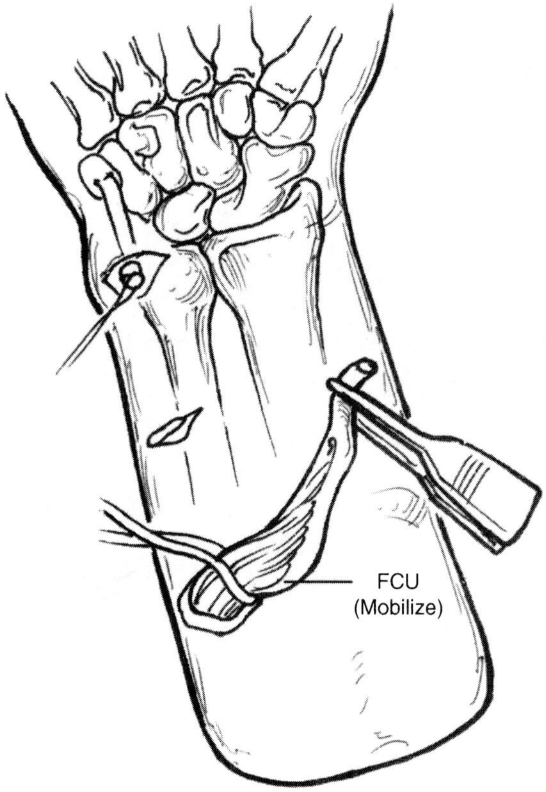

Figure 61–5

(**Fig. 61–4**). Bluntly dissect through subcutaneous incision to identify FCU tendon. Mobilize tendon in a circumferential fashion to protect underlying ulnar nerve and artery. Place Allis forceps around tendon and position wrist in flexion. Cut distal end of FCU tendon.

- Through a series of transverse incisions, mobilize FCU to midforearm level. Release fascial attachments to ulna to enhance available excursion. Protect adjacent ulnar neurovascular bundle. Pull FCU tendon into proximal incision (**Fig. 61–5**).
- Identify extensor carpi radialis longus (ECRL) and brevis (ECRB) via transverse incision proximal to wrist crease and just distal to the abductor pollicis longus (APL) and extensor pollicis brevis (EPB) muscle–tendon (M–T) junction. Incise fascia over second compartment and isolate individual tendons.
- Create subcutaneous tunnel between the second dorsal compartment and forearm incisions that contain ECU and FCU.

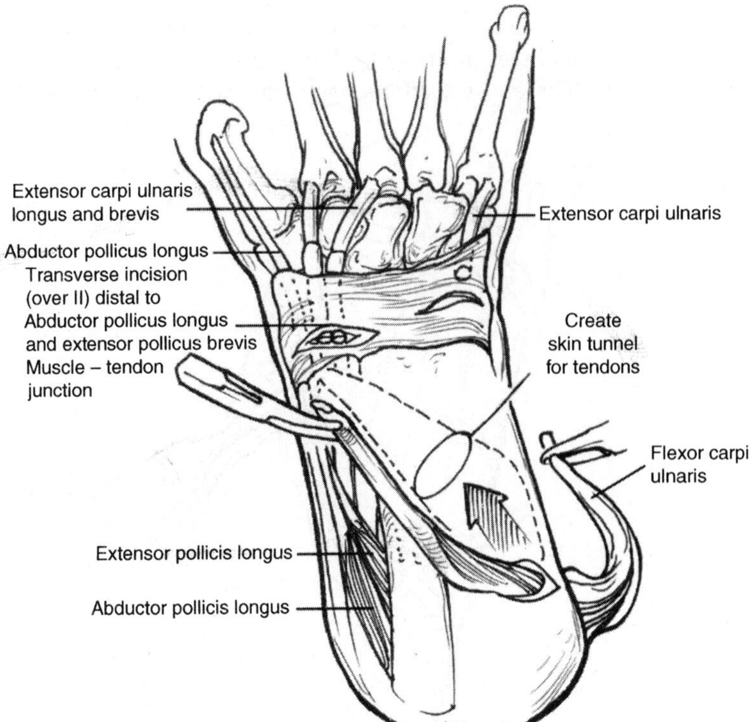

Figure 61–6

- Pass ECU and FCU through subcutaneous tunnel to incision over second dorsal compartment (**Fig. 61–6**). Weave ECU through ECRL and FCU through ECRB (**Fig. 61–7A,B**). Use tendon braider and Pulvertaft weave. Suture tenorrhaphy sites using nonabsorbable sutures in a horizontal mattress fashion. Tension tendon transfer to place wrist in ~20 degrees of extension.
- Close subcutaneous tissue and skin of all transverse incisions with absorbable suture.

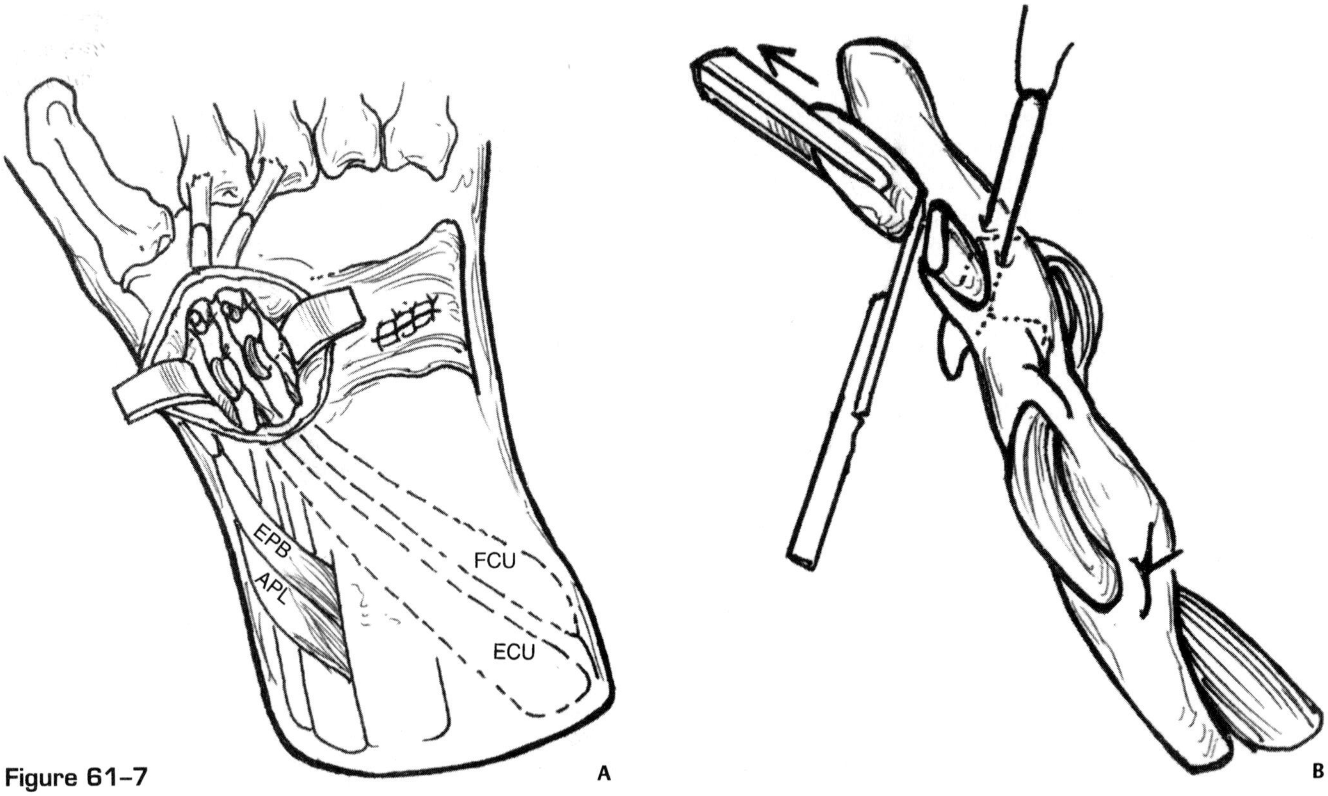

Figure 61–7

■ Pearls

Use both FCU and ECU as donor tendons. This will increase wrist extension moment and decrease ulnar deviation deformity.

- Mobilize FCU to midforearm prior to transfer. This will produce supination moment across forearm and lessen any concomitant pronation posture.

■ Pitfalls

Injury to ulnar sensory nerve during harvest of ECU

- Injury to ulnar neurovascular bundle during harvest of FCU
- Inadvertent laceration of extensor pollicis longus (EPL) during identification of ECRL and ECRB

Postoperative Care

- The extremity is initially immobilized in a compressive dressing and sugar-tong splint with the wrist in extension and forearm in supination.
- Elevation and finger motion are encouraged immediately following the procedure.
- Ten to 14 days after surgery, the sutures are removed and the splint changed to a short arm cast.
- Three weeks after surgery the cast is removed and a thermoplastic short arm splint is fabricated. Active and active-assisted motion of the wrist and forearm is instituted. The splint is worn part-time for 3 months.

Alternative Technique

- Wrist extension transfer may be combined with lengthening of either or both the wrist and flexor tendons.
- Lengthening of either or both wrist and flexor tendons without transfer; useful in patients with reasonable wrist extension that is overpowered by spastic wrist or finger flexors
- Alternative donor tendons, such as pronator teres, depending upon volitional control and strength
- Wrist fusion for uncontrollable spasticity and skin breakdown within the palm; may be combined with flexor digitorum superficialis to flexor digitorum profundus tendon transfer

Suggested Readings

Beach WR, Strecker WB, Coe J, et al. Use of the Green transfer in treatment of patients with spastic cerebral palsy: 17 years experience. J Pediatr Orthop 1991;6: 731–736

Keenan MAE, Kozin SH, Berlet AC. Manual of Orthopaedic Surgery for Spasticity. New York: Raven; 1993

Van Heest AE, House JH, Cariello C. Upper extremity surgical treatment of cerebral palsy. J Hand Surg [Am] 1999;24A:323–330

Wright T. Tendon transfer for wrist flexion deformity in cerebral palsy. Atlas Hand Clinics 2002;7: 133–151

62 Madelung's Deformity

Indications

Symptomatic adolescent with considerable Madelung's deformity

Technique

- Volar incision over the flexor carpi radialis (FCR) tendon beginning at wrist crease and extending 6 to 8 cm up the forearm (**Fig. 62–1**).
- Open FCR tendon sheath and retract tendon in radial direction. Incise the floor of the tendon sheath.
- Retract FCR tendon and sheath in a radial direction along with the radial artery.
- Retract carpal tunnel contents in an ulnar direction. Identify pronator quadratus (PQ) over metaphysis of distal radius.
- Incise PQ along radial margin and elevate from distal radius. Dissection is extraperiosteal to preserve osseous blood supply.
- Identify Vicker's ligament on the metaphysis of the radius and release from the radius in a proximal to distal direction up to the radiocarpal joint (**Fig. 62–2**).
- Create a biplanar dome osteotomy in the metaphysis. The concavity faces distal in the sagittal and coronal planes. Osteotomy is created with curved osteotomes (**Fig. 62–3**).

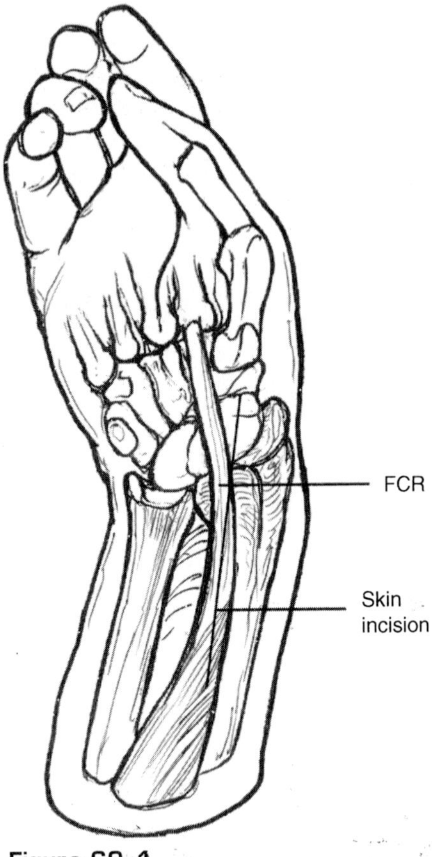

Figure 62–1

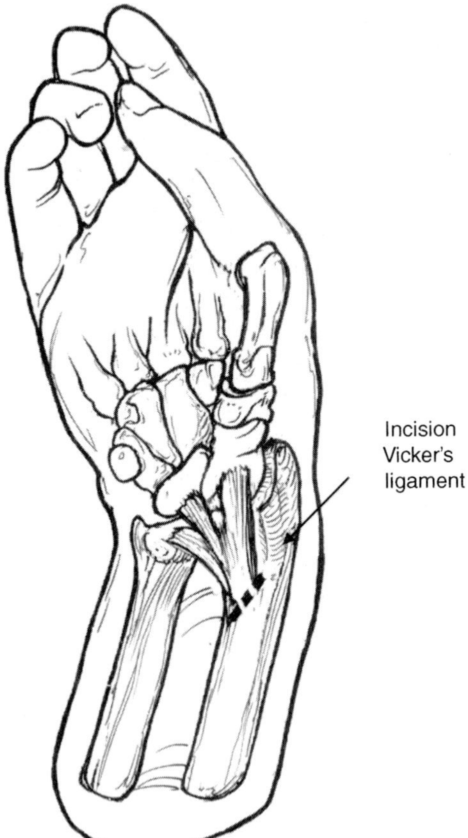

Figure 62–2

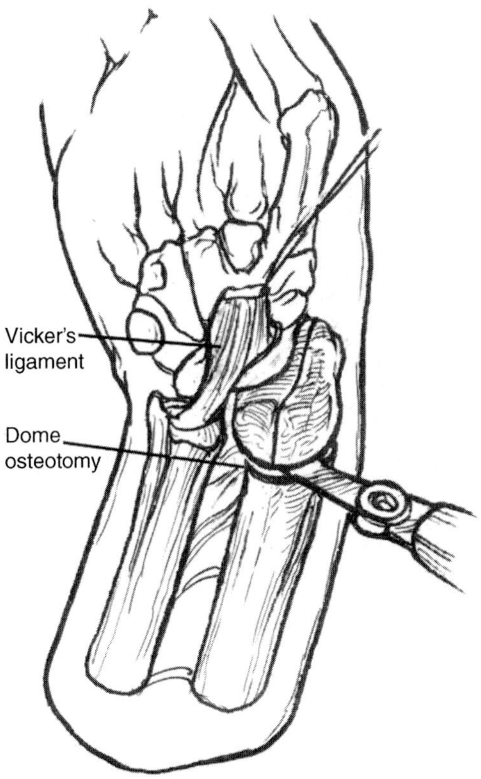

Figure 62–3

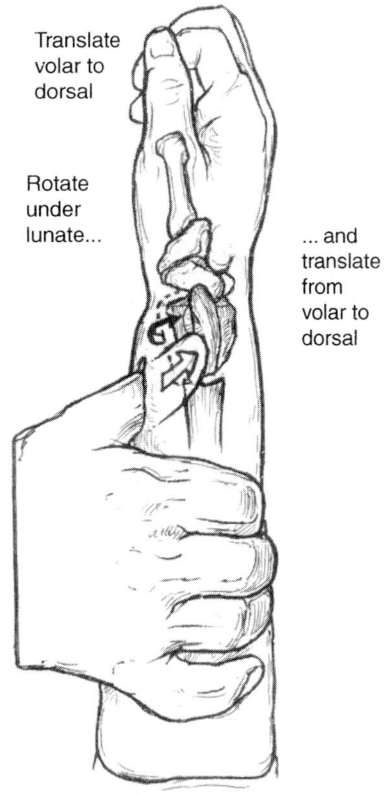

Figure 62–4

- Rotate the distal fragment to obtain better coverage beneath the lunate, and translate from volar to dorsal. Thumb pressure on the distal fragment facilitates correction (**Fig. 62–4**).

- Insert two percutaneous 0.062 in. pins from the radial styloid across the osteotomy site and into the proximal radius (**Fig. 62–5A,B**). Verify position by fluoroscopy. Cut pins beneath the skin.

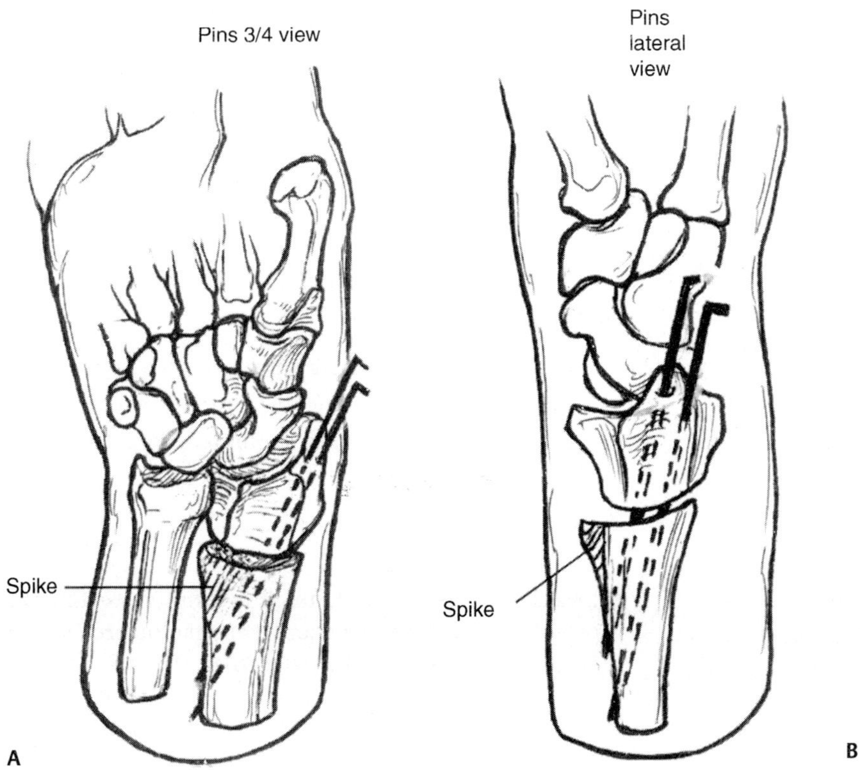

A **B**

Figure 62–5

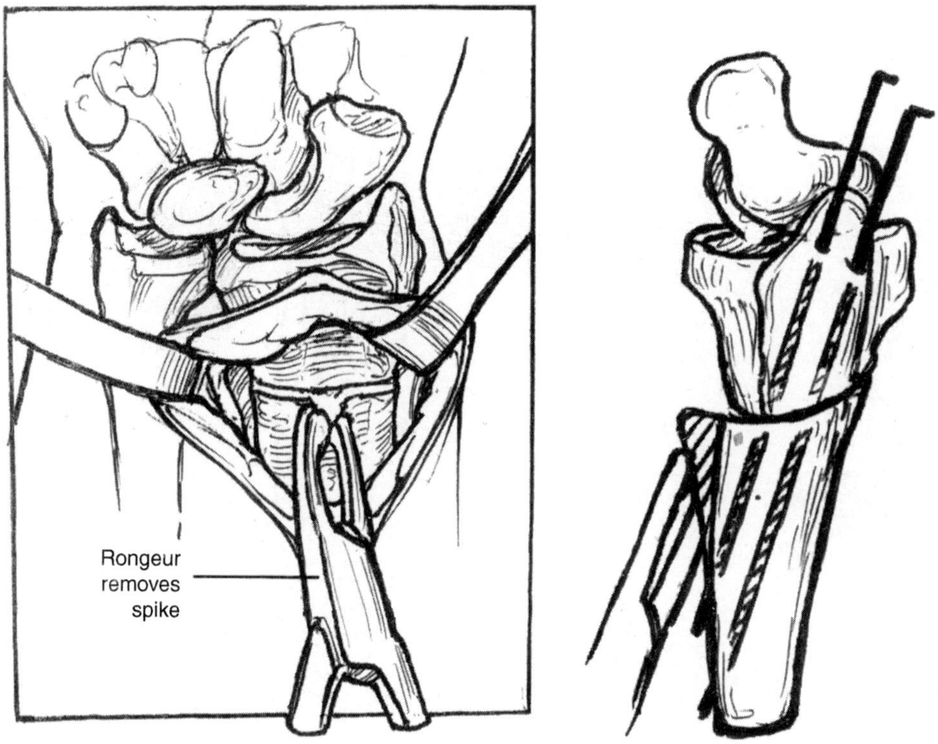

A B

Figure 62–6

- Remove protruding bone from the radius just proximal to osteotomy site using a rongeur (**Fig. 62–6A,B**).
- Close subcutaneous tissue and skin.

Pearls

Vicker's ligament begins on the volar, ulnar metaphysis of the radius and inserts primarily on the lunate. A volar approach exposes this ligament beneath the pronator quadratus.

- Thumb pressure on the distal fragment facilitates correction in both planes. A Steinmann pin can be inserted into the distal fragment to act as a joystick in severe deformities.

Pitfalls

Incomplete release of Vicker's ligament will prevent adequate rotation of the distal fragment.

- Occasionally, a reverse Madelung's deformity can occur with the growth disturbance affecting the dorsal ulnar aspect of the distal radius. The distal radius is angulated in a dorsal direction and the carpus is translated dorsally.

Postoperative Care

- The extremity is initially immobilized in a compressive dressing and sugar-tong splint with the wrist in extension.
- The forearm is positioned in neutral and the wrist extended. Elevation and finger motion are encouraged immediately following the procedure.
- Ten to 14 days after surgery, the sutures are removed and the splint changed to a long arm cast.
- Six to 8 weeks after surgery the Steinmann pins are removed. A thermoplastic short arm splint is fabricated. Active and active-assisted motion of the wrist and forearm is instituted. The splint is worn part-time for 3 months.

Alternative Technique

- Isolated release of Vicker's ligament in early deformity
- Ilizarov correction of the distal radius deformity
- Osteotomy of the radius combined with distal ulnar resection or Sauve-Kapandji procedure.

Suggested Readings

Ezaki M. Madelung's deformity. Hand Clin 2000;16: 713–721

Vickers D. Madelung deformity: surgical prophylaxis (physiolysis) during the late growth period by resection of the dyschondrosteosis lesion. J Hand Surg [Br] 1992; 17B:401–407

White G, Weiland A. Madelung's deformity: treatment by osteotomy of the radius and Lauenstein procedure. J Hand Surg [Am] 1987;12A:202–204

Section VI.11

The Wrist Joint: Ganglions

63 Excision of Dorsal Wrist Ganglion

Indications

Prominent lump that is painful, interferes with wrist use, or is considered cosmetically unacceptable

Technique

- Transverse incision over mass
- Place tag suture into the apex of the mass. This can be used to apply traction to the mass while dissecting around its margins (**Fig. 63–1**).
- Dissect to the base of the mass, identifying its stalk and origin.
- The origin is usually the scapholunate (SL) ligament or the midcarpal joint.
- Dissect parallel to the capsule, dorsal to the scapholunate joint to avoid damaging the scapholunate ligament (**Fig. 63–2**).
- Remove the mass with its stalk along with a small rectangle of capsule overlying the midcarpal joint (**Fig. 63–3**).
- Release the tourniquet and cauterize vessels, particularly those in capsule.
- Close skin. Apply bulky dressing with palmar splint.

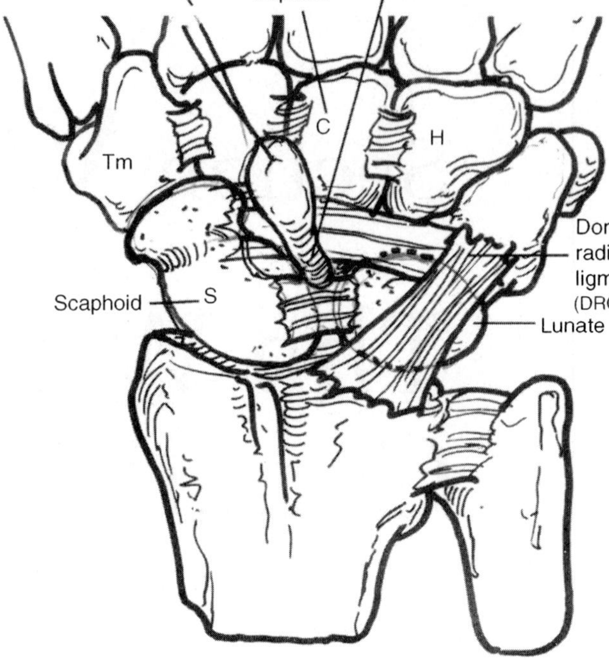

Figure 63–2

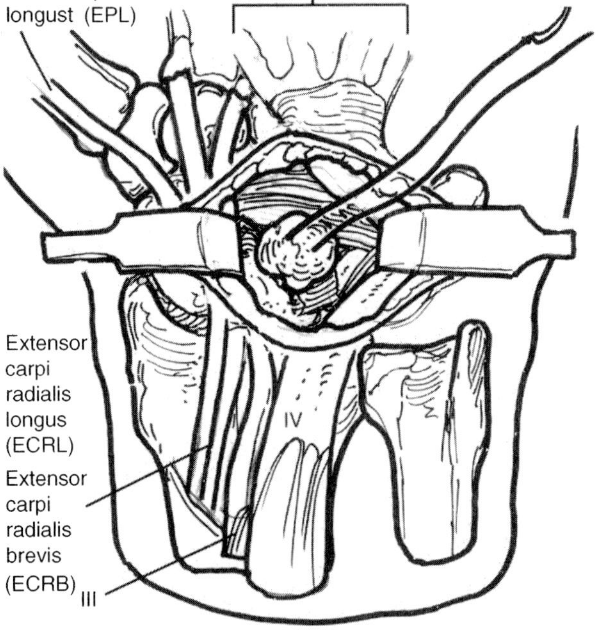

Figure 63–1

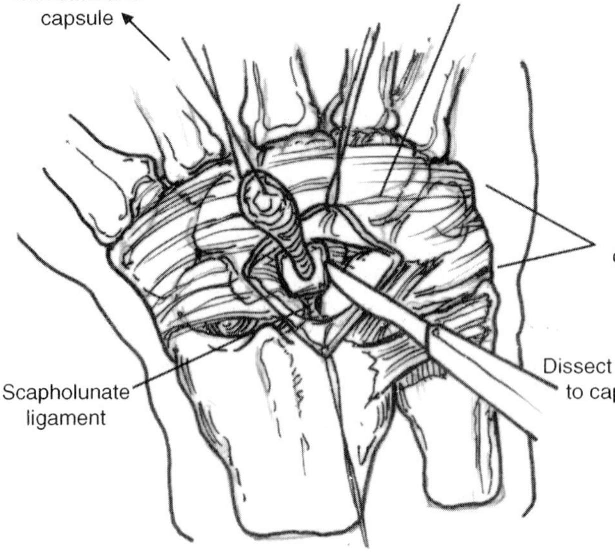

Figure 63–3

Postoperative Care

- Encourage finger motion.
- Splint off and sutures out in 10 to 14 days
- Progressive use

Alternative Techniques

Arthroscopic excision of dorsal ganglions

■ Pearl

Initially expect mid-wrist stiffness, especially loss of palmar flexion.

- Wrist discomfort is usually gone and motion acceptable in 8 to 12 weeks.

■ Pearl

Sharp dissection can be carried vertically along the cyst wall until the carpus is reached; dissection should then proceed horizontally to protect the intercarpal ligaments.

■ Pitfalls

Injury to the intercarpal ligaments

- Recurrence of the ganglion; 3 to 5%

Suggested Readings

Nahra ME, Bucchieri JS. Ganglion cysts and other tumor related conditions of the hand and wrist. Hand Clin 2004;20:249–260

Rizzo M, Berger RA, Steinmann SP, Bishop AT. Arthroscopic resection in the management of dorsal wrist ganglions: results with a minimum 2-year follow-up period. J Hand Surg [Am] 2004;29:59–62

64 Excision of Palmar Wrist Ganglion

Indications

Painful or cosmetically unacceptable mass on palmar aspect of wrist

Technique

- Brunner incision over mass (**Fig. 64–1**).
- Expose mass, usually in the interval between the flexor carpi radialis (FCR) tendon and the radial artery (**Fig. 64–2**).
- Identify the radial artery proximal to the mass. Dissect the radial artery away from the mass.
- Trace the mass and its stalk to its origin, usually the palmar wrist capsule.
- Excise the mass along with a small rectangle of palmar wrist joint capsule (**Fig. 64–3A–C.** C, capitate; R, raduis; L, lunate; S; scaphoid).
- Release the tourniquet and cauterize bleeding vessels. Pay particular attention to bleeding vessels coming from the radial artery.
- Close the skin and apply a bulky dressing with palmar splint.

Alternative Techniques

- Trace the cyst down to the stalk and excise the stalk only. The cyst will collapse and will not recur without the stalk. This technique reduces the risk of arterial injury.
- Arthroscopic excision of palmar wrist ganglion

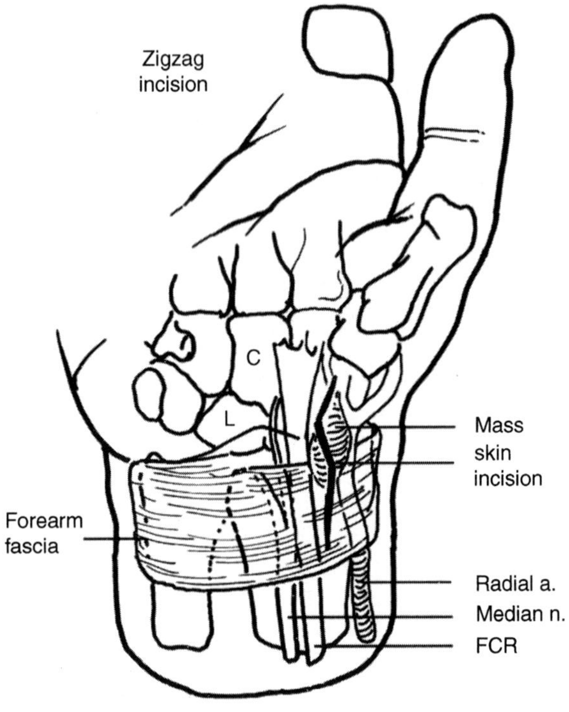

Figure 64–1

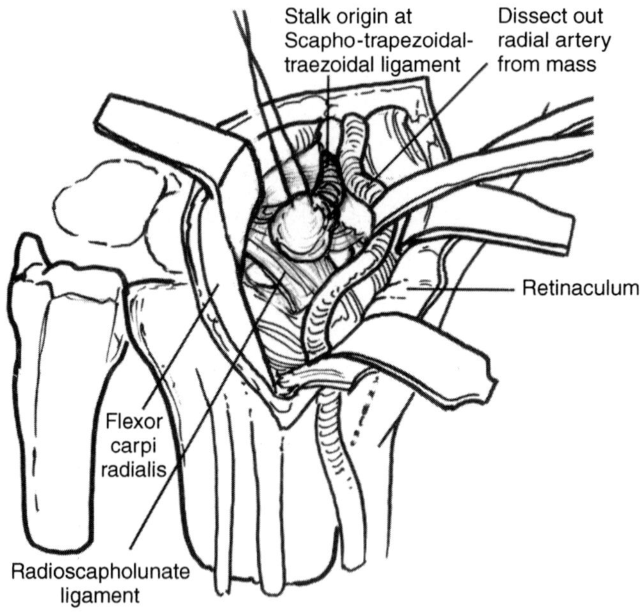

Figure 64–2

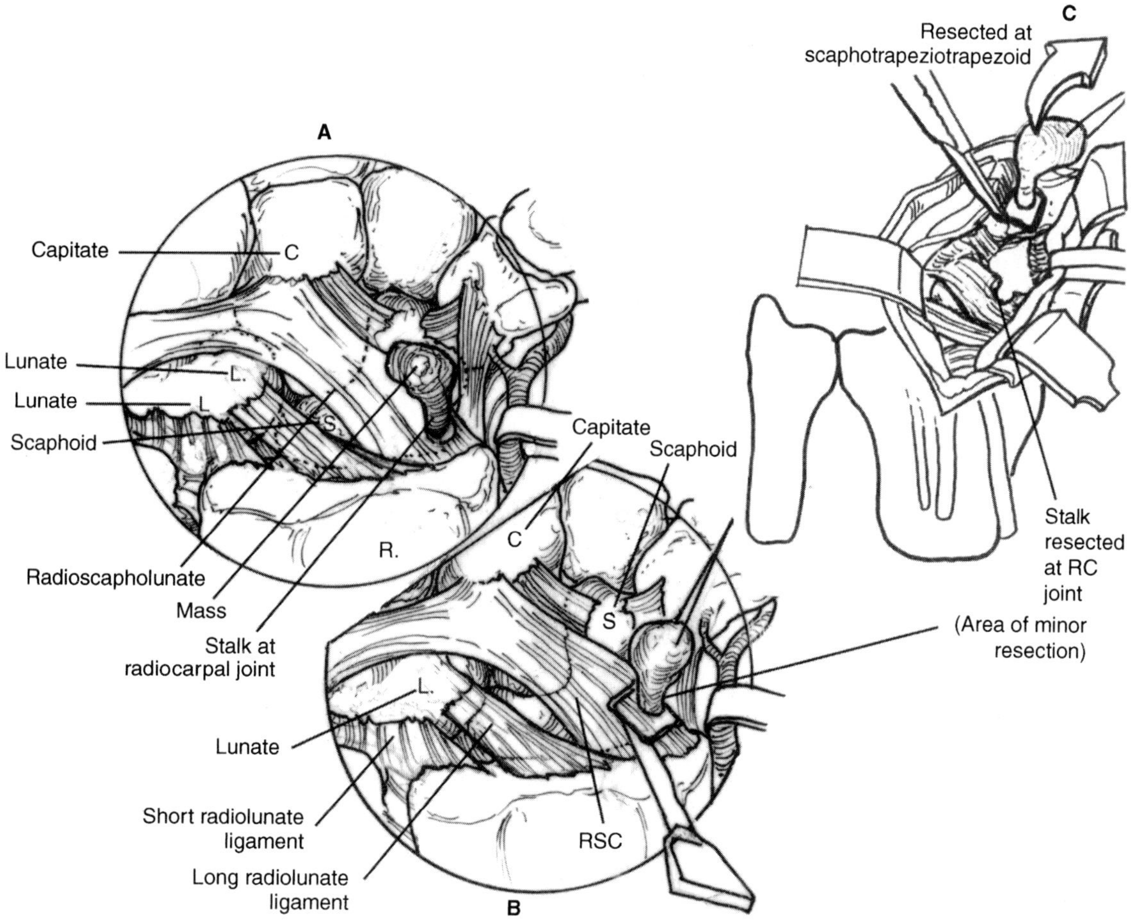

Figure 64–3

Postoperative Care

- Remove stitches and splint in 10 to 14 days.
- Encourage progressive use.

■ Pearls

Check an Allen's test preoperatively.

- Find the radial artery proximal and distal to the mass and alternatively dissect toward the center of the cyst. This reduces the risk of arterial injury.

■ Pitfalls

Injury to the radial artery

- Cyst recurrence: 3 to 5%

Suggested Readings

Nahra ME, Bucchieri JS. Ganglion cysts and other tumor related conditions of the hand and wrist. Hand Clin 2004;20:249–260

Rizzo M, Berger RA, Steinmann SP, Bishop AT. Arthroscopic resection in the management of dorsal wrist ganglions: results with a minimum 2-year follow-up period. J Hand Surg [Am] 2004;29:59–62

Section VII.1

The Carpometacarpal Joint: Thumb Carpometacarpal Joint Injuries

65 Ligament Reconstruction

Indications

Mild to moderate painful thumb carpometacarpal (CMC) joint arthritis recalcitrant to nonoperative management

- Also indicated for persistent instability after thumb CMC joint dislocation

Technique

- Plan incision along the dorsoradial aspect of the thumb at the junction between the glabrous and dorsal hair-bearing skin. Incision begins at midportion of the thumb metacarpal and extends to wrist crease. Extend the incision along the flexor carpi radialis (FCR) tendon for 2 cm (**Fig. 65–1**).
- Protect sensory branches of the radial and lateral antebrachial sensory nerves. Ligate the superficial branch of the radial artery. Avoid the palmar cutaneous branch of the median nerve.
- Elevate the thenar muscles in an extraperiosteal fashion from the thumb metacarpal and CMC joint. Identification of the CMC joint is facilitated by longitudinal traction on the thumb.
- Open the FCR tendon sheath at the wrist and isolate the tendon. Follow the tendon in a distal direction. Incise the transverse fascial fibers that form a separate fibro-osseous canal for the FCR tendon. Trace the tendon beneath the crest of the trapezium to its insertion point on the second metacarpal. Removal of a portion of the crest facilitates this dissection (**Fig. 65–2**).
- Isolate the first dorsal extensor compartment. Retract the tendons in a radial direction. Identify the extensor pollicis longus tendon and retract in an ulnar direction. Select a location between the tendons about 1 cm distal to the joint and perpendicular to the nail bed. This point serves as the initiation point for the bony channel created through the metacarpal base.

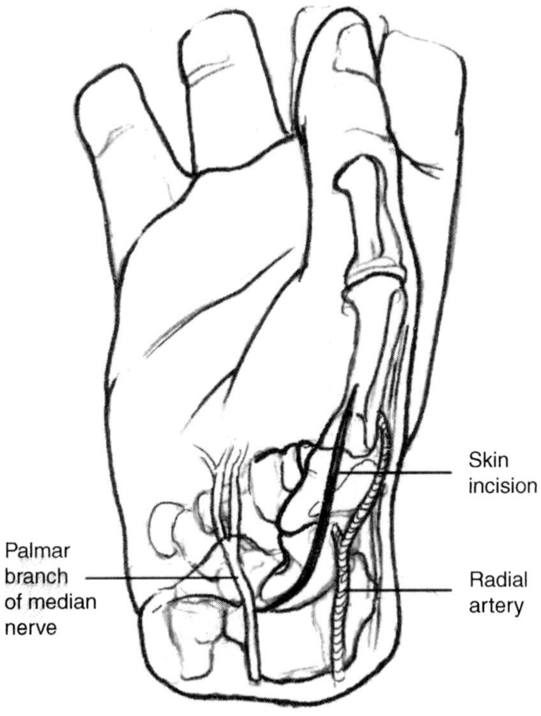

Figure 65–1

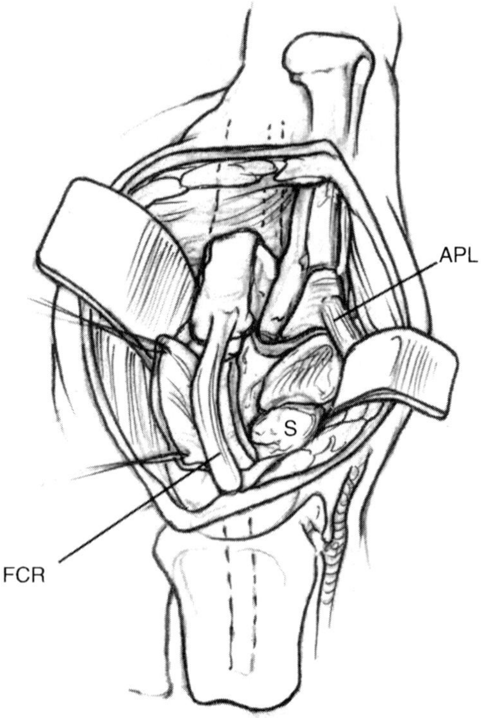

Figure 65–2

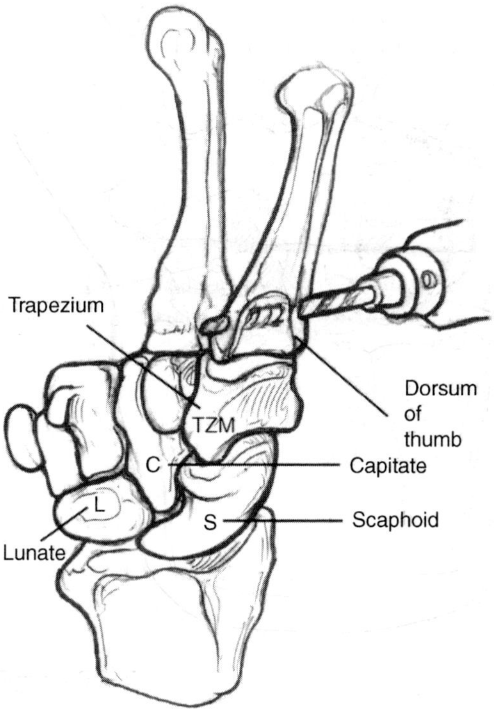

Figure 65–3

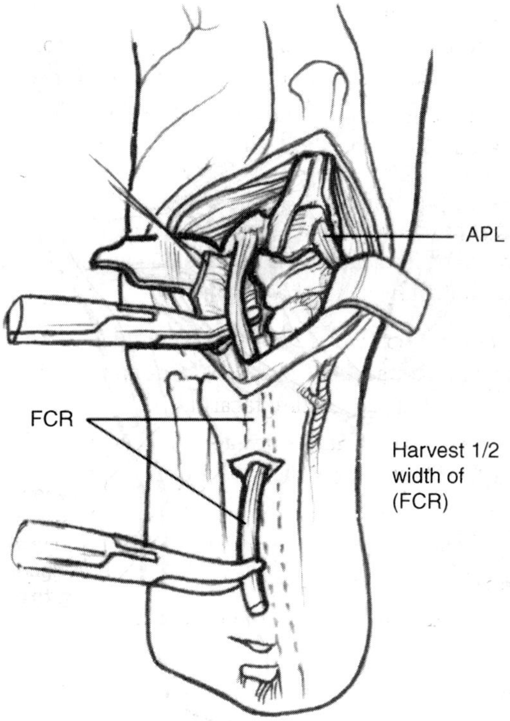

Figure 65–4

- Drill a small extra-articular bone tunnel from the dorsum of the metacarpal (perpendicular to the nail bed) to the volar beak of the metacarpal. Progressively enlarge the hole by using sequential drill bits. Make the drill large enough to accept one half of the FCR tendon. Curette any remaining bone within the channel (**Fig. 65–3**).
- Harvest the radial half of the FCR tendon 6 cm proximal to the wrist to the base of the index metacarpal. Multiple techniques are available for tendon harvest. Two transverse incisions (3 and 6 cm proximal to the wrist) allow safe harvest with minimal scarring (**Fig. 65–4**).
- Pass the free end of the harvested tendon graft through the drill hole from volar to dorsal. A tendon passer eases passage of the tendon. Fully reduce the thumb CMC joint and seat the metacarpal against the trapezium. Hold reduction with a percutaneous 0.045 in. wire inserted from the dorsoradial aspect of the thumb metacarpal into the second metacarpal or carpus. Angle wire from distal to proximal during insertion (**Fig. 65–5**).
- Draw the tendon taut and place a suture between the tendon and dorsal periosteum of metacarpal. Route the tendon in a radial direction across the dorsal capsule of the CMC joint and beneath the first dorsal

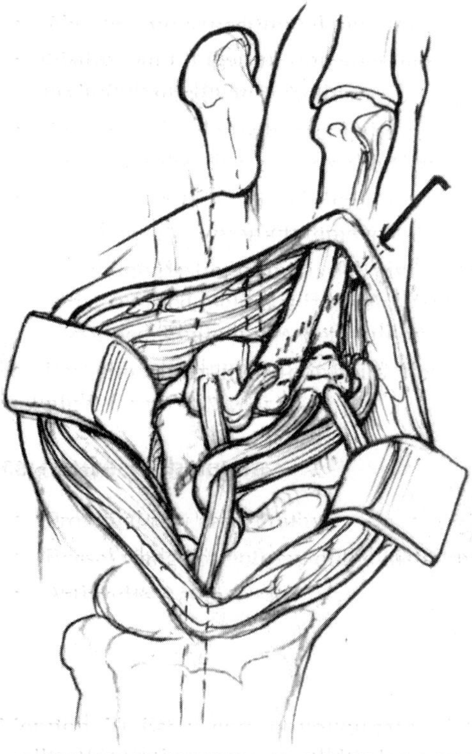

Figure 65–5

compartment. Pass the tendon around the remaining FCR tendon and back to the radial margin of the trapezium. Suture tendon to metacarpal periosteum.

- Repair the origin of the thenar musculature back to the metacarpal. Close the subcutaneous tissue and skin.

■ Pearls

CMC joint must be identified prior to drilling bone tunnel. If position of joint is unclear, place 25 gauge needle into joint and check with fluoroscopy.

- Removing a portion of the trapezial crest with a rongeur placed parallel to the FCR tendon facilitates dissection to the second metacarpal.
- Make bone tunnel large enough to accept tendon-pulling forceps (e.g., Carroll tendon passer; Jarit Surgical Instruments, Hawthorne, New York). Simply grasp tendon and pull through metacarpal.

■ Pitfalls

Injury to the radial sensory or lateral antebrachial cutaneous nerves

- Poor patient selection; patient should have early disease without considerable joint degeneration.
- Incorrect placement of bone tunnel

Postoperative Care

- Forearm-based thumb spica splint or cast; wrist in slight extension and thumb interphalangeal joint free
- Immediate thumb interphalangeal joint motion
- Immobilization for 6 weeks followed by Kirschner wire removal, splint fabrication, and active range of motion
- Pinch and grip strengthening are initiated 8 weeks after surgery.

Alternative Techniques

- Alternative tendon sources for ligament reconstruction such as the abductor pollicis longus (APL)
- Metacarpal osteotomy

Suggested Readings

Eaton RG, Lane LB, Littler JW Jr, et al. Ligament reconstruction of the painful thumb carpometacarpal joint: a long-term assessment. J Hand Surg [Am] 1984;9A: 692–699

Tomaino MM. Treatment of Eaton stage I trapeziometacarpal disease: ligament reconstruction or thumb metacarpal extension osteotomy? Hand Clin 2001;17:197–205

66 Closed Reduction and Internal Fixation of Bennett's or Rolando's Fractures

Indications

Base of the thumb metacarpal fracture with displacement or joint subluxation or both (**Fig. 66–1**)

Technique

- Regional anesthesia with intravenous sedation
- Fracture reduction with longitudinal traction, adduction of the thumb metacarpal base (i.e., abduction of the metacarpal head), and pronation of the thumb ray (**Fig. 66–2**)
- Direct pressure to the thumb metacarpal base toward the avulsion fracture (Bennett's fracture) facilitates reduction.
- Main focus is to reduce metacarpal subluxation and restore articular congruity to within 1 mm.
- Reduction verified using minifluoroscopy.

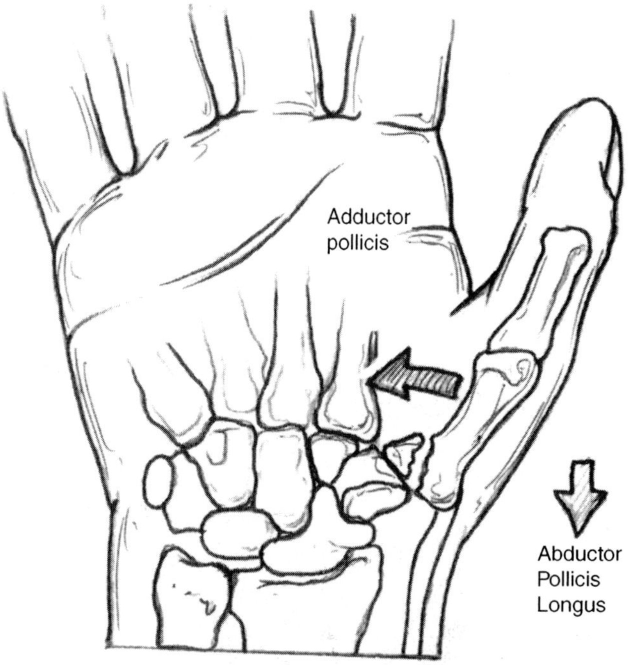

Figure 66–1

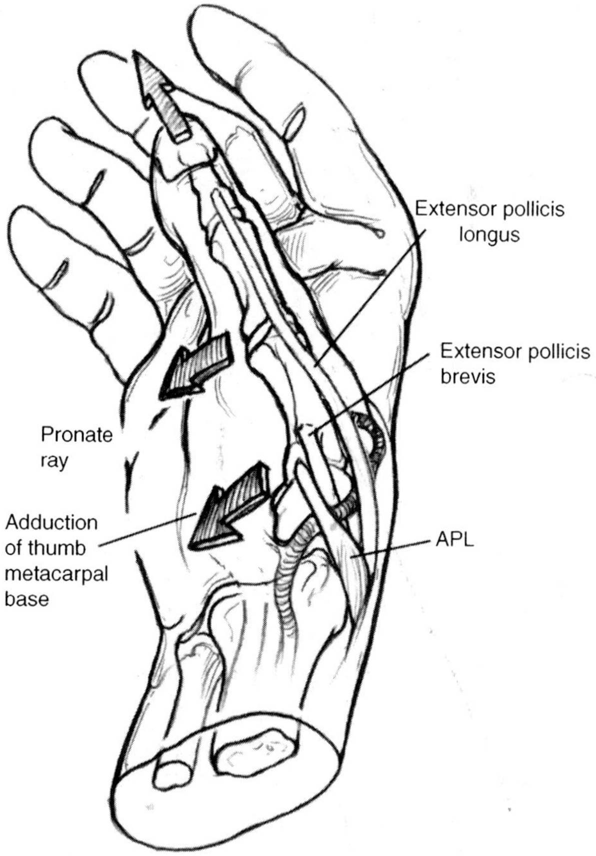

Figure 66–2

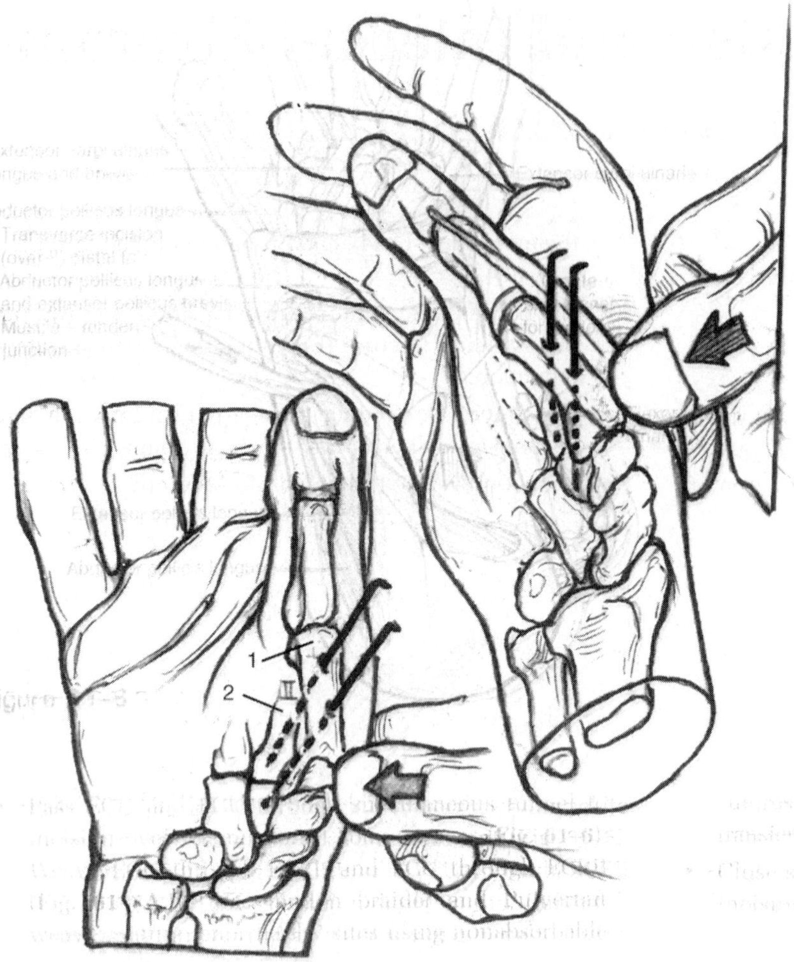

Figure 66–3

- Percutaneous fixation with two 0.45 in. (1.1 mm) trocar-tipped wires drilled through the thumb metacarpal and into the index metacarpal or carpus (**Fig. 66–3**).
- The ends of the wires can be left outside the skin or cut beneath the skin.

Pearls

The avulsion fracture (Bennett's fracture) remains nondisplaced and attached to the anterior oblique ligament. The abductor pollicis longus (APL) and adductor pollicis exert deforming forces upon the metacarpal shaft causing shortening and adduction.

- Pinning of a Bennett's fracture does not require direct fixation of the avulsion fragment. The pin maintains the metacarpal reduced on the trapezium.
- The Bennett's fracture fragment is ulnar and palmar. Open reduction requires a palmar surgical approach (**Fig. 66–4**).

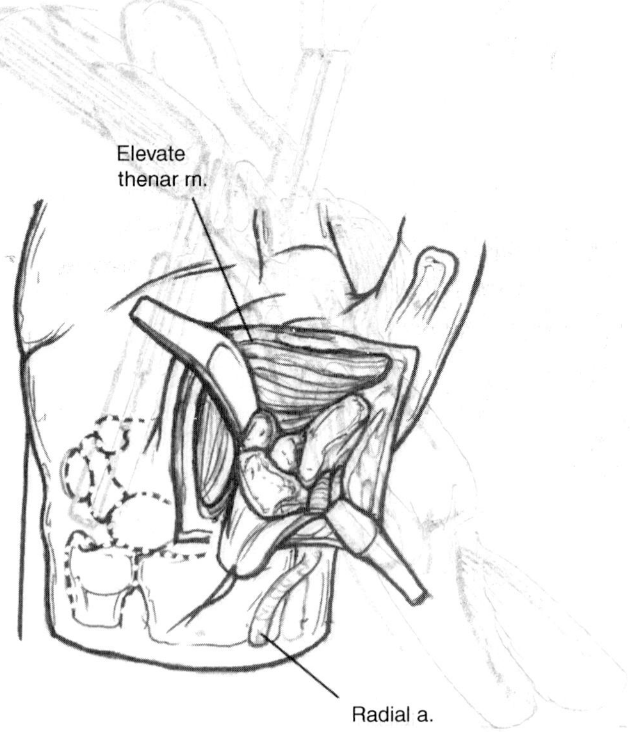

Figure 66–4

■ Pitfalls

Inadequate preoperative and intraoperative x-ray evaluation. AP and lateral x-rays of the thumb should be performed with the beam centered on the trapeziometacarpal joint. Placement of the palmar surface of the forearm and hand on an x-ray cassette and pronation of the wrist 15 to 35 degrees with the thumb remaining in contact with the cassette provides a true lateral image (Billing and Gedda view).

- A comminuted Rolando's fracture is difficult to treat by formal open reduction and internal fixation. Fracture fragments are small and often not amenable to internal fixation. Traction ± limited internal fixation is often a preferred alternative.

Postoperative Care

- Forearm-based thumb spica splint or cast. Wrist in slight extension and thumb interphalangeal joint free
- Immediate thumb interphalangeal joint motion
- Kirschner wire removal 5 to 6 weeks after surgery
- Range of motion and gradual return to normal activity
- Formal therapy usually not necessary.

Alternative Techniques

- Open reduction and internal fixation are reserved for large fragments (> 30% articular surface) that are irreducible. Require palmar approach. Rigid internal fixation preferred to allow early motion.
- CMC joint arthroscopy can be used to verify reduction.
- External fixation or skeletal traction instead of pin fixation. Usually reserved for comminuted Rolando's fractures. Can be combined with limited internal fixation.

Suggested Readings

Billing L, Gedda KO. Roentgen examination of Bennett's fracture. Acta Radiol 1952;38:471–476

Foster RJ, Hastings H II. Treatment of Bennett, Rolando, and vertical intra-articular trapezial fractures. Clin Orthop 1987;214:121–129

Leibovic SJ. Treatment of Bennett's and Rolando's fractures. Techniques in Hand and Upper Extremity Surgery 1998;2:36–46

Salgeback S, Eiken O, Carsam N, Ohlsson N. A study of Bennett's fracture. Scand J Plast Reconstr Surg 1971;5: 142–148

Section VII.2

The Carpometacarpal Joint: Thumb Carpometacarpal Arthritis

67 Metacarpal Osteotomy

Indications

Mild to moderate painful thumb carpometacarpal (CMC) joint arthritis recalcitrant to nonoperative management

Technique

- Incision along the dorsoradial aspect of the thumb at the junction between the glabrous skin of the palm and dorsal hair-bearing skin. Incision begins at mid-portion of the thumb metacarpal and extends to wrist crease (**Fig. 67–1**).
- Protect sensory branches of the radial and lateral antebrachial sensory nerves.
- Elevate the thenar muscles in an extraperiosteal fashion from the thumb metacarpal and CMC joint. Identification of the CMC joint is facilitated by longitudinal traction to the thumb (**Fig. 67–2**).
- Isolate the first dorsal extensor compartment. Retract the abductor pollicis longus (APL) tendon in a radial direction and the extensor pollicis brevis (EPB) tendon in a radial direction.
- Place subperiosteal reverse retractors around the thumb metacarpal ~1 cm distal to the CMC joint. Prepare wedge resection with apex based along volar aspect of metacarpal and base along the dorsal cortex.
- Cut bone parallel to joint surface using a fine-bladed microsagittal saw. Do not cut completely through the bone. Make second cut ~5 mm distal to the first cut

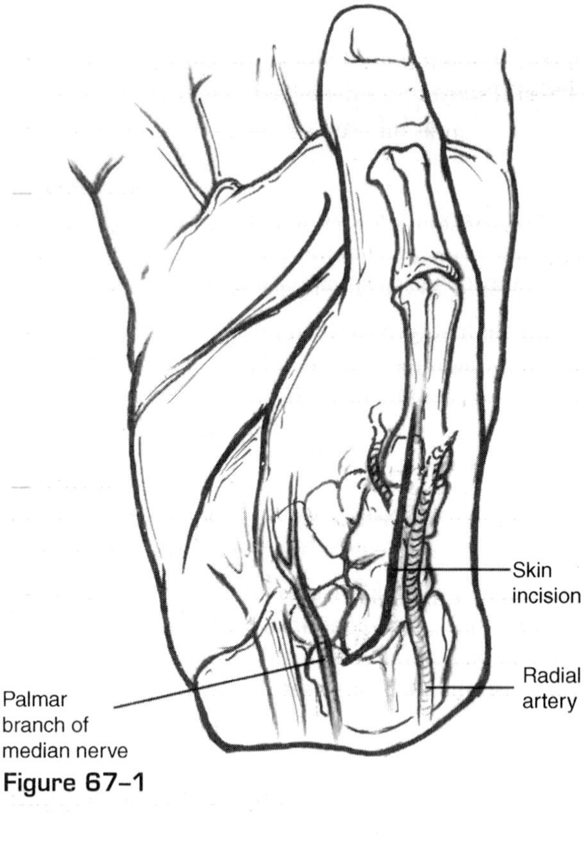

Figure 67–1

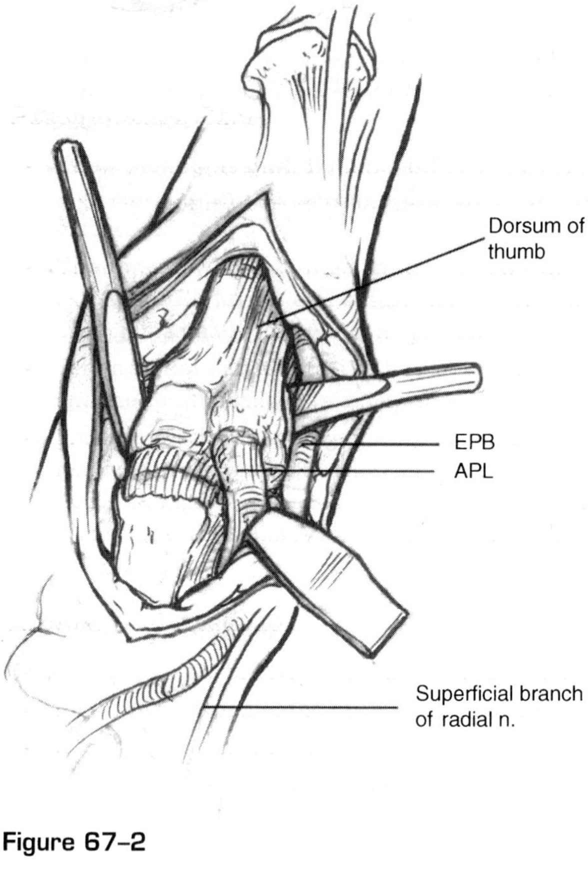

Figure 67–2

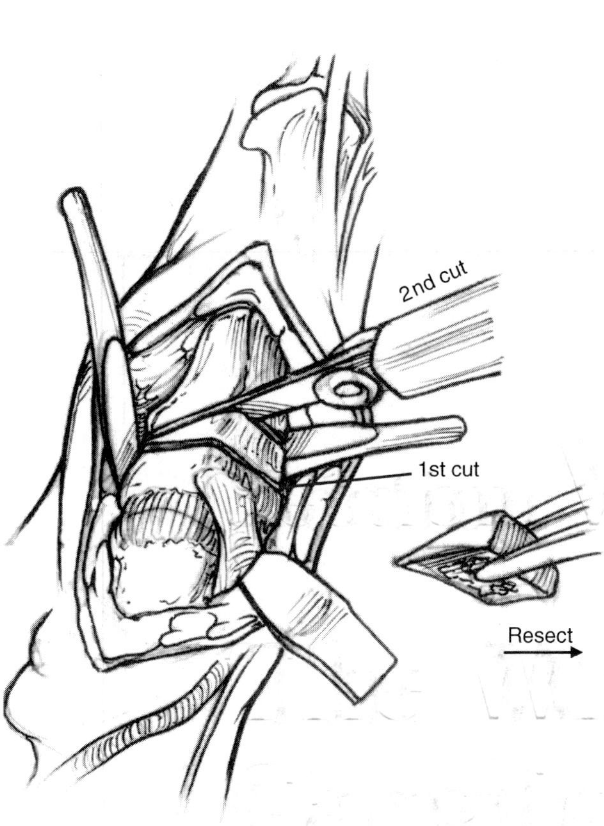

Figure 67–3

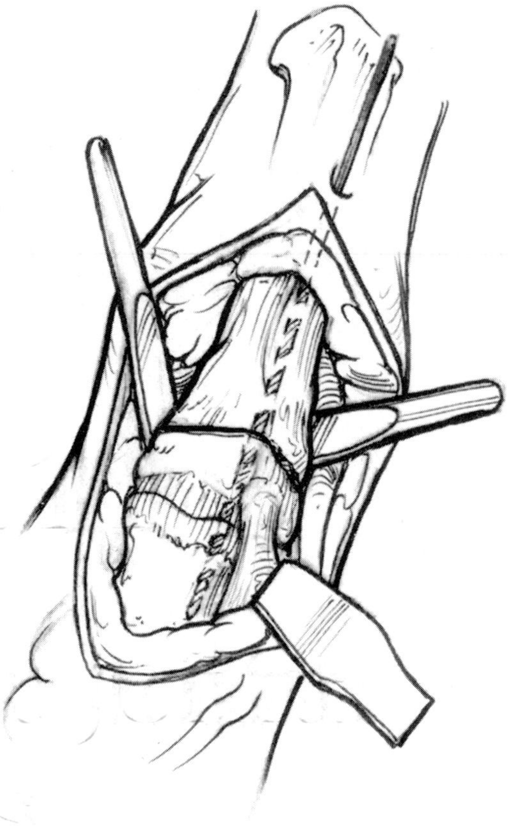

Figure 67–4

to delineate a 30 degree wedge of bone. Do not violate volar cortex (**Fig. 67–3**).

- Remove the wedge of bone and crack the remaining volar cortex. Reduce the osteotomy site until the triangular defect closes. Obtain provisional fixation with a 0.045 in. wire (**Fig. 67–4**).
- Add additional fixation using another wire, interosseous wiring, or a small plate and screws. Verify position of internal fixation using fluoroscopy.
- Repair the origin of the thenar musculature to the metacarpal using absorbable suture. Close the subcutaneous tissue and skin.

■ Pearls

CMC joint must be identified prior to osteotomy. If position of joint is unclear, place 25 gauge needle into joint and check with fluoroscopy.

- Perform incomplete osteotomy with first saw cut. This technique maintains a stable platform for second cut.
- Avoid violation of volar cortex during wedge resection. The volar cortex is cracked, which helps maintain some stability during wedge resection.

■ Pitfalls

Injury to the radial sensory or lateral antebrachial cutaneous nerves

- Failure to plan the osteotomy at the correct site and faulty technique during wedge resection

Postoperative Care

- Forearm-based thumb spica splint or cast. Wrist in slight extension and thumb interphalangeal joint free.
- Immediate thumb interphalangeal joint motion
- Length of immobilization varies with internal fixation technique. Rigid fixation can begin gentle motion at 2 weeks. Kirschner wire fixation requires 6 weeks of immobilization followed by removal of wires.
- Pinch and grip strengthening are initiated 8 weeks after surgery.

Alternative Techniques

- Ligament reconstruction
- CMC joint arthroplasty

Suggested Readings

Pelegrini VD. Extension metacarpal osteotomy in the treatment of trapeziometacarpal osteoarthritis. Atlas of the Hand Clinics 1997;2:183–202

Tomaino MM. Treatment of Eaton stage I trapeziometacarpal disease with thumb metacarpal extension osteotomy? J Hand Surg [Am] 2000;25A: 1100–1106

Tomaino MM. Treatment of Eaton stage I trapeziometacarpal disease: ligament reconstruction or thumb metacarpal extension osteotomy? Hand Clin 2001;17: 197–205

68 Thumb Carpometacarpal Joint Fusion

Indications

Mild to moderate painful thumb carpometacarpal (CMC) joint arthritis recalcitrant to nonoperative management. Arthritis must be limited to the trapeziometacarpal joint without involvement of the scaphotrapeziotrapezoid joint.

Technique

- Plan longitudinal dorsal incision from midshaft of thumb to scaphotrapeziotrapezoid joint. Incise skin and bluntly dissect through the subcutaneous tissue. Protect sensory branches of the radial and lateral antebrachial sensory nerves. Isolate first [abductor pollicis longus (APL) and extensor pollicis brevis (EPB)] and third [extensor pollicis longus (EPL)] extensor compartments (**Fig. 68–1**).
- Identify radial artery and its venae comitantes. Vessels course deep to the first compartment and at the level of the scaphotrapeziotrapezoid joint. Retract the vessels in a proximal direction.
- Retract the abductor pollicis longus tendon in a radial direction and the extensor pollicis brevis tendon in a radial direction. Identify the CMC joint and perform

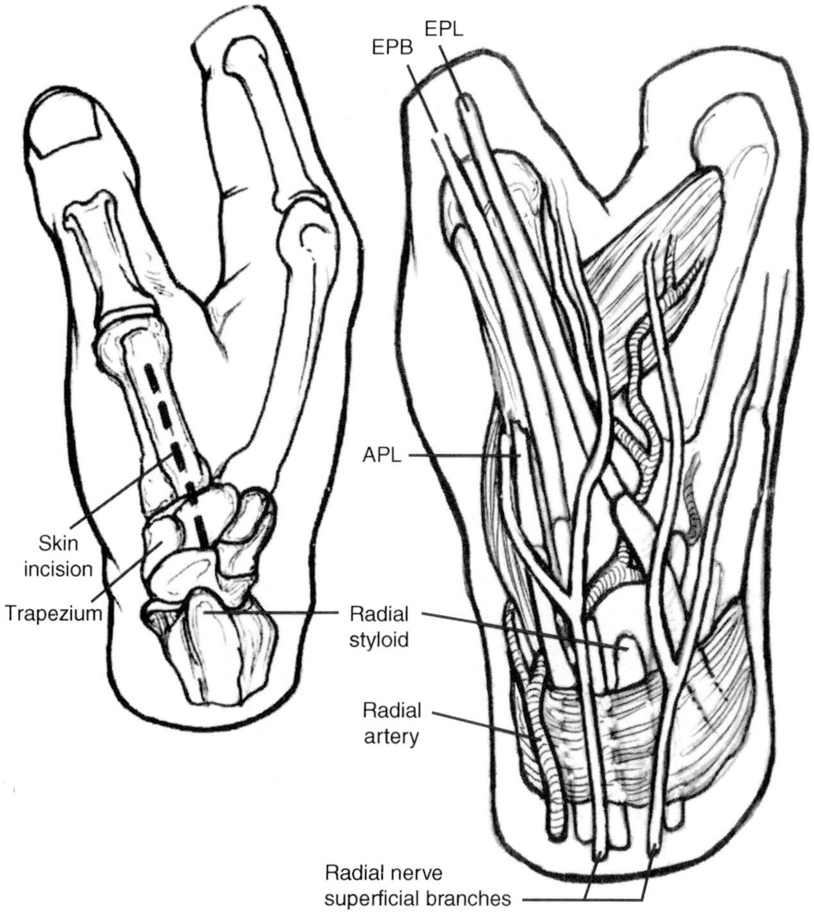

Figure 68–1

a longitudinal arthrotomy beginning at base of thumb metacarpal and ending over trapezium (**Fig. 68–2**).

- Elevate capsule in a radial and ulnar direction until entire base of thumb metacarpal and trapezium is exposed. Cut trapezium parallel to joint surface using a fine-bladed microsagittal saw (**Fig. 68–3**). Remove a slice of bone that includes articular surface and subchondral bone.
- Cut thumb metacarpal base to place thumb in the intended position of fusion. Standard position is 45 degrees to the coronal and sagittal planes of the palm. This requires a wedge resection with an apex along the ulnar side of the thumb. Remove enough bone to include the articular surface and subchondral bone.
- Position thumb with the resected surfaces in apposition. Check thumb alignment. Modify thumb metacarpal cut if necessary. Obtain provisional fixation via percutaneous 0.045 in. wire inserted across CMC joint (**Fig. 68–4**).

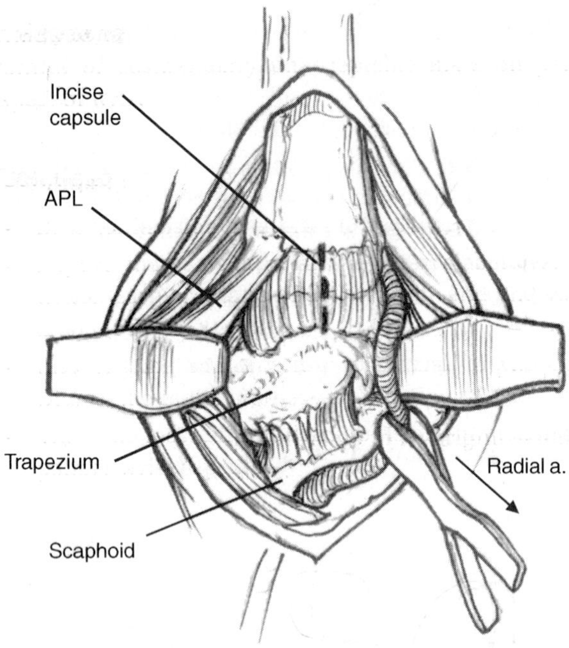

Figure 68–2

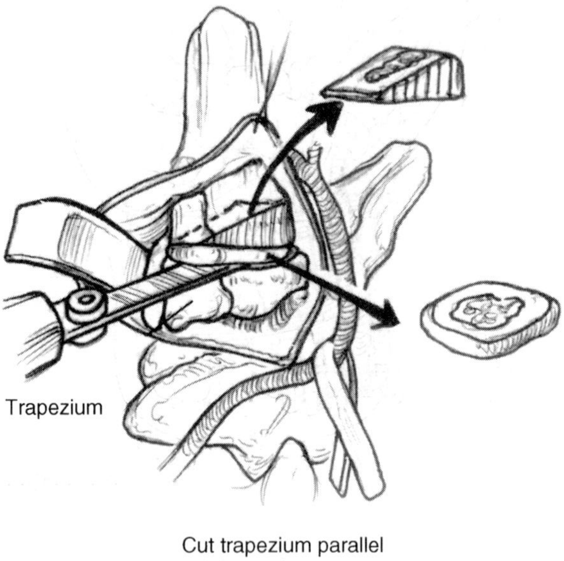

Figure 68–3

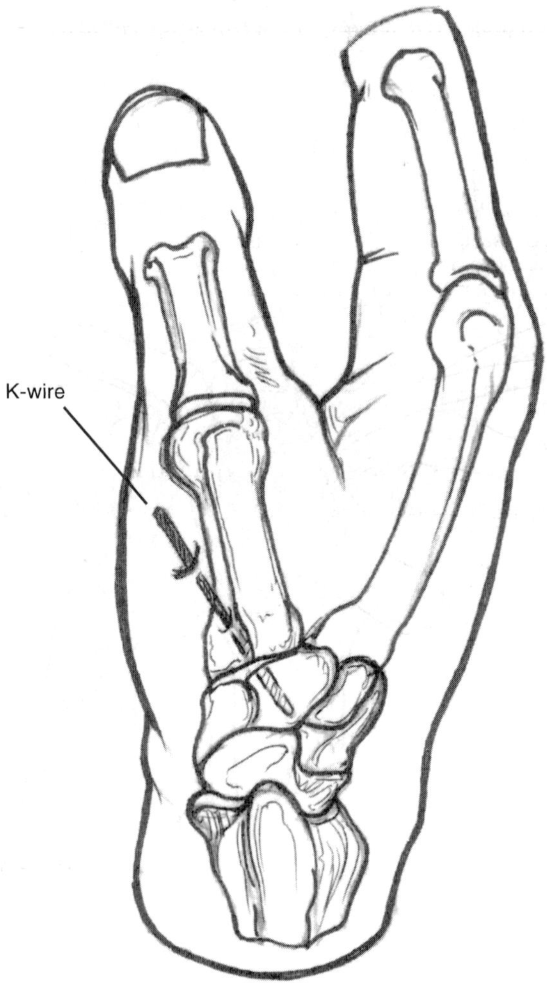

Figure 68–4

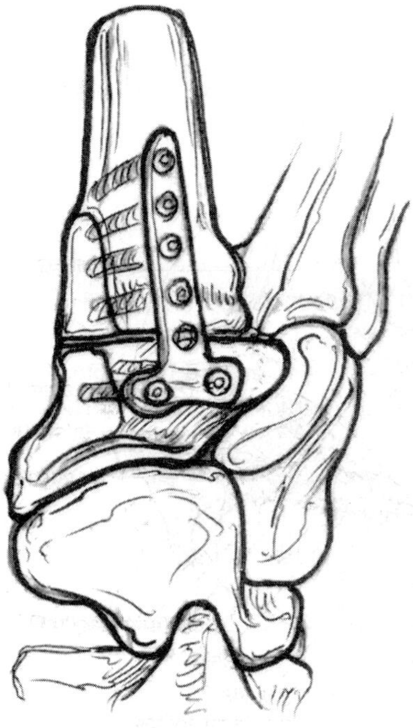

Figure 68–5

- Obtain rigid fixation with 2.0 mm or 2.4 mm minicondylar plate (**Fig. 68–5**). Cut plate to appropriate length to provide four to five screws into metacarpal. Contour plate so that it lies along the metacarpal and trapezium. Begin with fixation in the trapezium. Drill a hole to accommodate the blade portion of plate. Measure depth of hole and cut blade to correct length. Insert blade into hole and tap into position. Check alignment of plate and secure plate to metacarpal using bicortical fixation.
- Place screw into trapezium and additional screws into metacarpal. Verify position of internal fixation using fluoroscopy. If the fixation is rigid remove the wire. If the fixation is marginal leave the pin in place.
- Close subcutaneous tissue and skin with absorbable suture. Apply bulky compressive dressing and thumb spica splint with interphalangeal joint free.

■ Pearls

CMC joint must be identified prior to capsulotomy. If position of joint is unclear, place 25 gauge needle into joint and check with fluoroscopy.

- Cut trapezium parallel to joint surface and position thumb via metacarpal resection. The trapezium cut has a small margin for error.
- Provisional fixation with a percutaneous wire provides stability across the CMC joint and facilitates plate fixation.
- If unable to obtain satisfactory plate and screw fixation, use alternative fixation technique.

■ Pitfalls

Injury to the radial sensory or lateral antebrachial cutaneous nerves

- Failure to plan bony resection will result in malposition at fusion site.
- Failure to achieve bony apposition and rigid fixation will result in nonunion.

Postoperative Care

- Forearm-based thumb spica splint. Wrist in slight extension and thumb interphalangeal joint free
- Immediate thumb interphalangeal joint motion
- Length of immobilization varies with internal fixation technique. Rigid fixation can begin gentle motion at 2 weeks. Kirschner wire fixation requires 6 weeks of immobilization followed by removal of wires.
- Pinch and grip strengthening are initiated 10 weeks after surgery.

Alternative Techniques

- Alternative fixation techniques, including tension band, multiple Kirschner wires, staples, interosseous wiring, differential pitch screws
- CMC joint arthroplasty

Suggested Readings

Bamberger HB, Stern PJ, Kiefhaber TR, et al. Trapeziometacarpal joint arthrodesis: a functional evaluation. J Hand Surg [Am] 1992;17A:605–611

Eaton RG, Littler JW. A study of basal joint of the thumb: treatment of its disabilities by fusion. J Bone Joint Surg Am 1969;51A:661–668

Schwendeman LJ, Stern PJ. Trapeziometacarpal joint fusion. Atlas of the Hand Clinics 1997;2:169–182

69 Ligament Reconstruction with Tendon Interposition

Indications

Moderate to severe painful thumb carpometacarpal (CMC) joint arthritis recalcitrant to nonoperative management. Considerable joint degeneration precludes metacarpal osteotomy or ligament reconstruction without tendon interposition.

Technique

- Plan incision along the dorsoradial aspect of the thumb at the junction between the glabrous and dorsal hair-bearing skin. Incision begins at midportion of the thumb metacarpal and travels to wrist crease. Extend the incision along the flexor carpi radialis (FCR) tendon for 2 cm (**Fig. 69–1**).
- Protect sensory branches of the radial and lateral antebrachial sensory nerves. Ligate the superficial branch of the radial artery. Avoid the palmar cutaneous branch of the median nerve.
- Elevate the thenar muscles in an extraperiosteal fashion from the thumb metacarpal and CMC joint. Identification of the CMC joint is facilitated by longitudinal traction to the thumb.
- Open the FCR tendon sheath at the wrist and isolate the tendon. Follow the tendon in a distal direction. Incise the transverse fascial fibers that form a separate fibro-osseous canal for the FCR tendon. Trace the tendon beneath the crest of the trapezium to its insertion point on the second metacarpal. Remove the crest to ease tendon dissection. Retract the tendon in an ulnar direction (**Fig. 69–2**).
- Expose the articulations about the trapezium by a U-shaped capsulotomy based at the thumb metacarpal.

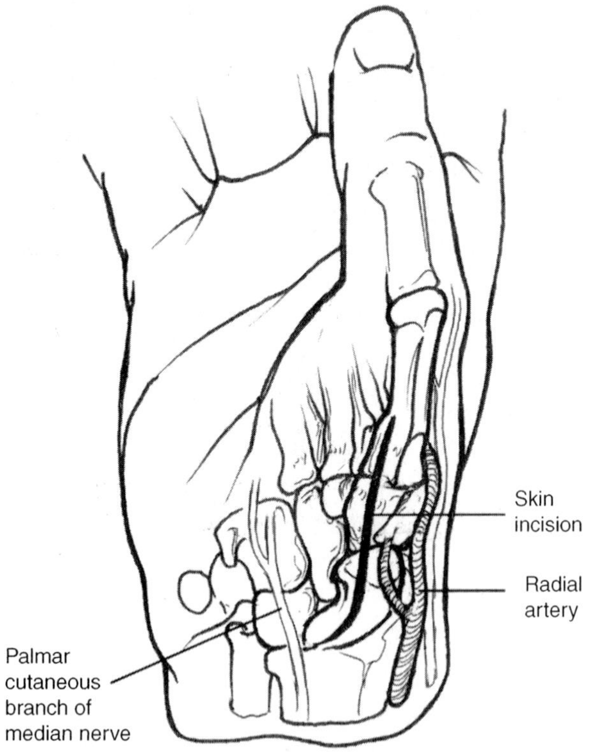

Figure 69–1

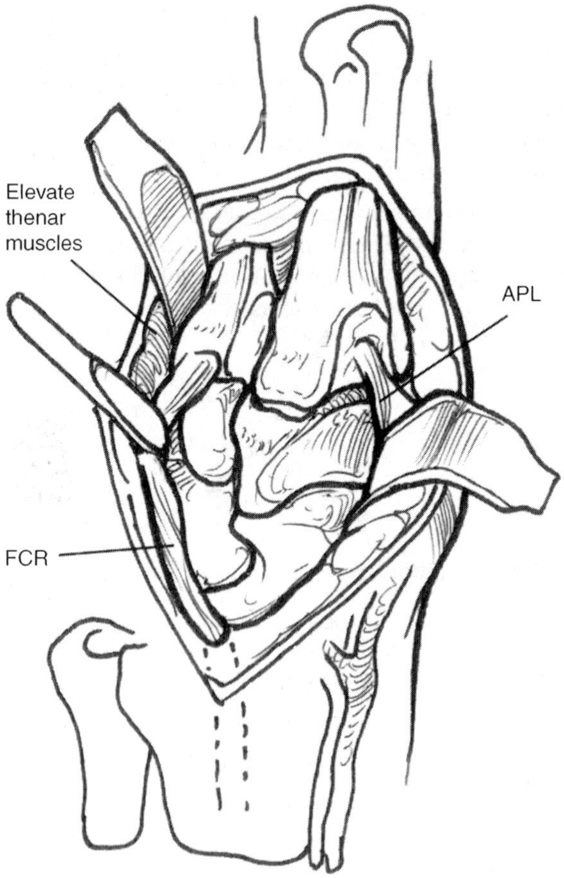

Figure 69–2

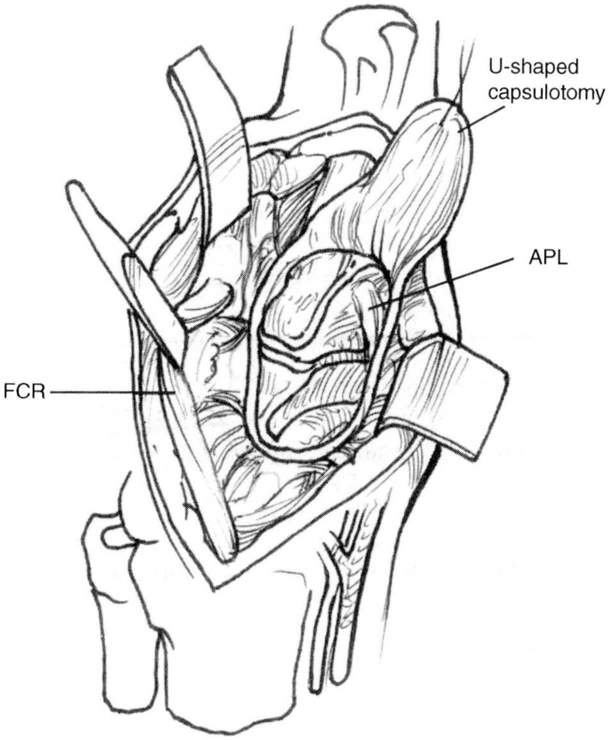

Figure 69–3

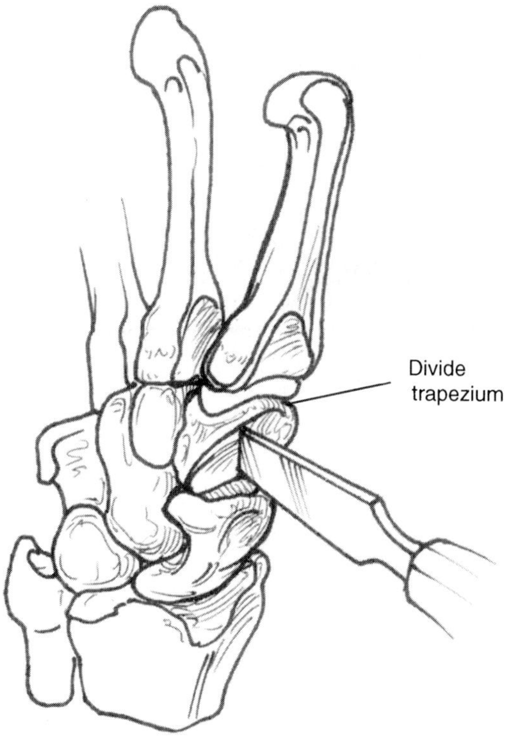

Figure 69–4

Incise the capsule sharply and elevate it from the trapezoid and scaphoid. Visualize the scaphotrapeziotrapezoid (STT) and CMC joints. Mobilize the entire trapezium by sharp dissection around its borders. Do not stray from the bone because the radial artery, adjacent tendons, and superficial nerves are in close proximity (**Fig. 69–3**).

- Divide the trapezium into a radial and ulnar half using an osteotome. Remove each section by sharp dissection and upward traction. Protect the FCR tendon during extirpation of the ulnar section (**Fig. 69–4**).
- Elevate the thumb metacarpal base from the wound and remove peripheral rim osteophytes with a rongeur. Inspect the scaphotrapezoid joint for degeneration. Remove any degenerated trapezoid by osteotomy using an osteotome or bur (**Fig. 69–5**).
- Isolate the first dorsal extensor compartment. Retract the tendons in a radial direction. Identify the extensor pollicis longus tendon and retract in an ulnar direction. Select a location between the tendons about 1 cm distal to the joint and perpendicular to the nail bed. This point serves as the initiation point for the bony channel created through the metacarpal base.

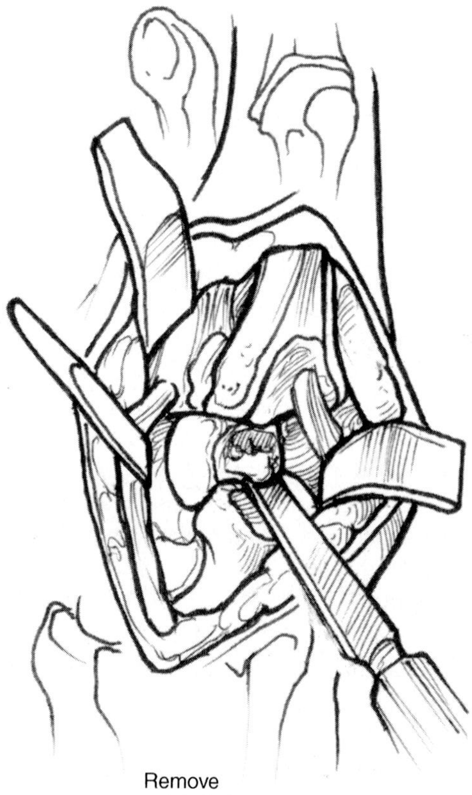

Figure 69–5

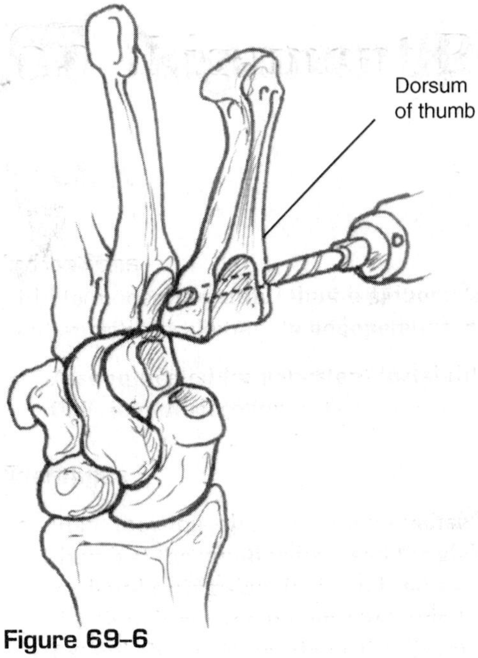

Figure 69–6

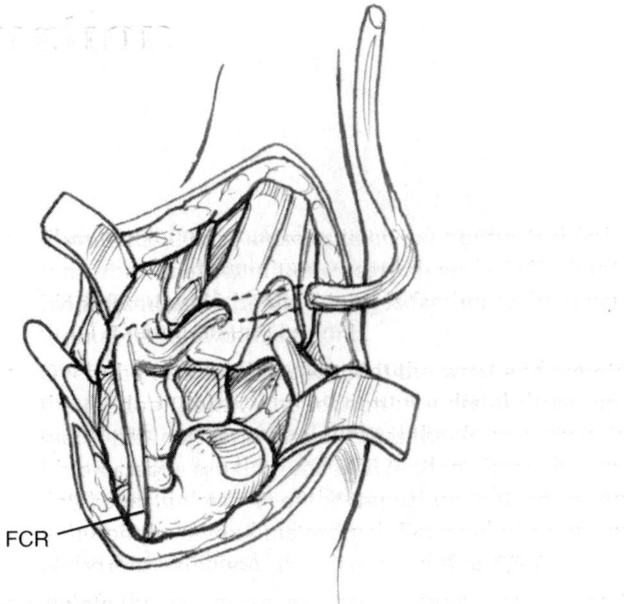

Figure 69–7

- Drill a small bone tunnel from the dorsum of the metacarpal (perpendicular to the nail bed) to the volar base of the metacarpal (**Fig. 69–6**). Progressively enlarge the hole by using sequential drill bits. Make the drill large enough to accept a tendon-pulling forceps (e.g., Carroll tendon passer; Jarit Surgical Instruments, Hawthorne, New York) and accommodate one half of the FCR tendon. Curette any remaining bone within the channel.
- Harvest the radial half of the FCR tendon from 8 cm proximal to the wrist to the base of the index metacarpal. Multiple techniques are available for tendon harvest. Multiple transverse incisions allow safe harvest with minimal scarring.
- Pass the free end of the harvested tendon graft through the drill hole from volar to dorsal using the tendon passer (**Fig. 69–7**). Apply longitudinal traction to the thumb to re-create the trapezial space and position the first ray. The thumb metacarpal base should align with the index metacarpal base. Avoid pulling too hard and overdistracting the trapezial space.
- Hold thumb position with a percutaneous 0.045 in. wire inserted from the dorsoradial aspect of the thumb metacarpal into the second metacarpal or carpus. Angle wire from distal to proximal during insertion.
- Draw the tendon taut and place suture between tendon and dorsal periosteum of metacarpal (**Fig. 69–8**). Route the tendon in a radial direction across the dorsal capsule of the CMC joint and beneath the first dorsal compartment. Pass the tendon around the remaining FCR tendon and back to the radial margin of the trapezium. Suture tendon to metacarpal periosteum.

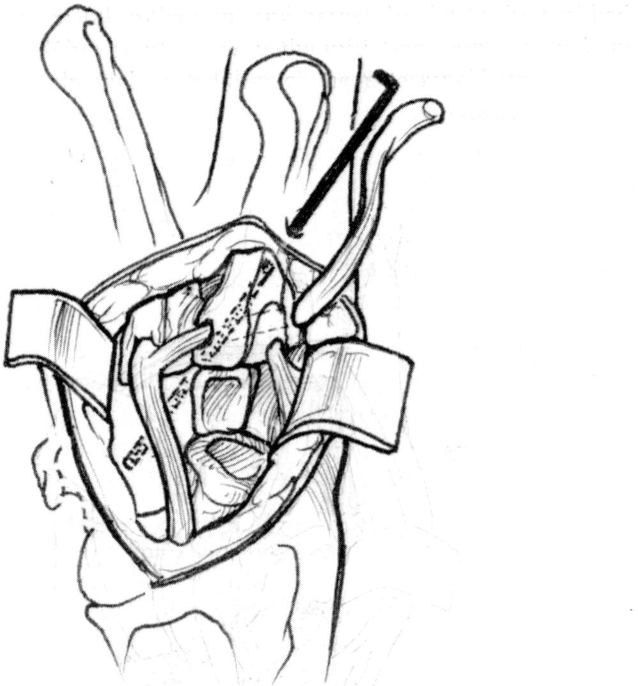

Figure 69–8

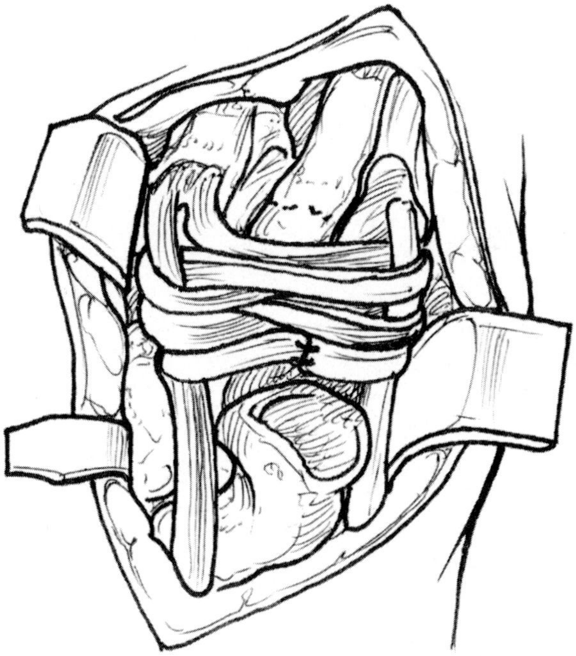

Figure 69–9

- Weave the remaining strip of the harvested FCR in a figure-of-eight fashion between the remaining FCR and abductor pollicis longus (APL) tendons (**Fig. 69–9**).
- Repair the origin of the thenar musculature back to the metacarpal. Close the subcutaneous tissue and skin.

Pearls

Volar approach allows complete identification and protection of FCR tendon during trapeziectomy.

- Remove the trapezial crest with a rongeur placed parallel to the FCR tendon to facilitate dissection of the FCR tendon to the second metacarpal.
- Carpectomy of the whole trapezium as a single unit can be performed; however, dividing the trapezium into radial and ulnar halves eases removal.
- Make bone tunnel large enough to accept Carroll tendon passer. Simply grasp tendon and pull through metacarpal.

Pitfalls

Injury to the radial sensory or lateral antebrachial cutaneous nerves

- Trapezium and CMC joint must be identified prior to removal of any carpal bones. If unclear, check with minifluoroscopy.
- Failure to remove the peripheral osteophytes about the base of the thumb metacarpal can lead to persistent pain between the thumb and index metacarpal bases.
- Failure to inspect the scaphotrapezoid articulation
- Excessive longitudinal thumb distraction during ligament tensioning results in lax ligament after traction released.
- Fracture of the bone tunnel through the metacarpal
- Failure to address concomitant metacarpophalangeal joint pathology, such as hyperextension or arthritis

Postoperative Care

- Forearm-based thumb spica splint or cast. Wrist in slight extension and thumb interphalangeal joint free
- Immediate thumb interphalangeal joint motion
- Immobilization for 6 weeks followed by Kirschner wire removal, splint fabrication, and active range of motion
- Pinch and grip strengthening are initiated 8 weeks after surgery.

Alternative Techniques

- Dorsal approach
- Alternative tendon sources for ligament reconstruction (e.g., abductor pollicis longus)

Suggested Readings

Burton RI. Ligament reconstruction tendon interposition arthroplasty. Atlas of the Hand Clinics 1997;2: 77–99

Burton RI, Pelligrini VD. Surgical management of basal joint arthritis of the thumb: II, Ligament reconstruction with tendon interposition arthroplasty. J Hand Surg [Am] 1986;11A:324–332

Tomaino MM, Pelligrini VD, Burton RI. Arthroplasty of the basal joint of the thumb: long-term follow-up after ligament reconstruction with tendon interposition. J Bone Joint Surg Am 1995;77A:346–355

Section VII.3

The Carpometacarpal Joint: Finger Carpometacarpal Joint Injuries

70 Closed Reduction and Internal Fixation of Reverse Bennett's Fractures

Indications

Base of the small metacarpal fracture with either or both displacement and joint subluxation. The entire ray is displaced with the radial intra-articular fragment of the metacarpal base remaining undisplaced on the hamate (H) (**Fig. 70–1**).

Technique

- Regional anesthesia with intravenous sedation
- Fracture reduction with longitudinal traction. Direct pressure to the small metacarpal base toward the avulsion fracture facilitates reduction
- Main focus is to reduce metacarpal subluxation and restore articular congruity.
- Reduction verified using fluoroscopy.
- Percutaneous fixation with two oblique 0.45 in. (1.1 mm) trocar-tipped wires drilled through the small metacarpal. One pin is directed into the ring metacarpal and the other is placed in an oblique direction into the carpus (**Fig. 70–2A–C**).
- Adjust pin position and length using fluoroscopy. The wires are either retained in a percutaneous position or preferably cut beneath the skin.

Pearls

Thirty degree pronation oblique x-ray view provides better visualization of injury than standard PA projection.

- The avulsion fracture (reverse Bennett's fracture) remains nondisplaced. The extensor carpi ulnaris (ECU) exerts a deforming force upon the metacarpal shaft causing shortening.

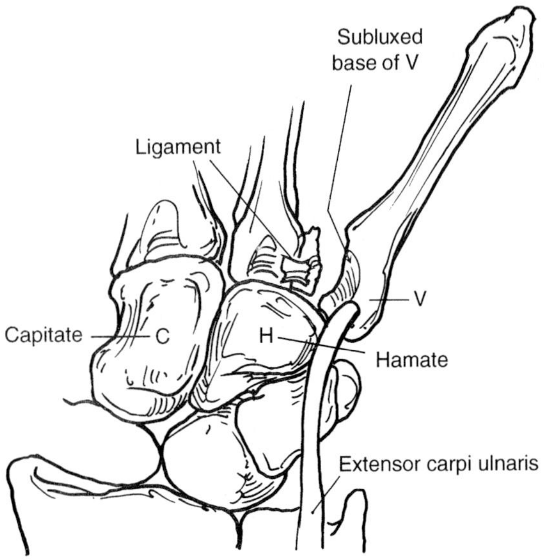

Figure 70–1

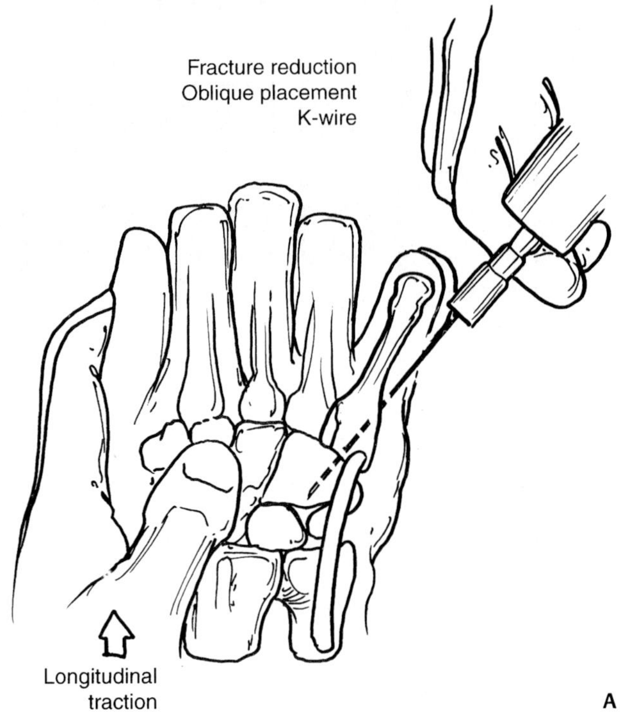

Figure 70–2

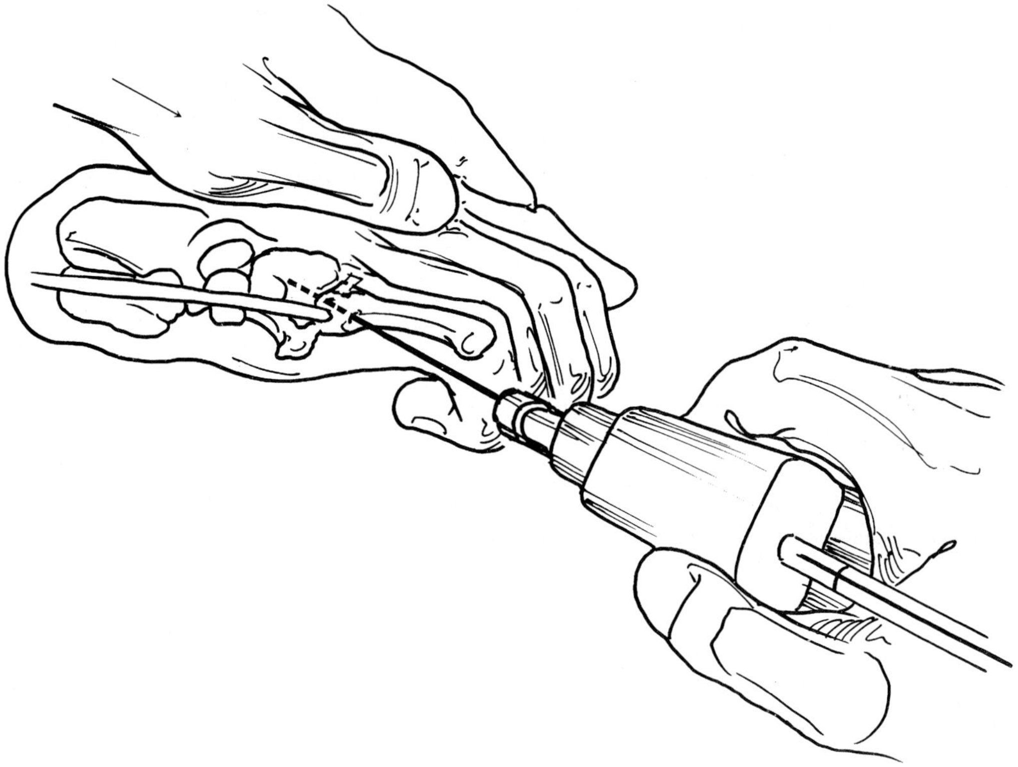

B

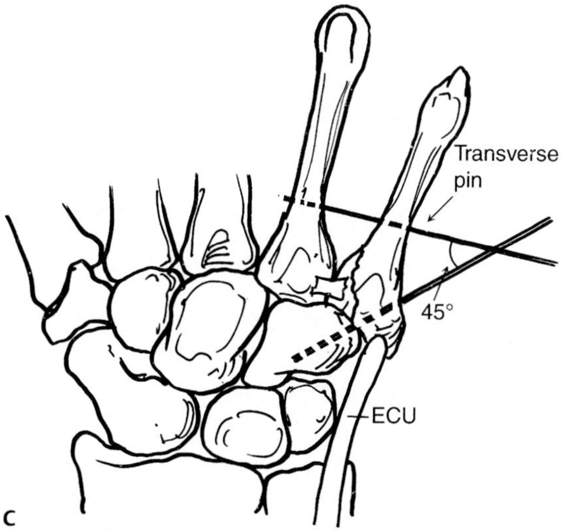

C

Figure 70–2 (*continued*)

- Pinning of a reverse Bennett's fracture does not require direct fixation of the avulsion fragment.

Pitfalls

Inadequate preoperative and intraoperative x-ray evaluation

- Inadvertent pin placement can damage dorsal ulnar sensory nerve or ulnar neurovascular bundle.
- Early pin removal can lead to repeat subluxation.

Postoperative Care

- Ulnar gutter spica splint or cast with wrist in slight extension and metacarpal phalangeal (MP) joints in flexion
- Wire removal 5 to 6 weeks after surgery
- Range of motion and gradual return to normal activity
- Formal therapy usually not necessary.

Alternative Techniques

- Open reduction and internal fixation are reserved for large fracture fragments or fractures that are irreducible.
- External fixation or skeletal traction instead of pin fixation; usually reserved for comminuted intra-articular fractures that require limited internal fixation.

Suggested Readings

Bora FW Jr, Didizan NH. The treatment of injuries to the carpometacarpal joint of the little finger. J Bone Joint Surg Am 1974;56A:1459–1463

Garcia-Elias M, Bishop AT, Dobyns JH, Cooney WP, Linscheid RL. Transcarpal carpometacarpal dislocations, excluding the thumb. J Hand Surg [Am] 1990; 15A:531–540

Rawles JG Jr. Dislocations and fracture-dislocations at the carpometacarpal joints of the fingers. Hand Clin 1988; 4:103–112

71 Open Reduction and Internal Fixation of Ring and Small Fracture-Dislocations

Indications

Dislocations of the ring and small carpometacarpal (CMC) joints with dorsal shear fracture of the hamate (H)

Technique

- Transverse or longitudinal incision over dislocated ring and small carpometacarpal (CMC) joints. Bluntly dissect through subcutaneous incision. Protect branches of ulnar sensory nerve. Identify extensor digitorum communis (EDC), extensor digiti quinti (EDQ), and extensor carpi ulnaris (ECU) tendons (**Fig. 71–1A,B**).
- Careful dissection and mobilization of dorsal ulnar cutaneous nerves. Retract EDC and EDQ in a radial direction and ECU in an ulnar direction. Identify ring and small CMC joints.
- Identification of hamate dorsal shear fracture (**Fig. 71–2**). Evacuation of fracture hematoma
- Longitudinal traction and direct manipulation of fracture to accomplish reduction. Provision fixation

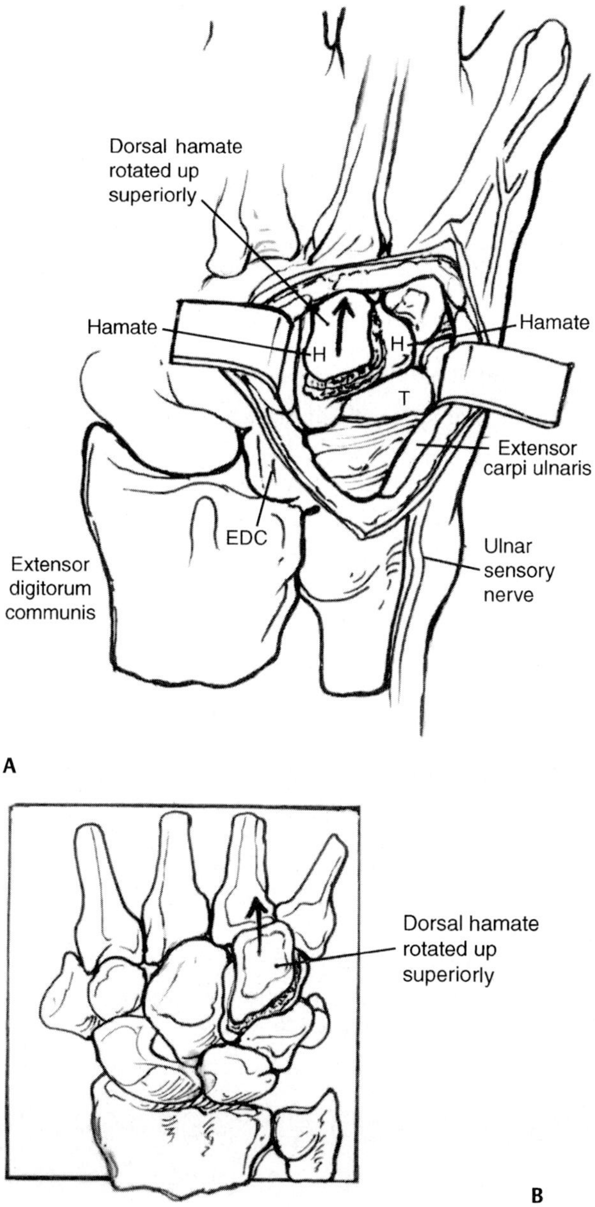

Figure 71–1

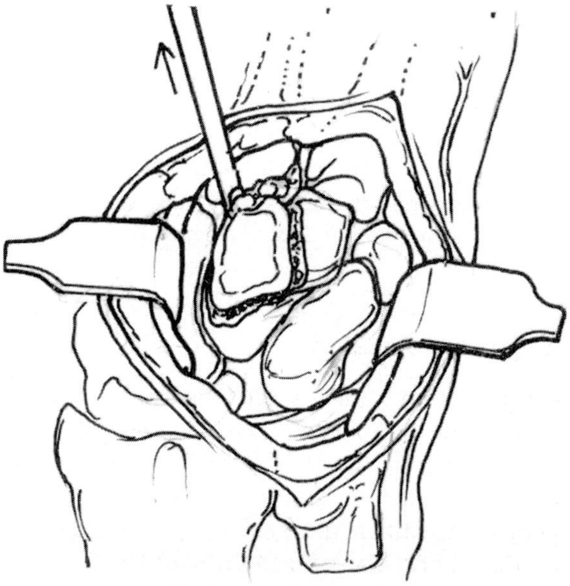

Figure 71–2

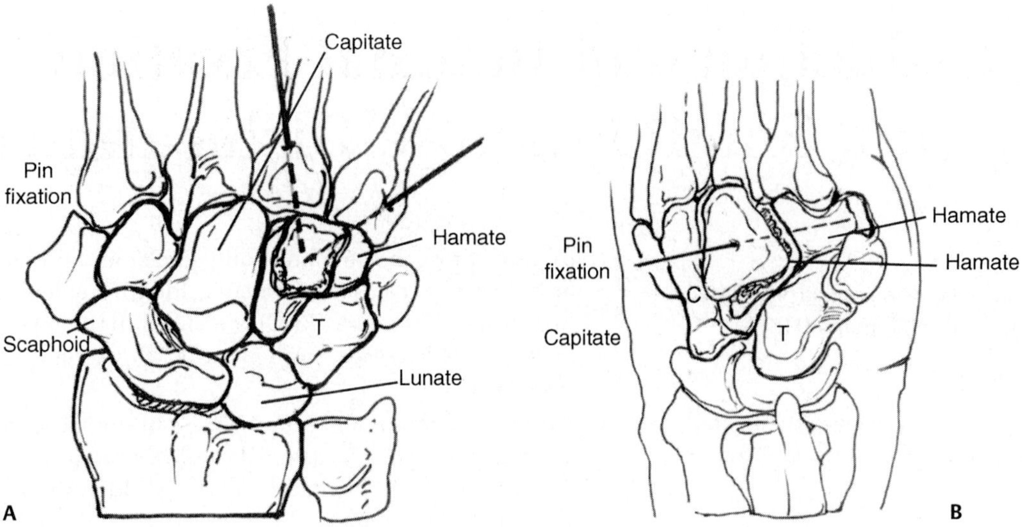

Figure 71–3

with 0.45 in. (1.1 mm) trocar-tipped wire drilled from dorsal to palmar (**Fig. 71–3A,B**). Plan wire position to allow for definitive screw fixation. Reduction verified using fluoroscopy.

- Definitive fixation with two 2.0 mm or 2.4 mm screws placed from dorsal to palmar into hamate. Countersink and lag to increase stability of fracture fixation.
- Remove wires and assess stability of fracture fixation. Rigid fixation requires no additional hardware.
- Percutaneously place a 0.045 in. wire through the bases of the fifth, fourth, and third metacarpals.

■ Pearls

Pronation, oblique radiographs facilitate identification of fracture configuration.

- Surgery is best performed within the first few hours after injury or delayed a few days to avoid period of maximum swelling that hinders exposure.
- Fluoroscopy is useful for fracture identification, confirmation of reduction, and screw position.
- Position a provisional wire to allow for removal and placement of second screw into same position.

■ Pitfalls

Inadequate preoperative and intraoperative x-ray evaluation

- Fragmentation of dorsal fragment using too large a screw

Postoperative Care

- Ulnar gutter spica splint or cast with wrist in slight extension
- Kirschner wire removal 5 to 6 weeks after surgery
- Range of motion and gradual return to normal activity
- Formal therapy usually not necessary.

Alternative Techniques

- Closed reduction and pinning for isolated CMC joint dislocation without hamate fracture
- Primary CMC joint fusion reserved for extremely comminuted intra-articular fractures that defy internal fixation.

Suggested Readings

Garcia-Elias M, Bishop AT, Dobyns JH, Cooney WP, Linscheid RL. Transcarpal carpometacarpal dislocations, excluding the thumb. J Hand Surg [Am] 1990; 15A: 531–540

Loth TS, McMillan MD. Coronal dorsal hamate fractures. J Hand Surg [Am] 1988;13A:616–618

Roth JH, de Lorenzi C. Displaced intra-articular coronal fracture of the hamate treated with Herbert screw. J Hand Surg [Am] 1988;13A:619–621

Section VII.4

The Carpometacarpal Joint: Finger Carpometacarpal Arthritis

72 Arthrodesis of Ring and Small Carpometacarpal Joints

Indications

Painful arthritis of the ring and small carpometacarpal (CMC) joints recalcitrant to nonoperative management, or chronic ring and small CMC joint dislocation

Technique

- Begin with 2.5 cm transverse incision ring and small carpometacarpal (CMC) joints. Bluntly dissect through subcutaneous incision. Protect branches of ulnar sensory nerve. Identify extensor digitorum communis (EDC), extensor digiti quinti (EDQ), and extensor carpi ulnaris (ECU) tendons (**Fig. 72–1**).
- Retract EDC and EDQ in a radial direction and ECU in an ulnar direction. Identify ring and small CMC joints. Use fluoroscopy if anatomy is distorted by injury.
- Remove osteophytes and excessive bone formation around CMC joints. Excavate any remaining cartilage from the base of the metacarpals and corresponding hamate (H) joints (**Fig. 72–2A,B**).
- Reduce any CMC joint malalignment or subluxation. Reduction verified using fluoroscopy.
- Percutaneous fixation with oblique 0.45 in. (1.1 mm) trocar-tipped wires drilled across ring and small CMC joints. Adjust pin position and length using fluoroscopy (**Fig. 72–3**).
- Bone graft any defects within CMC joint fusion mass. Bone graft is harvested from the distal radius. Iliac crest bone graft is alternative option.
- The wires are either retained in a percutaneous position or preferably cut beneath the skin.

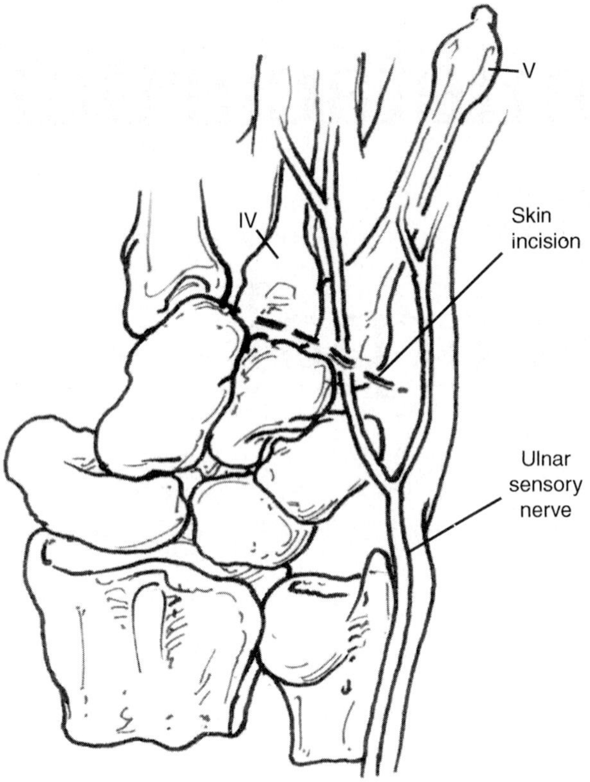

Figure 72–1

Pearls

Remove all cartilage to ensure successful fusion.

- Rigid fixation to eliminate micromotion across fusion site
- Bone graft any defect within fusion mass.

Pitfalls

Injury to ulnar sensory nerve during dissection

- Ring and small CMC joints must be identified prior to fusion. If unclear, check with minifluoroscopy.
- CMC joint malalignment can lead to scissoring during finger flexion.

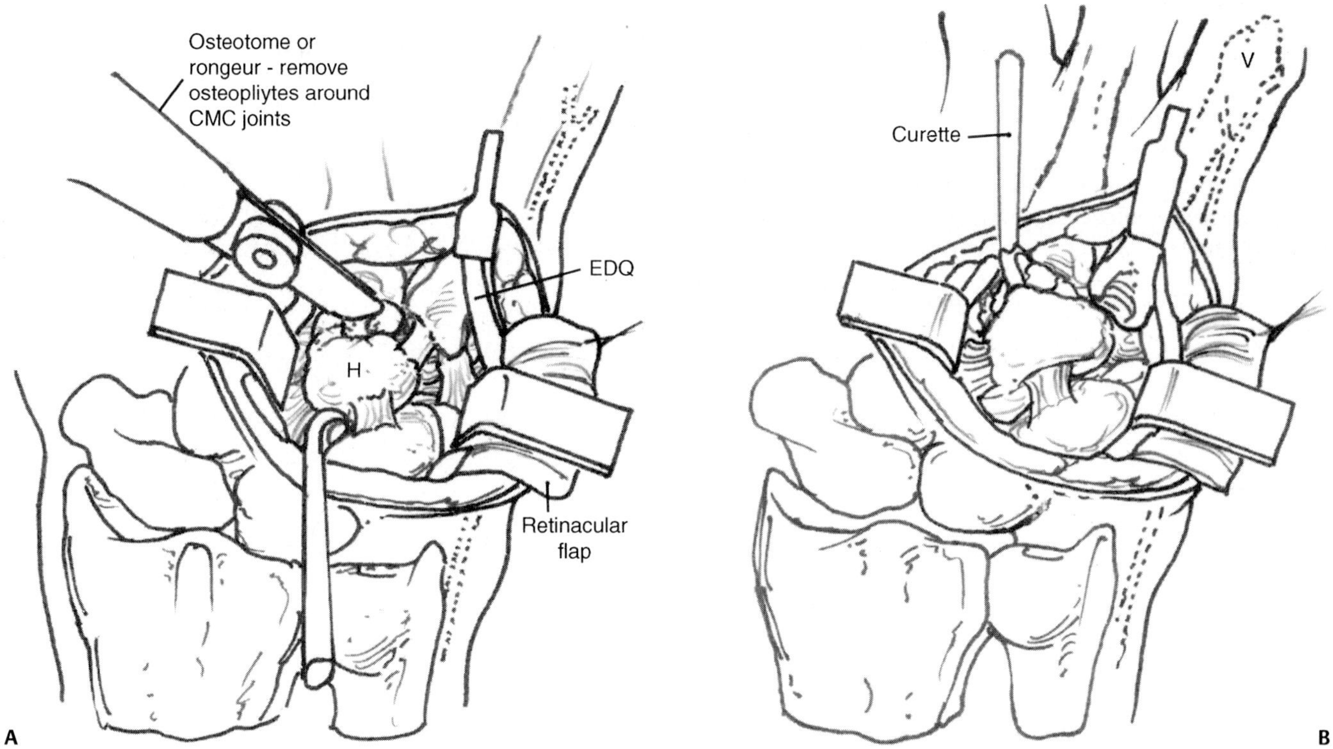

A B

Figure 72–2

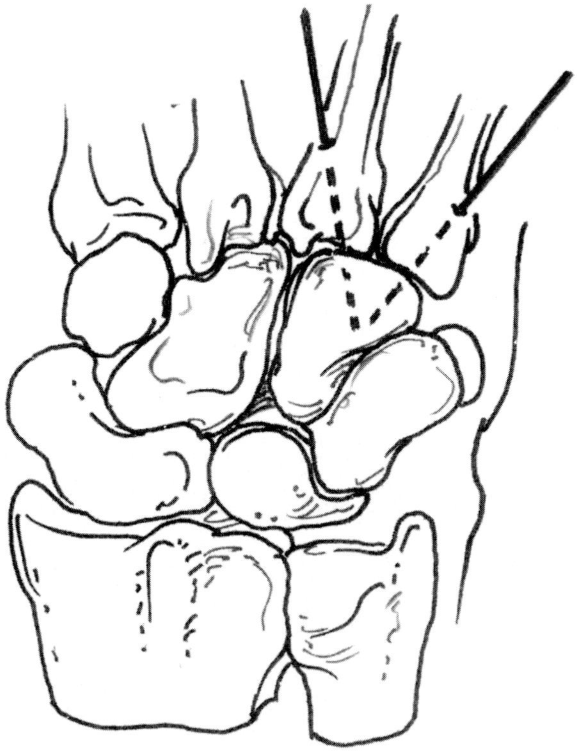

Figure 72–3

Postoperative Care

- Ulnar gutter spica splint or cast with wrist in slight extension. Place ring and small metacarpophalangeal joints in flexion. Interphalangeal joints not included.
- Wire removal 8 to 10 weeks after surgery
- Range of motion and gradual return to normal activity
- Formal therapy usually not necessary.

Alternative Techniques

- Screw or plate fixation across ring and small CMC joints using 2.0 or 2.4 mm implants
- External fixation across ring and small CMC joints; usually reserved for open injuries with a soft tissue deficit that requires immediate fusion or cases complicated by infection.
- Sliding bone graft technique using hamate bone as graft substance
- Soft tissue interposition arthroplasty
- Resection arthroplasty

Suggested Readings

Garcia-Elias M, Bishop AT, Dobyns JH, Cooney WP, Linscheid RL. Transcarpal carpometacarpal dislocations, excluding the thumb. J Hand Surg [Am] 1990;15A:531–540

Joseph RB, Linscheid RL, Dobyns JH, et al. Chronic sprains of the carpo-metacarpal joints. J Hand Surg [Am] 1981; 6:172–180

Rawles JG Jr. Dislocations and fracture-dislocations at the carpometacarpal joints of the fingers. Hand Clin 1988;4:103–112

Index

Page numbers followed by *f* or *t* indicate figures or tables, respectively.

B

C

D

G

H

I

K

R

T

U

V

W